Social Work and HIV

The Canadian Experience

Social Work and HIV

The Canadian Experience

Edited by
William Rowe and Bill Ryan

OXFORD
UNIVERSITY PRESS

OXFORD
UNIVERSITY PRESS
70 Wynford Drive, Don Mills, Ontario M3C 1J9
http://www.oupcan.com

Oxford New York
Athens Auckland Bangkok Bogotá Buenos Aires Calcutta
Cape Town Chennai Dar es Salaam Delhi Florence Hong Kong
Istanbul Karachi Kuala Lumpur Madrid Melbourne Mexico City
Mumbai Nairobi Paris São Paulo Singapore Taipei Tokyo
Toronto Warsaw
and associated companies in Berlin Ibadan

Canadian Cataloguing in Publication Data

Main entry under title:

Social work and HIV

ISBN 0-19-541301-6

1. AIDS (Disease) – Patients – Services for – Canada.
2. HIV-positive persons – Services for – Canada.
3. Medical social work – Canada. I. Rowe, William S., 1949– .
II. Ryan, Bill, 1955– .

RA644.A25S73 1998 362.1'969792'00971 C98-932371-4

Cover images: The NAMES Project—Canada/Le projet des NOMS—Canada is an independent charitable organization. Photographs of the Quilt Sections are provided without endorsement of any of the contents of the following pages.

Cover and Text Design: Brett Miller

1 2 3 4 – 01 00 99 98

This book is printed on permanent (acid-free) paper ♾.

Printed in Canada

Contents

Foreword

David Hoe

The Canadian social worker and HIV (human immunodeficiency virus) have now known each other for 14 years and the epidemic within the Canadian context is still being defined. For the social worker and people like myself who live with HIV/AIDS (acquired immune-deficiency syndrome) there is a vital need for development of knowledge and action regarding the psychosocial, economic, and political issues that frame how we think and respond.

HIV/AIDS demands that we lift previously unturned stones to understand fully the Canadian context. These stones, once lifted, cannot be put back without cost to personal integrity. Personal and professional values are challenged. It is the work of grasping wisdom, not only for the social workers, but also for those of us who live with the disease.

Much of the earlier evolution of social work practice with HIV was based on well-tried and trusted ways. At the same time much was left to fate. 'Being sure' was difficult. I am introducing the apparent difference between 'tried and trusted ways' and 'fate' because I believe that the work of the social worker and the experience of living with HIV have some commonalities when viewed between these two apparent poles. Early social work with HIV was, in many ways, left to fate. Social workers plunged into the lives of those of us living with the infection and our surrounding relationships. Systems were not in place, the disease was not well understood, and the environment was hostile—and this often included the social worker's work environment.

For many people who live with HIV illnesses, the experience can equally be described in similar terms. Much of the lived experience of the disease was a reflection of the paucity of knowledge, the lack of society's capacities to respond, and the fears that overtook the established health and social service systems. Social workers had as the most reliable resource their professional and personal intuition—intuition being the guide through fate and mystery. This continues today and will stay with us. This disease asks that we take ourselves to the point of our current experience and then some beyond that. It is at this point where integrity gets challenged and established. José Argüelles, an American visionary, says that integrity is the acceptance of our imperfections. This asks us to acknowledge that our capacities, at times, are not perfect. It also seems to me that it confronts any expectations we may have that we are, in our work and in our being, perfect.

Part of the struggle for many of us working with people with HIV has been the establishment of integrity with ourselves and with those with whom we have contact who are affected by the disease. If this be so, then HIV demands a personal and, for social workers, a professional look at imperfections. Absolutely, HIV

This essay has been adapted from the author's keynote address to the annual meeting of the Canadian Association of Schools of Social Work, Regina, June 1997.

holds up a mirror to the face of the soul and invites an examination of our imperfections.

If I, as a person living with HIV disease, accept this invitation to look at my imperfections, I sense that there is much for me to see. As though looking in a mirror my response will be determined by how long I can look into that mirror, what I see looking back at me, and what awareness I can develop from such an exercise. For social workers there is the duality of personal imperfections and 'humanness', on the one hand, and, on the other, their role as agents for society working through various institutions, many of which are now in crisis. Trust in our capacities to care for each other as people is in question!

I now believe I have a responsibility to my health to accept the recognitions of imperfections as a constant. I believe that in knowing the unalterability of an imperfection I receive the insight to create something new within myself, around myself, and for myself and with others.

For years my challenge was to accept the imperfections of inevitable physical deterioration and ultimate death. This may seem to be a sad state of affairs. It was not. Yes, there were moments of sadness. There were also moments of magnificent soulful anger and joy and there were moments that were profound in their ability to make me stop and be silent.

The search through imperfections for a truth is not halted by incidences of illness, or by various incapacities like being unable to climb stairs and care for oneself, or by the seemingly aging body in search of corpse-hood. Inner work and awareness do not stop. Throughout, the challenge is to build towards integrity.

Social workers with their duality have their own search. A commitment to that process will be the integrity that is brought to social work knowledge and practice. Employers of social workers are not the only ones who pay for that—life does also!

For those of us living with HIV our look at imperfections determines our relationship with the future. The future is always on the negotiating table. One time I remember being in hospital. My body was closing down and swiftly, it seemed, moving closer to its expiry date. A number of requests for attention were not taken urgently. Eventually, a visiting friend agitated the apparent complacency and doctors came by the squad, along with an impressive battery of electronic machinery. I was told they had about 15 minutes to intervene and I was asked if I wanted resuscitation. The word 'Yes!' came out. What was not said was 'Please can I have five minutes to think about it?' and 'Here is an opportunity for this struggle to end.' Those thoughts came in a split second, but the word 'Yes!' was said. This is not a dramatic tale for me, but it is a good example of negotiating the future. From somewhere came the capacity to renegotiate the future and to respond to a kind of a future that I wanted. I believe that was a rapid moment of examining my imperfections and then gaining awareness and moving on. It only took a few seconds.

Now, in the evolution of this disease, all of us are at an important moment. Much of social work has been in futures negotiation and this will increase. Until recently we have all lived with HIV disease during a time when the boundaries of life were reasonably clear. Illnesses had names, we were familiar with them, and they had their predictability. Life had little room for negotiation in the longer term, apart from dialogue with the human spirit, the economics and social comforts that may have been possible, and a few emerging treatments. It turned out that some of us eventually lived longer than others. Now those boundaries are becoming permeable with the arrival of new treatments.

All people living with HIV disease that I have known have developed a relationship with the boundaries of illness and death. Some of us now are sensing movement through these boundaries. A different life is seeping through. For those of us who are able to sense that permeability, our issues have shifted, and this impacts strongly on social workers. With the potential of some health and a longer life everything returns to the negotiating table and this is the world of personal and social change.

At the same time, this is not true for the majority of people living with HIV disease. It is not true for:

- those whose fate finds them living in economically poorer parts of the world;
- those who are addicted to other drugs—their boundaries can overwhelm the consciousness of a negotiable HIV boundary;
- those whose bodies react against the magic of the contemporary apothecary and the cleverness of computer-generated drugs;
- those whose bellies and throats react against even more pills to take;
- those who reject the notion of a permeable boundary: they do not want the daily ritual of more chemical taking, and without ritual, compliance with the treatment regimen is very doubtful;
- those who do not have the money, drug insurance, or the capacity to maintain health while on welfare.

These are some of the experiences I have encountered. Social workers, social work clients, social work education, and policy-making will be working to make sense of these imperfections. The above list is far from being complete. I invite you to lift the stones that you see, feel their weight, look at the dark damp undersides that have been exposed—the addict who steals morphine from other hospital patients to satisfy the addiction; the gay man who sees his services being less available because poverty and homelessness of others shoves his intimacy issues aside; aging, because of HIV, is now on a distant horizon for some of us. There are more. Some of them have been named: gay youth, health, and HIV for Aboriginal Canadians are some examples.

We know that death from AIDS is decreasing significantly where there is a good standard of living, where the political and health-care policies permit access to treatment and care, where the environment is committed to the belief that one's health can even surpass the state of health prior to HIV infection. It is that last belief that I invite you to embrace. Social workers have seen testing times. Their challenge has been to stay still and open at times when direction cannot be seen. It has been a challenge to be still, to be grounded, and to act with integrity. Through this has come inspiration. It has been done many times during this epidemic and there will be more to come. It is here where a good look at imperfections can bring changes to the integrity of social work and to the lived experience for people who are living with the disease of HIV/AIDS.

Now social workers are charged with a shifting set of HIV experiences. There are some who want to redefine life in relationships at the deepest levels of self, rework capacities and directions, redesign health-care and social service responses, or reaccept not wanting to change towards greater health possibilities or perhaps to reject the reality of new HIV treatments. I have been one of your clients and it is foreseeable that I will be a client again. The social worker who responded to my request for assistance provided what I wanted and established his readiness to respond to more complex issues as they arose. I am still reassured by his presence and he acts as a very strong reminder for me of the values and ethics that are embraced by the social work profession.

Social workers are therefore among the guides helping people living with HIV/AIDS through the mystery of illness. Counselling, practical aid, and advocacy are some of the ways that they serve. Together with those affected by the epidemic, social workers will enter a joint search for well-being through shared action in the development of advocacy for new treatments and human rights—for treatments that can be handled by those addicted to drugs; in being part of the upcoming discussions on safer sex as viral loads drop and transmission of the virus may shift; by continuing to be part of the development of the movement that deals with the new issues we turn up under the stones.

As I look back to those who have died I search for order, for my explanation of Why me? Why now? Again, I search for selfhood through such imperfections. My life tasks are different from six months ago. The previous quiet, content, almost esoteric tranquillity that soothed my mind and spirit through illness and potential death is being shifted by my agreement to take new medications. Now I feel as though I have been dropped in the middle of Manhattan and, subsequently, my imperfections are of a different kind. I now look at developing capacities in every aspect of life.

Honour your imperfections. Knowing them will take you to places that will stop this epidemic—and stop, it must! Honour your personal and professional history with HIV/AIDS and take your future further. Engage with the greater professional community to do some stone-turning. Finally, hold your vision of a community of life and safety that stands with integrity at the moments of illness and death. Define your community, for without community selfhood, with all of its imperfections, has little place to practise, and self is the place that will also be your future home.

This book, *Social Work and* HIV*: The Canadian Experience*, looks at the issues of social work in the Canadian context. It uses the wisdom gained from past stone-turning and brings us to areas demanding new understanding. All of the contributors call us to personal and professional accountability, to the values of social work practice and to further the creation of an improved society.

Acknowledgements

The editors wish to acknowledge that this work rests on the cumulative experience of hundreds of social workers and allied professionals who, since the beginning of the AIDS epidemic, have sought to provide compassionate and comprehensive care, prevention information, and policy development. As well, we wish to acknowledge the voices of those affected by HIV, unnamed, but evident in every part of this book.

We also wish to thank the contributors to this book who took time out from already impossible schedules to reflect on and share their experiences.

Finally, special appreciation goes to Cheh Cho, for his collaborative technical support in the production of this book.

Contributors

MICHÈLE BOURGON has been a professor in social work at the Université du Québec à Montréal since 1981. She has worked as a practitioner, educator, and researcher within the field of HIV/AIDS since 1990.

ANNE BOWLBY is currently Acting Manager of the Ontario Substance Abuse Bureau at the Ministry of Health. From 1986 to 1997, Anne worked for the Ontario Public Education panel on AIDS, the AIDS Section, and the AIDS Bureau of the Ministry of Health.

CHEH CHO is the Co-ordinator of the Direct Services Network at Maison CHESED House, an HIV/AIDS residence in Montreal's Jewish community. He is also a field instructor and sessional lecturer (currently completing his Ph.D.) at McGill University School of Social Work and has been involved in many HIV/AIDS-related, community-based projects since 1984.

DALE D'AMATTEO has worked in research at the Hospital For Sick Children, Toronto, for 14 years, the last 10 years with the HIV/AIDS Comprehensive Care Team. She is currently doing postgraduate work in public health at the University of Toronto.

MARIE-JOSÉE DROUIN has a Master's degree in sexology from the Université du Québec à Montréal.

DAVID FITZGERALD is presently employed with Pubic Health in Edmonton, and previously worked with an AIDS service organization in Edmonton, for seven years as Co-ordinator of Support Services and two years as the manager of a demonstration project developing a model of integrated community care.

SHIRLEY GROSSER is an Associate Professor who initiated the first HIV/AIDS education program in 1989 at the Faculty of Social Work, University of Manitoba. She designed, developed, and taught courses on HIV/AIDS in both the BSW and MSW programs at Manitoba, and in 1997 she collaborated with four other health sciences disciplines to design and launch the first interdisciplinary HIV/AIDS workshop in Manitoba.

MARC A. HAMEL received his MA degree in psychology in 1992 from the Université du Québec à Montréal. He is a clinical and research psychologist who has been actively involved in counselling and conducting studies with individuals living with HIV infection and AIDS. He is currently completing his doctoral studies at Concordia University.

DAVID HOE has worked in the fields of mental health, youth, and deaf and disabled children, as well as in cross-cultural social work as Director of Social Services in Iqaluit, Northwest Territories. For the last 10 years, David has focused his personal and professional interests in the field of HIV/AIDS. He is currently a policy adviser with Health Canada on HIV/AIDS and a consultant to community groups on organizational development, and is the past Executive Director of the AIDS Committee of Ottawa. He is a person living with AIDS.

LOIS JACKSON is Assistant Professor in the Health Education program of the School of Health and Human Performance at Dalhousie University. Her two main areas of research interest related to HIV/AIDS are the varied potential risks of HIV among female prostitutes and the social, behavioural, and psychological impact of HIV for HIV-positive women.

SUSAN KING is Associate Professor of Pediatrics at the University of Toronto and a specialist in Pediatric Infectious Diseases at the Hospital for Sick Children in Toronto. She is the Co-Director of the HIV/AIDS Comprehensive Care Program at the Hospital for Sick Children.

LYNNE LEONARD received her Master's degree in social work at the University of Warwick and is pursuing doctoral studies in the field of HIV prevention and women at the School of Social Work, McGill University. She is a Principal Investigator with the Community Health Research Unit at the University of Ottawa and Program Consultant for HIV/AIDS Policy, Co-ordination and Programs Division, Health Canada.

JOSEPH JOSY LÉVY is Director and Professor in the Department of Sexology at Université du Québec à Montréal. With a doctorate in anthropology, he is particularly interested in the sociocultural aspects of HIV infection. He is also a member of the provincial team of AIDS researchers funded by the Quebec Council on Social Research.

GLENN MARCOTTE is a social worker in an anonymous HIV testing centre at the CLSC-Métro in Montreal and is the liaison person for the CLSC-Métro with Chez Ma Cousine Evelyn. He has also been a street worker in Calgary.

JACK MCDONALD is Professor Emeritus, Faculty of Social Work, University of Calgary. He served as social worker for the Southern Alberta Hemophilia Clinic from 1978 to 1997. He became involved in the HIV epidemic in early 1983 and was active in clinical, community development, and applied social work research at the local, national, and international levels.

CAROL NERON has worked in the areas of HIV/AIDS, substance abuse, and violence against women. She is currently working as a social work consultant in Ottawa and has previously conducted research, published, and lectured on the topic of euthanasia, assisted suicide, and HIV/AIDS.

CLAUDE OLIVIER is a social worker with eight years' experience with community-based AIDS organizations. He is currently enrolled in the doctoral program at Memorial University of Newfoundland's School of Social Work.

JOANNE OTIS is Professor in the Department of Sexology at the Université du Québec à Montréal. Her research interests are primarily related to the psychosocial factors associated with risk-taking and in program evaluation, particularly in community settings. She is a member of the provincial team of AIDS researchers funded by the Quebec Council on Social Research.

WILLIAM ROWE is Director of the School of Social Work at McGill University and has also taught at Memorial University of Newfoundland and the University of Western Ontario. He has worked extensively in the fields of child welfare, corrections, health, and HIV/AIDS and was Chair of the Canadian Public Health Association AIDS Awareness Advisory Board, 1993–7.

BILL RYAN is a social worker and adult educator involved in HIV-related work since 1985 as a counsellor, teacher, and researcher. He has served on national and international committees and boards related to care and education over the years, and resides in Montreal where he teaches, administers programs, and counsels in issues related primarily to HIV and sexuality.

ROBYN SALTER-GOLDIE has been a social worker since 1976 and has worked with the HIV/AIDS Program at the Hospital for Sick Children in Toronto since it began in 1988. During this time, she has been providing psychosocial support for and with children and families with HIV/AIDS through counselling, resource development, advocacy, and research.

SHARON TAYLOR is currently Chair of the Department of Social Work at Lakehead University. Her interest in confidentiality issues related to HIV developed from students' field placements with the AIDS Committee in Thunder Bay, Ontario.

LILLIAN WELLS is Professor and Associate Dean, Faculty of Social Work, University of Toronto. She has been involved in teaching and research related to HIV/AIDS since the mid-1980s.

JUDY WEISER, Director of the Photo Therapy Centre in Vancouver, is a psychologist and art therapist specializing in counselling (and consulting about) HIV-infected/affected Aboriginal people and families, particularly street-involved Native youth.

Introduction

William Rowe and Bill Ryan

> *AIDS. Probably the single most powerful word of our era for evoking intense individual and societal responses. The reasons for this are often cited: fear, death, stigmatization, prejudice, discrimination, illness, suffering.* (Somerville and Gilmore, 1992: xi)

In Canada it was recognized early that the spectre of the human immunodeficiency virus (HIV) would place demands on issues in health and social policy that would quickly outstrip our capacity to respond effectively and humanely. Legal, ethical, and policy issues in public health, drug use, homosexuality, sex education, confidentiality, discrimination, health, and social security came under intense scrutiny and were most often found wanting.

The story of social work and HIV in Canada began somewhat slowly and quietly. In many ways, it depended on where you were and who you were working with as to when the epidemic first began to challenge social workers. For many, the epidemic had to hit home, affecting either social workers or their families before they began to take notice from a professional point of view.

For many, in the early 1980s, the nascent HIV epidemic was reflected only in the information from the United States about a disease that seemed to be affecting mostly gay men and possibly some other groups. Social workers whose practice included work with the gay community, health, and in some instances human sexuality saw a few cases. These social workers had little information or preparation and simply used the traditional skills they had available to respond in the best way they could. A great deal of fear and confusion existed in those early days—fear of contagion, confusion about transmission routes and the natural history of the disease.

In Canada, as in other countries, the initial response to the AIDS crisis was spearheaded by community-based organizations. Social work professionals were variously involved with these groups, but it was not until the mid- to late 1980s that HIV found its way into the lexicon of social work practice in Canada. The Canadian Conference on AIDS in 1988 helped focus attention on the growing number of infected and affected individuals in Canada. The eloquence of activists like Jim St James and Kevin Brown helped to put an articulate and an empowered face on the epidemic. The Canadian Association of Social Workers and the Canadian Association of Schools of Social Work sponsored projects in curriculum development and continuing education to help accelerate the response of the social work profession to the crisis. These events coincided with the establishment of the federal government's National AIDS Strategy, which focused on research, prevention, care, treatment, and support. Canadian social workers were present in large numbers at the International AIDS Conference held in Montreal in 1989 and demonstrated a number of practice and policy innovations that secured them a place in the global response to HIV.

By 1990, the Canadian Association of Social Workers had developed a resource kit entitled 'Preparing for HIV and AIDS' and the Canadian Association of Schools of Social Work had developed other materials to help infuse HIV information into the curriculum. Social workers became involved in AIDS work at various points and their contributions are now widespread, ranging from prevention through care and treatment to policy developments.

In 1993, the second phase of the National AIDS Strategy began. This second phase was concerned with enhancing the partnerships and health promotion and creating supportive social environments for people living with HIV. Health Canada created a series of practice modules to help people working in the fields of HIV and AIDS to communicate information and practice techniques. The Canadian Association of Social Workers was commissioned to develop *Module 6—Psychosocial Care* in the *Comprehensive Guide for the Care of Persons with HIV Disease*. This project brought together social workers from across the country whose years of experience and broad consultations with their colleagues and people from the HIV-affected community developed a highly acclaimed practical guide.

In the winter of 1996, a special edition of the CASW journal, *The Social Worker*, was dedicated solely to social work and HIV and demonstrated that social workers in Canada are now contributing at all levels of practice, research, and policy development in a sustained and creative fashion. This book, the first of its kind in Canada, is another milestone in social workers' response to HIV.

Social Work and HIV: The Canadian Experience is not a practitioner's guide *per se*. Much of that hands-on practical approach is nicely articulated in *Module 6* of the *Comprehensive Guide*. Rather, this book has gathered together some of the voices of experience to illustrate the kind of thinking that social workers have generated over the past few years. It is not meant to be an exhaustive work but rather a representative one that can help new social workers coming into the field of HIV to appreciate more fully the challenges and opportunities the field holds. Some of these voices are familiar in the Canadian landscape; others may be heard for the first time. The book is divided into three parts: Prevention, Care, and Practice, Policy, and Politics. All of the contributors were asked to think about the current and unfolding issues in their particular sector concerning HIV and AIDS and to use vignettes and case illustrations where possible to help provide the fullest picture.

The book begins by examining prevention, an area often neglected in the social work field because many have tended to believe that prevention is the purview of health and education. It is clear, of course, that some of the most creative prevention programs stem directly from the community-based initiatives in which some social workers were directly involved or served as facilitators. Part One does not simply provide the ABCs of prevention; rather, the chapters look at both theory and practice and describe practice innovations, some of which are unique to the Canadian experience.

Part Two, Care, covers a wide variety of topics and helps to illustrate the breadth of social work involvement in HIV care and treatment. These chapters provide a rich narrative of the social work experience in HIV care. Behind each story are a thousand more, each with its own unique impact. The reader is encouraged to make the links between what the authors have presented and his/her own practical experience to help set the stage for an even greater social work response in the Canadian context.

Part Three, Practice, Policy, and Politics, focuses on some of the perplexing issues that have surfaced in relation to the HIV epidemic in Canada. HIV and AIDS have served as a lightning rod at times, at other times as a lens. As a lightning rod, the disease has forced the social work profession to consider issues that for many years remained in the comfortable confines of academic and professional debates. But it has also provided a new lens through which social workers view their practice and their role to clients and communities. Few of these issues are resolved or possibly even resolvable, but HIV has forced us to reconsider a number of ethical and legal positions in a highly charged life-and-death atmosphere.

One of the most difficult tasks in the past decade of dealing with HIV has been developing and sustaining networks for social workers to become informed, to share their practical wisdom, and to debate questions of practice. Our hope is that this book may serve as a communication tool to link isolated practitioners, as well as inspire new generations of social workers to consider the implications of HIV for social work practice.

REFERENCE

Somerville, M., and N. Gilmore. 1992. 'Foreword to the Canadian Edition', in D. Kirp and R. Bayer, eds, *AIDS in the Industrialized Democracies: Passions, Politics, and Policies*. Montreal and Kingston: McGill-Queen's University Press.

Part One

Prevention

Commonly, social workers in Canada have been unclear as to their specific role in prevention activities and prevention programs concerning HIV and AIDS. Many have deferred to the health professions, specifically public health and the AIDS service organizations, which, on the surface, have appeared better suited to the task. Social workers have identified more readily with care, support, treatment, and advocacy roles in terms of the AIDS epidemic. In addition, many workers have questions concerning the effectiveness of prevention programs, given the relentless spread of the epidemic on a global basis and the continuous number of new infections in Canada despite widespread information and awareness campaigns.

As of December 1996, the number of cumulative deaths from HIV and AIDS worldwide had reached 6.4 million, the number of AIDS cases was just over 8.4 million, and the number of HIV infections was estimated at 30 million. In Canada the number of newly diagnosed AIDS cases began to level off in 1993 and to decline steadily thereafter. The Bureau of HIV/AIDS and STD (sexually transmitted disease) estimated that as of the end of 1996 a total of 50,000–54,000 Canadians had been infected with HIV since the onset of the epidemic. The number of new infections per year seems to have remained constant for the past few years, between 3,000 and 5,000. The majority of the increase in HIV infections appears to be occurring among injection drug users (IDU) and young gay men. Available data also suggest that there are dramatically increasing numbers of HIV infections among non-IDU heterosexuals (especially women and Aboriginal peoples).

The good news is that, because of new medications, AIDS cases and AIDS deaths appear to be declining in Canada. The bad news, of course, is that the incidence of new HIV infections has remained the same or increased slightly since the early 1990s. This means that the number of Canadians living with HIV is increasing. Rising prevalence means there is an increased need for care and support for persons living with HIV and potential increased risk of HIV transmission in Canada overall. This information clearly means that prevention must be a central part of any National AIDS Strategy. Prevention strategies must be employed by all human service professionals.

In July 1996, a large number of prevention specialists from around the world gathered together for the HIV 'Prevention Works' symposium in Vancouver. Following are some points about prevention that were supported by over 95 per cent of the participants.

1. HIV prevention works.
2. Well-designed HIV prevention interventions have demonstrated that risky sexual and drug-using behaviours can be changed to reduce the spread of HIV.

3. The participation of individuals infected with HIV in communities affected by the epidemic is critical to an effective, humane, and ethical response.
4. Prevention strategies must take fully into account that the epidemic is focused disproportionately on individuals who are marginalized in society and under-served by formal institutions and programs.
5. The populations hardest hit by the epidemic are already facing other health, social, and economic challenges. In concrete terms this means that HIV prevention strategies need to address poverty, must work to end violence against and any exploitation of women and children, and must promote the rights of ethnic minorities, refugees, migrants, drug users, sex workers, and the poor.
6. The key aspect of HIV prevention is a non-judgemental approach to individuals and communities most affected by HIV and AIDS. Equality within couples, families, and communities is important to people to be able to protect themselves against HIV infection.

The above points, while endorsed by a wide group of individuals experienced in HIV prevention, should be ideas and strategies that are very familiar to social workers and should leave no doubt that social workers have a central role to play in HIV prevention. As stated in the *Comprehensive Guide for the Care of Persons with HIV Diseases*:

> HIV infection is caused by a virus. It is also caused by poverty, by discrimination, by fear, by power imbalances in relationships, by low self-esteem, by the inability to make healthy personal choices, by drugs and other substances that cloud people's judgement, and by social attitudes that keep people from talking openly about sex and sexual orientation and from negotiating safer sex practices. (CASW, 1997: 139)

Clearly, the above is a prescription for social work involvement, and social workers would recognize the issues, the clients, and the processes inherent in these words. As such, this first section is devoted to prevention, which is largely multidisciplinary in perspective. Only by looking at prevention in all its complexity can we begin to see strategies emerge. Social workers will recognize the imperative of a critical analysis related to race, class, gender, and sexual orientation. This analysis provides a lens through which the social worker's traditional role in advocacy is challenged. If vulnerable populations are to be empowered to protect themselves from HIV infection, it will be due, in large part, to societal change impacting on the social determinants of health.

Chapters 1 and 2, compiled by a team from the Department of Sexology at the Université du Québec à Montréal, provide some important contributions to the literature. The first chapter, 'Sexual-Health Education and Promotion: The Heavy Burden of Preventing HIV Infection', critically examines the range of theories that have provided the basis for sex education and health promotion. Reviewing approaches that focus on the individual, interpersonal, social group, and societal levels, the authors help us to understand better both the failure and the promise of prevention programs. This chapter, rich in theory, is complemented by Chapter 2, which gives concrete examples of how theory has been put into practice. As such, they should be viewed as being two parts of a whole.

In Chapter 2, 'Putting Theory into Action: Prevention Programs in Canada', Joanne Otis, Joseph Lévy, and Marie-Josée Drouin review examples of prevention programs in Canada. The authors discuss programs that are demonstrably effective as well as those that have shown less promise so that readers can better appreciate the practical complexities of prevention programming.

In addition to the information and insight provided by these two chapters, English-Canadian social workers will get an uncommonly rare exposure to some of the creative programs that have been embraced in Quebec but have seldom been written about, or even discussed, in English Canada.

In Chapter 3, 'Social Workers and HIV Prevention: A Neglected Dyad', Lynne Leonard, after critiquing the position of social workers *vis-à-vis* social work and HIV prevention in Canada, presents a creative transtheoretical model for prevention activities. The model is consistent with modern social work's view of the client in a social context where structural analysis of class, gender, and culture in light of equality and oppression must guide effective practice. Leonard's model demonstrates how clients can become empowered to overcome the obstacles to health promotion in their lives and social contexts.

In Chapter 4, 'The Challenge of Risk Reduction Practices', William Rowe and Glenn Marcotte look at the controversial new prevention programs based on 'risk reduction' strategies borrowed from the field of addiction research. The authors review the tenets and principles of risk reduction methods and describe a unique program for clients with difficult life circumstances that is based on this philosophy.

Finally, while it is recognized that the majority of social workers may be new to HIV prevention activities, it is clear that social work practice and social workers bring a unique and critical element to HIV prevention and will form an important part of the solutions so desperately sought.

REFERENCE

Canadian Association of Social Workers. 1997. *Comprehensive Guide for the Care of Persons with HIV Diseases*. Ottawa: CASW.

Chapter 1

Sexual-Health Education and Promotion

The Heavy Burden of Preventing HIV Infection

JOANNE OTIS, JOSEPH LÉVY, AND MARIE-JOSÉE DROUIN

Since the beginning of the epidemic, in Canada as in the rest of the world, the burden of preventing HIV infection has rested almost exclusively on sexual-health education and promotion. As the dynamics of such infection have become better understood, these strategies have been adjusted and refined: the earliest efforts were aimed only at improving knowledge of modes of transmission and means of prevention, whereas today the most promising educational strategies combine community mobilization and empowerment at the levels of both the individual and the collectivity. They take into account not only individual risks but the social vulnerabilities associated with, for example, discrimination, poverty, and power relations.

Nevertheless, the epidemic continues to grow, which has allowed many to conclude that prevention based on these educational strategies has failed. Defending these efforts in Berlin in 1993, Lamptey et al. (1993) confirmed their value with respect to supporting individuals in modifying their risky sexual behaviours or in adopting and maintaining safety practices, as well as in creating more favourable attitudes towards safer sex. In their view, the real problem is the absence of the explicit political and societal will required for these experiments to be applied on a broader scale. Thus, the apparent failure of prevention does not mean that educational strategies are ineffective; rather, it reflects the inadequacy of their implementation in a socio-economic context that will make success even more difficult to achieve in the future (Barrett, 1994; references for Chapters 1 and 2 are at the end of Chapter 2).

In the next decade, the challenge of preventing HIV infection through sexual-health education and promotion will be all the greater because, rightly or wrongly, the advent of new therapies, with all their implicit promises, offers a less dramatic image of HIV and AIDS. This shift in image, from a fatal disease to one that is chronic or even curable, is bound to affect the way we approach prevention and hence education in the area of sexual health. Should we be doing more? Doing a better job? Or doing things differently?

This chapter in no way pretends to answer these questions. However, it may contribute to the discussion. It will present a number of approaches, models, and theories offering a direction for sexual-health education and promotion. In the following chapter, certain features of effective programs of education and promotion of sexual health will be discussed, along with the conditions facilitating or, on the contrary, impeding the implementation of such programs. Some experiments with various target groups will be described to illustrate not only the richness and diversity but also the frustrations of the responses to the HIV epidemic, both in Quebec and on the national level. This assessment will be followed by a number of reflections aimed at reorienting sexual-health education and promotion with respect to the new challenges to be faced in the field of HIV prevention.

SOME APPROACHES, MODELS, AND THEORIES TO GUIDE OUR ACTIONS

The approaches, models, and theories that have directed educational activities in the field of HIV prevention reflect both the advances that have been made in understanding the transmission dynamics of infection and the various disciplines that have taken up the mandate of prevention. Experts in public health (epidemiologists and professionals in behavioural science), on the one hand, and community-based organizations, on the other, often with very different ideas and financial resources, have had to learn to improvise as planners, project managers, and evaluators of so-called education and health-promotion programs for both the general public and more vulnerable groups. Thus it is not surprising that the majority of the dominant approaches come from the public-health and health-education sectors. These approaches, models, and theories can be grouped in three categories: individual, interpersonal, and community (Glanz, 1991; Lazes, Caplan, and Gordon, 1987; Lewis, 1991; Rimer, 1991; Valdiserri, 1989).

Ten years ago, most preventive education programs took a primarily individual approach, since the epidemiology of HIV and the urgency of the epidemic put the emphasis on modification of risk behaviours and adoption of safer behaviours. Use of condoms in all sexual relations with persons of unknown HIV status became the central aim of all intervention. To lead individuals to adopt this behaviour, programs sought to improve understanding, attitudes, and technical skills with respect to condom use. But this approach found only limited success, and it became clear that adoption of such behaviour was also influenced by the peer norm and the cooperation of the sexual partner; education programs thus were obliged to look at the interpersonal, emotional, and circumstantial dimensions and to put more emphasis on social skills (Botvin, Schinke, and Orlandi, 1995; Gaudreau, 1997; Maticka-Tyndale, 1997; Otis et al., 1997a). It was also necessary to realize that condom use was only one in a much more complex repertory of protection strategies that individuals have developed intuitively in response to the threat. More recently, the observation that the HIV epidemic reflects social and economic factors such as discrimination, power relations, and poverty has underlined the importance of tackling these factors at the community and even the sociopolitical and legislative levels, which has reasserted the value of community perspectives.

Today the challenge of preventing HIV infection requires that sexual-health education and promotion integrate the individual, interpersonal, and community perspectives. In fact, such integration is desired and upheld at the federal level by the 'National Guidelines for Sexual Health Education' (Health Canada, 1994).

DIRECTING ACTION AT THE INDIVIDUAL LEVEL

To promote changes at the individual level, educational activities have been guided by various approaches drawn primarily from psychology and the behavioural sciences. Though not exhaustive, Table 1 presents a number of these, grouped according to type: cognitive and decision-making theories, theories appealing to fear, emotions, and motivation, and theories of learning.

Table 1 Approaches, Models, and Theories Emphasizing the Individual Level

1. *Cognitive and decision-making theories*
   - health-belief model (Rosenstock et al., 1994)
   - theory of protection motivation (Rogers, 1983)
   - theory of reasoned action (Ajzen and Fishbein, 1980; Fishbein, 1979)
   - theory of planned behaviour (Ajzen, 1991)
   - theory of interpersonal behaviour (Triandis, 1979)
2. *Theories appealing to fear, motivation, and emotions*
   - theories of fear (Averill, 1987; Janis, 1967; McGuire, 1968; Rogers and Mewhorn, 1976; Sutton, 1982)
   - theory of locus of control (Wallston and Wallston, 1978)
   - theory of learned helplessness (Abrahamson et al., 1978)
   - theory of attribution (Heider, 1958; Weiner, 1993)
3. *Learning theories*
   - theory of operant conditioning (Skinner, 1969)
   - social cognitive theory (Bandura, 1977)
   - self-efficacy theory (Bandura, 1986, 1990)
   - relapse prevention theory (Marlatt and George, 1984)
   - self-regulation theory (Leventhal et al., 1983)
   - transtheoretical model (Prochaska et al., 1994)
   - AIDS risk reduction model (Catania, Kegeles, and Coates, 1990)
   - experiential taxonomy (Steinaker and Bell, 1979)

COGNITIVE AND DECISION-MAKING THEORIES

In general, cognitive and decision-making theories are based on the proposition that individuals are rational actors and processors of information, and that as soon as they know certain behaviours are risky, they will make choices to avoid them. These choices may be influenced, on one hand, by the perception of the gravity of HIV infection and the individual's own vulnerability to contracting it, and, on the other, by favourable attitudes towards the preventive behaviours to be adopted. These attitudes are the product of valuing the positive consequences and minimizing the negative consequences of adopting such behaviour. Some of these theories recognize the influence on such decisions of people important to the individual; their approval is a favourable factor, as is the perception that a given behaviour is valued by the social group to which the individual belongs.

Although these theories have been criticized for neglecting the influence of motivations and emotions, two of them have produced particularly convincing results: the theories of planned behaviour (Ajzen, 1985) and interpersonal behaviour (Triandis, 1979). The first recognizes the individual's perception of the psychological or environmental barriers that may prevent him from adopting a certain behaviour, barriers affecting the perception of control that the individual believes he exercises over the behaviour in question. These perceived barriers are often of an interpersonal or emotional nature, and they direct educational strategies towards the development of skills in the areas of communication and management of highly emotional situations. The theory of interpersonal behaviour, for its part, suggests that we take into account the moral responsibility to protect oneself and others; this moral dimension is absent from the other models, but it is nevertheless important in the context of preventing HIV infection.

THEORIES APPEALING TO FEAR, MOTIVATION, AND EMOTIONS

Theories appealing to fear, motivation, and emotions (unlike cognitive and decision-making theories) recognize a variety of processes internal to the individual that are capable of motivating a change in behaviour or of explaining why, in certain cases, he or she adopts inappropriate or dysfunctional behaviours such as denial, avoidance, flight, fatalism, etc.

Theories of fear arousal assume that the fear of contracting HIV is an emotion leading to a state of unease that the individual will seek to reduce. The management style adopted will depend on the intensity of the emotion; if the fear threshold is too low or too high, it will lead to inappropriate management styles; if the threshold is optimal, it can engender a rational, appropriate response leading to self-protection.

Among theories relating to motivations and emotions, two are especially relevant because they allow reflection on social vulnerability to HIV infection. Individuals with an external locus of control (with a constant overall perception that they are not in control of their fate) are often characterized by fatalism, passivity, depression, low self-esteem, and life conditions that are often precarious (low socio-economic status and income)—all factors associated with increased vulnerability to HIV infection. Other individuals who do not necessarily have this personality trait will develop a feeling of 'learned helplessness' through repeated exposure to events or situations that they are not able to control. Faced with the threat of HIV/AIDS, they will tend to transpose that feeling to this situation, assuming it to be beyond their power and, as it were, uncontrollable. This inability to take charge will have repercussions for the belief that a given preventive measure (such as condom use) can be an effective and useful defence against the threat.

The attribution theory also takes up these notions of locus of control and the controllability of events and situations. In a way, attributions are the causes that individuals generate to give meaning to their world. When an event occurs, assigning causes makes it possible to manage this event effectively. In fact, the actual nature of causal attributions (internal or external to the individual, general or specific, controllable or uncontrollable, permanent or temporary) will lead to the expression of various emotions (anger, shame, pride, guilt, gratitude, etc.) and changes in the expectations of success possible when the same situation arises in the future. The nature of the emotions experienced and the expectations of success, in turn, should lead to the adoption of reasoned behaviour. Although attributions are more closely related to the search for causes, they may also include the justifications, reasons, or excuses that an individual provides for a behaviour, emotion, or situation. The study of attributions relative to the prevention of HIV infection can assist us in understanding the meaning and explanations that individuals give to this phenomenon and in describing the emotions and behaviours that result from this quest for explanation or meaning.

As a whole, these theories (fear arousal, motivation, emotions) have not been widely used in the field of preventive education, except for fear theories in persuasive communication approaches. In fact, they have found little success. By contrast, the theories of learned helplessness, locus of control, and attribution have been underexploited, especially when one considers the importance now accorded to the emotions, the factors associated with social vulnerability, and the empowerment of vulnerable groups.

LEARNING THEORIES

Theories of learning, especially those developed by Bandura, have served as the basis for the development of many preventive education programs that have been found effective. In general, learning theories stress the environmental conditions capable of leading to the adoption and maintenance of a behaviour. Identifying these conditions makes it possible to direct action. No doubt the simplest of these theories is the theory of operative conditioning, since it postulates nothing about the cognitive processes involved. It rests exclusively on the appropriateness of a stimulus (a situation), a response (a behaviour), and a reinforcement agent represented by the positive or negative consequences generated by the response. The value of this theory for preventive education is simply its recognition of the importance of the circumstantial, even limited nature of a risk behaviour or a safety measure.

Bandura's social learning theory (hereafter social cognitive theory), on the other hand, is much richer because it takes into account cognitive processes and suggests a sequence in the structuring of educational activities. First, it is important that the information be provided in such a way as to raise awareness of the existence of the problem and to improve understanding of the health risks. Then it is necessary to develop the appropriate social skills and to promote the process of self-regulation required for these new concerns to be transformed into effective preventive action. It is important to provide opportunities to put these new skills into practice and at the same time to offer the corrective feedback for the individual to develop a strong, rooted belief in his self-efficacy with respect to the behaviour in question. A number of strategies may be used to this end: direct experience, indirect experience (modelling), verbal persuasion, and arousal of positive psychological states (e.g., pride, trust, etc.). Finally, meaningful sources of social support and reinforcement must be identified in the environment.

Social cognitive theory is the basis for most of the learning theories used in the field of HIV education and prevention. For example, according to the theory of relapse prevention, a return to risk practices would be associated with a weakening of the belief in self-efficacy as a result of a series of failures that the individual attributes to his own lack of skills or to the presence of too many external obstacles to maintaining a safer behaviour.

The concept of self-efficacy is particularly important in two more recent theories that treat the adoption of a particular behaviour as a process rather than an end point. According to Prochaska et al. (1994), individuals are situated along a five-stage continuum running from risk practices without the will to change to the adoption and maintenance of safety practices. Movement from one stage to another will be repetitive and strongly influenced by the individual's motivation to change and belief in personal efficacy. Catania et al. (1990) have suggested a similar model (three stages: perception of risk, intention to change behaviour, adoption and maintenance of the chosen behaviour) in which belief in self-efficacy plays a major role. These two models are particularly relevant to prevention of HIV infection because they accept the dynamic nature of the process through which desirable behaviours are or are not adopted, and suggest certain factors that should be taken into account to facilitate movement from one stage to the next. Although these models have only recently been applied to preventive education, they seem promising.

The theory of self-regulation puts forward the hypothesis that people generate implicit theories with respect to their bodies and their health, representations that are themselves constructed through social learning (direct and indirect experience, etc.). This hypothesis links self-regulation theory to theories about social representations developed within an entirely different paradigm. Several authors have studied the social representations of AIDS and its prevention, and in their view preventive education would benefit from greater concentration on this angle (Desaulniers, 1994; Gaudreau, 1994; Paicheler, 1997). Thus, whereas self-regulation theory suggests approaching representations of the disease from the angle of risk perception, expression of fear, and social learning (concepts closer to determinist models), the approaches founded on social representations assume a process of simultaneous reference both to external social influences that have already been integrated and to values, beliefs, opinions, attitudes, emotions, knowledge, and personal experience (a more constructivist perspective) (Gaudreau, 1994).

In our opinion, a combination of these paradigms offers the most promise for sexual-health education and promotion. In fact, most of the theories or approaches used until now to direct action at the individual level have had as their goal the adoption and maintenance of safe behaviour, on the hypothesis that modifying the predictors of such behaviour will lead to its adoption. This determinism often neglects the learning process itself and the ways it can be facilitated. Of all the theories described, only Bandura's social cognitive theory includes explicit postulates in this regard. Thus, other more interactive or constructivist approaches should be considered. Without dictating the content of educational programs, such approaches could allow the people involved to define that content and to take a more active role in their own learning. In this regard, the experiential approach suggested by Steinaker and Bell (1979) merits consideration. Encouraging the formation of persons in their totality, the experiential approach actively involves the learner in the learning process on the cognitive, socio-affective level as well as the behavioural level. The process of meaningful learning becomes rooted in the lived experience of the learner (perception of his/her own needs, concerns, and desires for change) because he/she must take charge of his/her own learning process, understand personal experience, take responsibility for choices, and manage his/her actions autonomously (Côté, 1990).

The experiential approach to education aims not only at the acquisition of knowledge and the development of skills, but also at the development of personal attitudes and values leading towards responsible habits of action. Furthermore, it rests on the assumption that the process of consciousness-raising associated with meaningful learning takes place in distinct stages that are not linear but concentric. The experience acquired at one stage is reinvested to promote a deepening of experience and an appropriation of learning that becomes more and more personal.

The process of integrating learning experiences consists of five *progressive, cumulative* stages and substages. The first stage (opening up) creates the intention to develop responsible habits—for example, with respect to sexual well-being and prevention. The second stage (participation) transforms experience through the personal involvement of the learner: conscious and thoughtful participation permits a personal representation of the knowledge and skills that are the objects of the process. The third stage (identification) produces change at the level of personal attitudes and values, change that has a meaning for the person. These new attitudes and values will determine the feelings, preferences, and priorities that will influence the individual's judgement of situations and his decision-making process as to the choices possible in action. The fourth step (interiorization) seeks to expand learning, permitting resolution of various situations involving decisions about sexual well-being and prevention, following the principle of generalization of learning, which promotes the emergence of responsible habits in the person's life. These habits involve an intention and a sense of self-efficacy that manifest themselves as often as necessary in everyday life. They also involve the capacity to reflect on the relevance/appropriateness of an action, depending on the importance and priority of the values at play in a given situation and the consequences of the action. This process permits the adoption of appropriate behaviours. In the final stage (dissemination), learning produces an internal change in self-image, leading the learner to want to tell others about the modifications his own habits have undergone. This new mode of being manifests itself in the concern to serve as a model for others (Côté, 1990).

In terms of content for preventive education, this approach resembles most of the theories presented above. Nevertheless, it suggests that we proceed *differently* in leaving everything to the experience of the individual and the meaning she or he gives to it. This kind of approach should be considered in our efforts at education in the area of sexual health. However, we must remember that it requires a different kind of investment on the part of interveners: instead of trainers, they become animators; instead of guiding forces, they become facilitators, agents of change. The power passes from the educator to the educatee, and this approach can only promote empowerment for the individual. Will interveners prove equal to this challenge? Perhaps they will have to.

In future, programs seeking modifications at the level of the individual may have to rely on some combination of the theories outlined here, while respecting the principles on which each is based. Among cognitive and decision-making theories, the theories of planned behaviour and interpersonal behaviour are probably the most promising. Theories of motivation and emotions are interesting because they allow room for the expression of emotions and recognize their influence on behaviour. Some of them also allow reflection on social vulnerability. Bandura's social cognitive theory remains an extremely useful theory of learning, but perhaps we will have to learn how to use it from experiential approaches.

GUIDING ACTION AT THE INTERPERSONAL LEVEL

Not many approaches, models, or theories are concerned with interpersonal dimensions, and few of them have been specifically applied to education about sexual health in the field of HIV prevention. Table 2 lists some of these approaches, the first considering interactions with peers and the immediate social circle (theories of social influence, social support, and stress management), the second dealing more with interaction with partners (sexual scripts, the IMB [information-motivation behavioural] model, theories of interpersonal communication, and feminist theories), and the last discussing interaction between professionals/interveners/educators and patients/clients/educatees. In general, these theories are based on the assumption that individuals are social beings who acquire their sense of power and skills through interaction with others. This interpersonal environment affects their evaluation of threats, provides the necessary information and the services or resources they need, and influences both their behaviour and, eventually, their health (Lewis, 1991). These theories come from psychology, sociology, and the sciences concerned with communication.

THEORIES OF INTERACTION WITH PEERS AND THE IMMEDIATE SOCIAL CIRCLE

According to theories of social influences, others (peers, the immediate social circle) have an impact on changes in an individual's beliefs, attitudes, or behav-

Table 2 Approaches, Models, and Theories Emphasizing the Interpersonal Level

1. *Theories of interaction with peers and the immediate social circle*
   - theories of social influence (Festinger, 1950; Moscovici, 1985)
   - models of social support and stress management (Evans and Cohen, 1987; Lazarus, 1966)
2. *Theories of interaction with partners*
   - sexual scripts (Adelman, 1992; Simon and Gagnon, 1986)
   - theories of interpersonal communication (Edgar, 1992; Metz and Fitzpatrick, 1992)
   - information-motivation behavioural (IMB) model (Fisher and Fisher, 1992, 1993)
   - feminist theories stressing gender-based power relations (Holland et al., 1992)
3. *Theories of interaction between educators and educatees*
   - models of interaction between professionals and patients/clients/educatees (Joos and Hickam, 1991)
   - social pedagogy of intervention (Bouchard, 1997)

iours in two ways: normative (change being motivated by the desire to win others' approval) and informative (change beginning with the perception that the group consensus reflects an objective reality). In both cases, the durability of the change will depend on the credibility and attractiveness of the source of social influence (more durable) or the power it exerts on the individual (less durable). These latter principles are related to those of persuasive communication (discussed below). In preventive education, theories of this kind support the use of several methods based on peers (modelling, peer training, etc.). On the other hand, the management style that an individual adopts in response to a threatening situation will depend in particular on the support of his/her immediate circle. With respect to HIV prevention, this principle, backed up by theories of social support and stress management, encourages the development of support groups and peer aid networks—educational strategies that have been widely used and are relatively effective.

THEORIES OF INTERACTION WITH PARTNERS

Approaches focusing on interaction with sexual partners, particularly regarding condom use, are still at a developmental stage but nevertheless interesting to examine.

According to Miller et al. (1993), studies in the negotiation of safer sex should take into account the dynamic nature of sexual interaction, which is subject as much to individual processes (desires, goals, intensity of sexual excitation, etc.) as to the interpersonal processes in which individuals influence one another. Their theory of personal communication requires consideration of four elements: (1) the goals of each partner (e.g., desire to avoid conflict, maintain intimacy, etc.); (2) the perceived obstacles, intrinsic and extrinsic, to safer sex; (3) the plans and strategies that might be and are used to negotiate safe sex (direct and indirect, verbal and non-verbal methods based on some kind of power—charm, self-assertion, aggression, manipulation, seduction, coercion, violence, etc.) (Otis et al., 1997b); (4) how these strategies and practices fit into sexual scripts.

Sexual scripts are ordered sequences of behaviour, usually with social and cultural roots. According to several authors, efforts at education and prevention must be more explicit about the opportune moments to propose and negotiate condom use. Identification of the sexual scripts specific to a particular group makes it possible to suggest the moment(s) in the sexual choreography when this kind of proposition will be accepted as normative. Although sexual scripts can be fairly stereotyped, some authors (Adelman, 1992) urge us to recognize that they can also be improvised. Thus it is not only a matter of suggesting to individuals a propitious moment in the sexual sequence for negotiating condom use, but also of supporting them in the development of more creative strategies—for example, based on play or humour.

In the Canadian context, Fisher and Fisher (1992, 1993) have recently proposed a model of preventive education based both on cognitive and decision-making theories and on sexual scripts. Their IMB model assumes that behaviour is actually a complex series of steps, rather like a scenario. The behavioural skills envisioned in this model are explicitly presented. The individual must be able:

- to accept one's own sexuality;
- to obtain the relevant information (and to assess it accurately);
- to set a personal prevention agenda;
- to negotiate safer sex;
- to eliminate situations where negotiation is not possible;
- to perform certain public actions (buying condoms in a drug store, asking for an HIV antibody test);
- to find ways of reinforcing oneself and one's partner;
- to evaluate the quality of one's actions and adjust them as necessary by changing one's own sexual scripts.

Application of this model to sexual-health education and promotion is particularly innovative because it integrates safer sex not only within the sexual choreography but within the entire range of actions to be performed by the individual as well as in the interpersonal context.

Nevertheless, in the educational context, consideration of the interactions that take place within the love/sex dyad cannot ignore the existence of power relations based on gender, which vary widely with the values and norms of a given culture but too often fail to promote the sexual health of women (Holland et al., 1992; Amaro, 1995). The influence of power relations based on gender, characterized by the domination, control, and pressures exerted by the male partner, express themselves in the sexual scripts and communication styles used by one partner or the other to negotiate safer sex (Otis et al., 1997b; Arroyo et al., 1997). The tensions to which these relations give rise must be addressed in every educational intervention, emphasizing the specificities of masculine and feminine identities, social and sexual roles, sexist stereotypes, etc. On the other hand, power relations based on gender also lie at the root of the increased vulnerability of certain women to HIV infection because of their impact on the social conditions under which these women live: economic dependence, poverty, violence and abuse of all kinds. From the perspective of female empowerment, on the individual as well as the collective level, the theme of gender-based power relations cannot be avoided.

THEORIES OF INTERACTION BETWEEN EDUCATORS AND EDUCATEES

Several models, drawn from social psychology in particular, address the role played and the place given to one or the other of the people involved in interactions between educators and educatees. Some of these models are cognitive in nature. The educator provides the information (essential and specific) and checks the understanding of the educatee, whose role is, as it were, passive. In our view, this kind of interaction is too common in preventive education, and in many cases accounts for the failure of such efforts. Other models put more emphasis on the social influence of the educator and his/her ability to persuade the educatee. Because of the educator's privileged position, he/she is in a position of power as the credible and legitimate expert, the one with the power to dispense rewards or reprimands. Although he/she listens to the educatee, it is his/her mandate to guide the latter towards a predetermined goal, and persuasive strategies often reflect the power that the educator is willing or able to exercise. This potential power relationship between educator and educatee can both promote and hinder learning. It is not clear that interveners in the field of preventive education are always aware of the effects this relationship can have in their educational interactions.

While some models focus only on the educator's capacities for listening and empathy and his/her ability to create an atmosphere of trust (personal interaction models), others are based mainly on the ability to establish a climate for negotiation. Models of conflict resolution and negotiation (Kleinman, 1980; Leventhal, 1985) centre primarily on the educatee. The educator is there to create the conditions under which exchange can take place. She or he provides the basic information and should communicate to the educatee respect, understanding, and acceptance. The educatee is allowed to present his or her perspective on the problem, to express desires and expectations. Later, the educator helps the educatee to establish personal priorities and a mutual action plan is developed. These theories in which the educator is above all a guide and facilitator are akin to principles of adult education. In a context where educational activity ought to promote empowerment, the kind of interaction between educator and educatee that these theories suggest is certainly desirable.

Bouchard (1997) presents a new vision of the educator-educatee relationship in his reflections on partnership and the social pedagogy of intervention in the prevention of AIDS. In his view, partnership involves attitudes, values, beliefs, and know-how consistent with appropriation and self-determination. This partnership is achieved through reciprocal learning, a kind of pedagogical interdependence in the reciprocal development of educator and educatee, intervener and learner. The relationship is not one of helper and helpee, but rather of giver to giver, in which each party learns from the other's knowledge and experience. This reciprocity of learning is fundamental to what Bouchard calls the social pedagogy of intervention. It implies a model of educational practice that facilitates the effect of pedagogical synergy between *authors* and their equality with respect to the division of power and knowledge. According to Bouchard, 'it is no longer a question of training subject-agents of prevention whose only initiative is to follow the instructions laid down by others, nor subject-actors responsible for playing the role determined by prevention specialists, but rather of training authors able to draw on their capacity for autonomy and their power to transcend themselves both individually and collectively.'

In a context where educational activity ought to promote empowerment, the type of interaction suggested by the theories of conflict resolution, negotiation, and above all the social pedagogy of intervention could serve as the basis for a new way of approaching education in the field of sexual health and prevention of HIV infection. Moreover, this vision of educator-educatee interaction is entirely compatible with the experiential approaches described above.

In the next few years it will be imperative for the development of models or theories of an interpersonal nature to be integrated into the conception and implementation of programs. Several of the theories presented here depart from the traditional paths; perhaps they will allow us to do a *better* job . . . and to do it *differently*.

DIRECTING ACTION AT THE COMMUNITY LEVEL

When changes of every kind are desirable on the level of communities or social systems, various approaches, theories, and models, mainly from sociology or anthropology, can be used to support the design and implementation of preventive educational activity. Table 3 presents some of these. They fall into two groups, depending on the source initiating the change: an agent external to the community (persuasive communication, diffusion of innovations, social marketing) or the community itself (theories of community organization).

PERSUASIVE COMMUNICATION

Since preventive education on a broad public scale was first attempted, persuasive communication in particular has been widely used. Its principles are based on a matrix that McGuire (1985) defines as consisting of, on one hand, the 'inputs' to be considered and, on the other, the process and the expected results. Briefly, the inputs are the source of the message and its characteristics (credibility, attractiveness, power), the message itself and the nature of its appeal (cognitive, emotional [fear, responsibility], etc.), the channels of communication to be used, the charac-

Table 3 Approaches, Models, and Theories Emphasizing the Community Level

1. *Theories of persuasive communication* (McGuire, 1985; Petty, Gleincher, and Jarvis, 1993)
2. *The theory of diffusion of innovations* (Rogers and Shoemaker, 1971; Rogers, 1983)
3. *Social marketing* (Kotler, 1982; Lovelock and Weinberg, 1984)
4. *Theories of community organization*
   - social planning (Glanz, 1991; Rothman, 1979)
   - precede-proceed model (Green and Kreuter, 1991)
   - organizational development (Glanz, 1991)
   - locality development (Glanz, 1991; Rothman, 1979)
   - social action (Glanz, 1991; Rothman, 1979)
   - emergent change methodology (Schoonbroodt and Gélinas, 1997)

teristics of those receiving the message, and the target aimed at (knowledge, attitudes, values, behaviours, etc.). The process and the results can be summed up as follows: exposure to the message, grasp of its content, interest in and understanding of the message, message retention, decision-making, action, and re-evaluation of action. Although several large public campaigns have been developed following these principles, their effects are often limited to increases in knowledge and sensitivity—only rarely do they include changes in attitudes or behaviour.

THE THEORY OF DIFFUSION OF INNOVATIONS

The theory of diffusion of innovations (which also explains the process of communication) puts forward the hypothesis that the distribution patterns and adoption rates for a particular innovation are a function of the attributes of the innovation itself and the characteristics of the adopter. In general, the innovations with the best chance of being adopted are compatible with the values of the system and the adopter; they have a certain flexibility (its components are separable or sequential) and are reversible; they have advantages over other products or services; they offer more benefits than drawbacks; and they involve little risk at the time of adoption. The process of developing a new product consists of six steps:

1. recognition of a problem or need;
2. research, first basic, then applied, into the product and the potential adopters;
3. development of the new idea according to the needs of various adopters;
4. commercialization (production, marketing, and distribution);
5. distribution and follow-up on adoption;
6. evaluation of effects and consequences.

According to this theory, there are five stages to adoption: awareness of a problem, interest in the suggested innovation (solution), trial, decision, and adoption. In the present context, this theory can be especially relevant for following the evolution of the combination therapies approach and its dissemination to doctors and to people living with HIV or recently infected. It can also help us to understand certain groups' resistance to condom use, a behaviour with some characteristics that run counter to the most successful innovations.

SOCIAL MARKETING

While emphasizing communication, social marketing is a process of planning and implementation similar to that in the theory of diffusion of innovations. Once the nature and size of the potential market are known, various segments of it are identified and targeted; then, if necessary, different strategies are developed for these segments. A key concept in social marketing is the 'marketing mix'. It is important to highlight the benefits of the product on offer and to consider the price the individual is prepared to pay for it (this notion of costs/benefits, advantages/disadvantages, is consistent with several cognitive theories). Then thought must be given to distribution (where, when, and how), and the whole communication strategy must be developed and put into play: personal communication, media activities, public relations, promotion and information at various service points—what is called the 'communication mix'. This approach has been widely used, especially in developing countries, and has certainly contributed to the worldwide growth in condom sales (Lamptey et al., 1993).

THEORIES OF COMMUNITY ORGANIZATION

The three approaches described above involve an external agent who seeks to initiate or support a change. In contrast, theories of community organization assume that the motivation for change comes from within the community. Nevertheless, these theories of community organization often take different views of the nature of the interaction between the initiators of the project and the individuals to whom it is addressed.

Social planning is the process by which experts seek to resolve a social problem through rational strategies and changes controlled by the experts themselves. It is result-oriented. (Organizational development is similar, except that it refers to the planning and implementation of this kind of change within an organization.) In Canada at the national level and in Quebec, government anti-AIDS strategies correspond in a way to this approach, in which priorities are defined, a priori, by experts who are often selected on the basis of their involvement (basic research, treatment, epidemiology, or education) in the prevention and control of HIV infection. While the community perspective is taken into account, the final decisions are made by the experts, especially where the allocation of financial resources is concerned.

Green and Kreuter's precede-proceed model (1991) was not specifically intended to be applied in this kind of social planning, but it is in this way that it is most frequently used in the field of sexual-health education. This model involves a series of five diagnostic stages, a single implementation stage, and three evaluation stages. Its great strength lies in the systematization of each stage, permitting consideration of all the elements involved in establishing a program promoting sexual health. It looks at all the stakes involved—individual, interpersonal, organizational, administrative, and political—as well as the interactions between these various factors.

By contrast, locality development is more oriented towards the process by which a community focuses on the development of its own skills and feelings of competence in order to improve social conditions. It is based on mutual assistance and problem resolution through consensus, and is particularly effective when the interests of all parties are compatible and reconcilable. With this kind of approach, the agent of change begins by facilitating the development of conflict-resolution skills and becomes a co-ordinator when the time comes to take action.

Social action, for its part, is the approach by which a disadvantaged segment of a society organizes itself to demand a redistribution of resources. Consensus does not exist between the various social classes in the community. The targeted segment appears to be the group victim of powerful economic and political interests. Social action is task-oriented and focuses on the establishment of strategies to ensure that their demands and protests are heard. Feminist movements have favoured social action. In addition, this critical approach is related to the consciousness-raising developed and practised by Paulo Freire in the 1970s. In social action, the agent of change is not simply a resource, but also a critical facilitator.

The last two theories of community organization (locality development and social action) rest on very different paradigms from social planning and promote the empowerment of individuals and of the community. In the context of Quebec, Schoonbroodt and Gélinas (1997) have developed an approach consistent with the principles of the last two models. It, too, is oriented towards empowerment, although they prefer the term 'appropriative management', which they define as 'the process by which a person, group, or collective becomes conscious of the diversity of its representations, its stakes, its resources and its constraints, and translates these into decisions for his/its future' (Gélinas et al., 1995). 'This process aims at the appropriation, by social actors, of the symbolic tools that can help them to understand and take on the problems of everyday life, the conflicts and paradoxical situations' (Schoonbroodt and Gélinas, 1997).

To further this process, they suggest the methodology of emergent change, which has many ontological foundations (soft systems methodology, social representations, concept of complexity, etc.). This methodology is made up of four repeated, non-linear steps. 'Problemation' consists in identifying, with the actors, the situation posing the problem in order to lead them to express what it is they want to change and what means they see of bringing this about. The intervener does not interfere in this process of identifying the problem or objects of change. At the stage of 'conceptualization' the intervener becomes the analyst. He identifies the different visions and develops various conceptual models. These models are based on scientific knowledge, but should reflect the constructions of meaning that the actors give them. At the stage of 'deliberation', the models thus generated are compared with the actors' reality. The scientific, theoretical, and experiential worlds come together: the proposed models are transformed, evolve. At the 'contextualization' stage the actors decide on the action to be taken and carry it out. Let us recall that this is a dynamic process and allows for movement back and forth between stages, in any order, as required and depending on the context. This methodology has not yet been applied to education in the area of sexual health. However, the challenges of preventing HIV infection are such that we should perhaps consider doing things differently. This approach offers a path worth exploring if interveners can accept this involvement, this co-construction towards self-determined change, in which the object of change may be something quite different from the choice to use a condom.

If the notion of social vulnerability is now accepted and supported by the scientific community concerned with HIV/AIDS, community mobilization and empowerment become the favoured strategies. Community approaches based on communication remain useful, but are not sufficient to bring about profound change at the individual and community levels. Nevertheless, they can play a role in creating an environment that is more favourable, more tolerant, more open to differences, and can help to support and reinforce the other educational strategies that are implemented. Locality development and social action are more necessary than ever, especially in a context where we must deal with discrimination, poverty, and power relations of all kinds.

EFFECTIVENESS CRITERIA AND CONDITIONS OF IMPLEMENTATION

After 15 years of efforts to prevent HIV infection, the accumulation of experience in the area of sexual-health education and promotion makes it possible to identify certain criteria that appear to be associated with success (Kirby et al., 1994; Samson, 1995; Health Canada, 1994; Botvin et al., 1995). These are presented in Table 4. Without discussing all of them, some in particular are worth underlining.

Intervention in the area of preventive education must be rooted in the best possible understanding of the needs, values, and norms of the group in question. Whatever methods are used, analysis of these stakes, whether preliminary or ongoing, is essential to the implementation process. Furthermore, the planners or agents of change must provide and put in place adequate strategies to reach the target population. Vulnerable groups often have no contact with captive settings, and the only way to reach them is through street work and outreach (Gillis, 1994). These strategies in themselves set the limits for education in the area of prevention.

In terms of objectives, successful programs have been oriented explicitly towards the modification of risky sexual practices and their individual, interpersonal, or social determinants. Nevertheless, identification of this criterion of effectiveness is closely related to the determinist paradigm within which most interventions have been planned, and it would be useful to evaluate the impact of new educational activities more deeply rooted in interactive and constructivist

Table 4 Effectiveness Criteria for Education in the Area of Sexual Health and Prevention of HIV Infection

1. Sensitivity to psychological, sexual, cultural, and social needs; respect for developmental characteristics (age and experience), environmental context, and cultural norms.
2. Theoretical grounding favouring learning and taking into account 'person-environment' interaction.
3. Establishment of adequate strategies to reach the target population.
4. Objectives explicitly oriented towards reduction of risky practices and adoption and maintenance of safety precautions.
5. Course contents:
   - specific knowledge of how HIV/AIDS is transmitted
   - favourable attitudes towards safer sex
   - motivation and ability to judge situations
   - social skills concerning management of sexuality and safer sex
   - change in or reinforcement of individual values
   - change in peer-group norms
   - preventive behaviours re: alcohol and drug abuse
   - discrimination
   - solidarity
   - community resources and social support
   - creation of a favourable environment
6. Educational methods: interactive and experiential (use of peer groups, modelling, etc.).
7. Linkage and complementarity of resources, integrative approaches:
   - community participation and support (CLSC [Centre local de services communautaires], parents, etc.)
   - policy development
   - environmental change
   - media reinforcement
   - social action
   - integration with health services and reinforcement of these services
   - involvement of important political and religious bodies and their leaders
8. Training and support for various participants (parents, interveners, community leaders, etc.).

perspectives and centred on learning and appropriation rather than results. In fact, this proposition is consistent with the group of pedagogical methods found to be most effective: that is, the more interactive and experiential methods (discussion groups, role-playing, games and simulations, use of peers, modelling, personal testimony, direct experience, etc.). The choice of one or another of these pedagogical methods should be determined by very specific criteria depending on the nature of the health problem in question, the characteristics of the target group, and administrative considerations. Green et al. (1980) offer a fairly exhaustive inventory of these criteria in relation to certain pedagogical methods oriented towards communication, training, or community organization. Effectiveness, however, depends more on the degree of cognitive involvement and emotional engagement made possible by the educational approach proposed than on the length and intensity of programs, as Green et al. suggest.

The last two effectiveness criteria identified in Table 4—intervention that is tightly linked to other structures in the environment (services, resources, organizations, sociopolitical institutions, etc.) and the training of the various interveners involved—are very important. Not only are these criteria of effectiveness, but they make up an important part of the conditions required for the implementation and pursuit of education and prevention efforts in a given community.

However well articulated a program may be, it still must be implemented to a degree sufficient to bring about the change it seeks. Too often, educational and preventive interventions have been found ineffective when the extent of their implementation has not been taken into account in the evaluation design. Many factors—personal, organizational, and interorganizational—affect the implementation of a program (Denis and Champagne, 1990).

On the personal level, the characteristics of all the actors involved, at every possible level, play a major role. Their values, attitudes, motivations, and feelings of competence *vis-à-vis* both themselves and the orientations of the program; the perceived incentives, both internal and external, to become involved; the clarity of the organizational expectations; their technical competence; their active participation in the development and implementation of the program—all of these factors can either facilitate or hinder the implementation of the project.

On the organizational level, the characteristics of the setting for a prevention program will influence the intensity of implementation. For example, does the setting recognize the existence of the problem or the presence of the target clientele? Do the orientations of the proposed program correspond to the mission of this setting, its values, and its priorities for action? How does the hierarchical structure ensure that interveners get the time, the resources, and the support they need from the decision-makers? What are the working dynamics among the various actors involved in this setting? Every one of these questions will bring to mind instances where each of us has encountered resistance to implementing some activity that, however well conceived and well suited to the needs of our clientele it may have been, was incompatible with the aims of the organizational setting.

On the interorganizational level, given the importance of close links between the setting for a program and other services or resources, the existence and quality of the partnership, the mechanisms in place to facilitate and reinforce it, and the clear definition of the roles and mandates of everyone involved in a concerted action are all factors affecting the quality of the program, once established.

In the Canadian context, despite the existence of policies, national strategies, and guidelines and the availability of various written programs, pedagogical tools of all kinds, and audiovisual materials designed for various target groups, there is a large gap between what is encouraged at the bureaucratic level and what is actually implemented at the local community level; the factors outlined above may explain some of this gap. Moreover, even when a program has proved effective (often because it was a pilot project receiving generous funding), the conditions for its continuance remain precarious because the current funding structures do not always permit these efforts to be sustained or repeated. Once again, from the perspective of empowerment, perhaps we have to learn to do things differently, if sexual-health education and promotion are to carry the responsibility for preventing HIV infection.

Chapter 2

Putting Theory into Action

Prevention Programs in Canada

JOANNE OTIS, JOSEPH LÉVY, AND MARIE-JOSÉE DROUIN

In Canada, the responsibility for preventing HIV infection is shared by many different structures, which means that it is difficult to co-ordinate their efforts in an integrated overall action plan. On one hand, provincial organizations may be supported by different federal government authorities, whether in the area of sexual-health education and promotion or in the area of preventing HIV infection; on the other hand, many initiatives are first developed with provincial support, which varies widely, in form and amount, between provinces, depending on the structures in place. In this context it becomes particularly difficult to attest to the richness and diversity of Canada's response to HIV infection, especially since most of the experiments in the area of sexual-health education and promotion have not been evaluated or made available through formal publication. Furthermore, although various federal, provincial, or regional policies provide direction in terms of priorities defined on the basis of epidemiological data and grant funds according to these priorities, in practice, action often takes a different form, depending more on the receptivity and sensitivity of a given setting, the conviction and will of the human resources in place, the ease of joining a given group through already existing structures, etc. These facts explain why, at present, the most vulnerable individuals and groups have rarely been reached, while others have been overexposed to a message they do not strongly identify with.

In this chapter we will describe a number of experiments—some successful, others less so—in order to share the lessons that may be drawn from these actions with various target groups: teenagers reached in the school setting, young offenders reached in halfway houses, street youth, women, men having sex with other men, and interveners. Success can be measured on one or several of various indicators such as: changed behaviour, changed values, reduced risk, lower seroprevalence, more tolerance towards people with HIV, etc. Activities undertaken with injection drug users and prostitutes are treated in Chapter 10; but there is no published information on any systematic educational activity concerning ethnocultural communities or people with disabilities (physical or intellectual)—an absence that reflects the insufficiency of prevention efforts directed at these groups.

EDUCATIONAL ACTIVITIES WITH TEENAGERS IN SCHOOL

Although teenagers represent less than 1 per cent of all declared cases of AIDS both in Quebec and nationally, intervention efforts on their behalf are justified for several reasons, especially epidemiological: for example, the proportion of declared AIDS cases among people aged 20–9 (20 per cent), which suggests that many of them were infected during adolescence, and the high prevalence among those aged 15–24 of sexually transmitted diseases (STDs), which have several risk factors similar to those associated with HIV infection (premature sexual relations, unprotected sex, etc.). Other arguments rely more on the high potential for influencing behaviours before they become deeply rooted in the individual's scripts. Adolescence is a time of discovery and new learning in various spheres (friendship, love, sexuality, alcohol, drugs, etc.), many of them interrelated. The possibility of guiding this learning and creating the conditions under which these new experiences will be positive offers a unique opportunity to act before problems arise. Furthermore, the school setting not only makes teenagers far easier to reach than other target groups, but also offers the best possible conditions for a gradual learning process, keeping pace with their psycho-socio-sexual development.

In Canada the guidelines for sex education vary from one province to another, and AIDS education is not always clearly integrated into them. For example, in the late 1980s some provinces, such as Ontario, made AIDS education compulsory through limited curricula, not integrated into sex education; it often took the form of seminars or a handful of sessions oriented primarily towards improving knowledge (Chandarana et al., 1990; Scott et al., 1990).

SKILLS FOR HEALTHY RELATIONSHIPS

In 1991, based on new findings concerning adolescent sexuality and prevention of HIV infection, the Skills for Healthy Relationships program was introduced in four provinces for students in grade 9. The 20 hours required for this program were taken from courses in family economy (New Brunswick), sciences (Manitoba), personal and social development (Nova Scotia), and physical and health education (Ontario). A program of such broad scope would not have been possible without significant financial support and the involvement of a whole team of experts. Under the aegis of the Council of Ministers of Education, its development and evaluation were subsidized by Health Canada and carried out by the Social Programs Evaluation Group at Queen's University. Unlike earlier experiments on the national level, this program was based on solid theoretical premises, notably the information-motivation-behavioural skills model, combining certain cognitive and decision-making theories with the integration of learning experiences within sexual scripts as suggested by Fisher and Fisher (1992, 1993). It emphasized four components: acquisition of adequate knowledge, development of responsible attitudes and intentions, consideration of motivational factors providing the necessary support from peers and parents, and acquisition of skills (Warren et al., 1994). It consisted of 31 learning activities, 25 of them to be done in class under the direction of the teacher and in small groups led by student team leaders, and six at home with parents participating. These activities were supposed to achieve the following objectives:

> to persuade young people who are not yet sexually active to delay the moment when they do become active, to modify the behaviour of other

young people so that they return to abstinence, to encourage young people who are having sexual relations to take more precautions, to promote an attitude of tolerance towards homosexuality, and of compassion towards people living with HIV, among students. (Warren et al, 1994)

The results of the rigorous evaluation of this program (quasi-experimental design, pre-test, post-tests, with a non-random control group) indicate that, two years after it ended, the students who participated in it had a better understanding of HIV, AIDS, and STDs than those in the control group, more favourable attitudes towards homosexuality and people living with HIV, stronger intentions regarding communication with partners (talking about previous sexual experiences, refusing sexual relations, discussing condom use), and a greater feeling of competence about obtaining or buying condoms. On the other hand, the program does not seem to have had any impact on rates of sexual activity among young people or constancy of condom use (Warren and King, 1994). Following this evaluation showing its relative effectiveness, the program was reworked in depth and its developers suggest that, after implementation, reinforcement activities should be offered to students on a regular basis to maintain knowledge and encourage behavioural changes. At present, this program is offered in various provinces and the Northwest Territories, following local training workshops for teachers. Meeting the majority of the criteria presented in Table 4 in Chapter 1, it is certainly one of the most promising programs on the national level in Canada.

In Quebec, sex education programs have been the primary vehicle for activities aimed at preventing HIV infection. Since 1989, concerted action by the health and education networks has led to the introduction of an optional but specific segment on AIDS within the framework of the Personal and Social Education (PSE) course. This course was compulsory in both primary and secondary schools and includes sex and health education, themes that allow for the inclusion of a segment relating to AIDS (Hamel, St-Onge, and Desaulniers, 1994). Furthermore, starting in 1992, the Ministerial Policy on Health and Welfare reinforced these efforts and contributed to the creation of a favourable atmosphere by including the promotion of condom accessibility in the school setting. In fact, a recent study directed by the Quebec AIDS Co-ordination Centre (CQCS) (Fournier, 1997) indicates that the rate of students with access to condoms has risen from 55.4 per cent in 1994 to 70.0 per cent in 1996 in Quebec's public secondary schools, the principal means of access being through the school's health service (89.3 per cent of schools where condoms are available) and through condom machines (31.3 per cent of schools where condoms are available). These efforts appear to have contributed to the reduction in STDs and the increase in the adoption of safer practices among Quebec teenagers (Otis, 1996).

Unfortunately, the reforms currently under way in Quebec's health and education networks raise serious concerns about how to prevent HIV infection in the school setting; on one hand, the inclusion of PSE courses in future secondary-school programs is now in question; on the other, the hours when school nurses are present are being reduced. These formal structures and resources, supported politically at the provincial level, were a great asset, and their loss represents another obstacle to future activities in the area of sexual-health education and promotion. Now these activities will depend on the leadership and goodwill of regional and local authorities, which may mean unequal access for students to these educational activities. In this context, a number of Quebec experiments are worthy of mention.

LIFE-SAVERS

For several years, a dynamic, constantly changing program has been operating—without any subsidy—in a multi-ethnic school on the South Shore of Montreal (Caron, 1996; Caron, Otis, and Pilote, 1998). Life-Savers is a program based on peer training, a strategy especially well suited to a multi-ethnic context in which the message must be in keeping with the values of various cultures. Every year, several grade 10 students are chosen on the basis of various criteria (leadership, popularity among their peers, ethnic representativeness, regardless of academic record) and receive 20 hours of training in organizing activities and in prevention of STDs and AIDS. The themes covered in this training are: STDs and AIDS, people living with HIV, homosexuality and homophobia, sexuality and values related to sexuality, options related to sexual activity (abstinence, sex without penetration, sex with condoms), decision-making, condoms, communication, planning and organizing prevention activities. In the course of this training, in addition to gaining knowledge and skills, each two-student team must develop an activity around one or another of the following subjects: abstinence, condoms, assertiveness techniques, the conditions for an enriching sexual relationship, and equality in relationships. Later, these activities will be offered to students in grades 8 and 9. During the training the teacher provides guidance as to the content of the activities to be developed, but leaves the students plenty of freedom as to how this content will be incorporated in various activities. At the end of the training, she/he ensures that all the activities further the development of responsible attitudes, norms, skills, and intentions—factors that, according to the theory of planned behaviour (Ajzen, 1985), promote the adoption of safe behaviours.

This program has recently been evaluated (quasi-experimental design, pre-test, post-test, with a non-random control group), and demonstrated its capacity to modify the attitudes and intentions of students exposed to the activities presented by their older peers, especially with regard to condom use. The program's impact on condom use has not been measured because more than 80 per cent of the students in this school have never had sex (Caron, Otis, and Pilote, 1998). The fact that such a program could be implemented in a relatively traditional multi-ethnic setting, and has been able to deal with both abstinence and condom use among students who, for the most part, were not sexually active, points to the concerted and continued efforts that have been made with parents, the parents' committee, the teachers, and the administration, who have been involved on an ongoing basis in developing the program.

PUTTING SEX OFF UNTIL LATER

The latter experiment stands in odd contrast to another peer-training program now operating in a similar setting in the Montreal area: '*Remettre à plus tard les relations sexuelles*' (Djandji, 1996). Borrowed from Grady Memorial Hospital in Atlanta, this program, based on the work of pairs of previously trained students in grades 10 and 11, is aimed at delaying the first sexual experience. Addressing young people in grades 7 and 8, it uses information about the psychological and physiological consequences of unwanted sexual relations to pursue the following objectives: to lead young people to recognize the various kinds of pressures that influence their sexual behaviour; to recognize their rights in interpersonal relationships; to know how to resist peer pressure; and, finally, to identify the risks associated with premature sexual relations. The underlying premise of this program is that young people of this age lack the intellectual, psychosocial, and moral maturity to become sexually active.

The difference between the two experiments underlines the degree to which prevention of HIV infection through sexual-health education and promotion in the school setting is subject to the actual values of the setting as well as the presuppositions and notions regarding young people's needs and sexuality held by the decision-makers and planners. For example, without being explicit, the program discussed by Djandji takes a traditional view of the allocation of sexual roles, of which it is important to be aware (Desaulniers, 1996). It also demonstrates the scope of the efforts that must be made, a priori, to make those involved in conducting the program aware of certain realities rather than clinging to values that, at a certain moment, no young person will be capable of sharing. In offering only one choice—whether abstinence or condom use—we marginalize some and make others guilty; either way, neither group is given the skills necessary to make their own choice.

COLLEGIALITY IN ACTION

Also valuing peer involvement, the *Collégialité dans l'action* program (Fafard et al., 1996), implemented in the Chaudière-Appalaches region, relied on peer helpers to further the promotion of sexual health in a secondary school. After 18 hours of training as assistants in the area of sexual health (birth control, pregnancy, STDs, HIV/AIDS, etc.), young people aged 14–16, most of them nominated by their peers, became clearly identified as resource people to whom other students could turn at any time for information, for someone to talk to, for advice, or for a referral, as needed. In addition, the peer helpers had the mandate to develop and implement various extracurricular informational and consciousness-raising activities. Assessment of this experiment indicates that almost 10 per cent of students familiar with the project had consulted a peer helper and that most of them felt better following this intervention. The extracurricular activities undertaken, though original, were less numerous than had been hoped, not because the young people lacked initiative but rather because the school environment was not conducive to some activities. In fact, the administration and staff supported the broad principles of the project; however, when the young people proposed activities, several of them were refused because their specific content was incompatible with the decision-makers' values and ways of looking at things.

This experiment, although it gave young people the power to define the action and objects of change, ended in half-failure for several reasons. The planners of the intervention (public health and the school nurse) were not sufficiently familiar with the organizational culture of the setting; on the other hand, because the setting itself did not play an active role in its development and implementation, it supported the project without really understanding the stakes surrounding the mobilization of young people in the development of activities promoting sexual health. Besides this major constraint affecting the extent to which this project could be implemented, the recourse to peer helpers and the mobilization of young people in action may not have had any impact on the adoption of safety measures by the students at this school; nevertheless, these strategies appear to have contributed to the creation of a more favourable atmosphere for the promotion of sexual health and for young people to take charge of their own health.

SEXUAL WELL-BEING—MINE AND OTHERS'

More recently, in 1995–6, an innovative experiment was tried in 11 secondary schools in the Quebec City and Chaudière-Appalaches regions among students with learning and behavioural difficulties (ages 16–18). Compared to their peers in regular schools, students with behavioural and learning problems are more vulnerable to HIV infection (Otis et al., 1996), but often their curricula do not include any training in sex education or prevention—a major gap that the planners of the *Mon bien-être sexuel et celui de l'autre* program hoped to fill. The woman who conceived the program, herself a teacher for 25 years and a sexologist-educator, developed the course following the experiential approach of Steinaker and Bell (1979). Aimed at helping young people to develop healthy and responsible habits with respect to sexual well-being and the prevention of STDs, AIDS, and pregnancy, 18 75-minute sessions (two sessions in every nine-day cycle) were offered. The planned activities touched on various themes, such as relations between girls and boys, the pleasures of sex, abusive control of partners, communication, STDs and various protection strategies available, teenaged father- and motherhood, and self-assertion. The pedagogical methods used were highly interactive (interactive presentations, discussion groups, role-playing, debates, values clarification, mental imaging, demonstration, imitation-recall, practice exercises, various audiovisual materials, keeping a personal journal, etc.) (Baillargeon, et al., 1996). The originality of this program consisted in the integration of prevention in the larger context of sexual well-being, defined by the students themselves, who established their own objectives for change; the suggested activities were intended only to facilitate the process of bringing these changes about. That the activities allowed for a concentric—that is, progressive and cumulative—learning process was confirmed when the program was evaluated.

The evaluation was based on a pre-test/post-test design (without a control group) and on information (qualitative as well as quantitative) collected from students, teachers, school nurses, and administrators. The program was greatly appreciated by the students and the teachers involved. Moreover, at the end of the program the young people's knowledge had grown significantly, and their perception of the risk of contracting an STD or HIV was stronger. Attitudes towards abstinence and especially condom use were more favourable. In terms of belief in their self-efficacy, these students felt more capable of ensuring that their needs were respected in the sexual sphere and of respecting those of their partners, of asserting themselves and communicating with their partners, of controlling their sexual impulses, and of using condoms, even if they judged their partner to be low-risk and despite the presence of certain barriers (difficulty buying condoms, negotiating their use, and actually using them). Their sexual values were more positive and their communication style seemed centred more on self-assertion and less on passivity. In addition, the program had a significant positive impact on behaviours in the last month: more of their sexual encounters were protected by oral contraceptives and condoms. These results were observed among boys as well as girls (Otis et al., 1997c). Even though the evaluation design was weak and the sample was small (n=209), the results favour similar experiments based on the experiential approach.

LOVE 15–16 THEATRE WORKSHOP

Along similar lines, and also in the Quebec City region, the preventive intervention *Chantier-théâtre amours 15–16* (Ouellet and Lindsay, 1991) took its inspiration from the principles of the experiential approach to promote communication between partners about their sexuality and responsibility in terms of preventive practices. Adopting an interpersonal perspective and consisting of three sessions, this intervention presented to grade 11 students three sketches depicting the daily life of a teenaged couple, each session followed by class discussion. The sketches put particular emphasis on the sexist stereotypes present in communication and on the cognitive biases to which they give rise in terms of norms, expectations, and behaviours that are socially constructed according to gender. Evaluation of this intervention with respect to students' attitudes towards safety measures and communication raises very interesting questions. On the basis of a design combining qualitative and quantitative approaches, it seems that the intervention reinforced the girls' attitudes *vis-à-vis* these two themes, while the boys' attitudes were weakened. According to the author of the evaluation (Drolet, 1996), the workshop provoked a lively confrontation between the sexes, consolidating traditional sexist stereotypes among the boys, who felt threatened by changes in this area, and reinforcing a change already under way among the girls towards self-assertion in the area of responsible sexuality. What could be seen as a negative impact among the boys was in fact strongly positive, because it was linked to a heightened awareness that brought them into closer contact with their discomfort and difficulty in talking openly with their partners. The problem with this intervention was its short duration.

The strength of the experiential approach is precisely that it provokes these periods of destabilization, of heightened awareness, in such a way that they can be reinvested later in the learning process. The *Chantier* intervention was simply a release mechanism and did not provide follow-up activities permitting a reappropriation of the experience of heightened awareness. The lesson to be drawn from this intervention is that the experiential approach is capable of shaking up deeply rooted stereotypes and creating an opening for change. But it must be given the chance to work! Thus this kind of pedagogical method does seem to be worth pursuing, but within a more comprehensive course that allows for the reinvestment of these new experiences in a more progressive and cumulative learning process, as the *Mon bien-être sexuel et celui de l'autre* did.

HIV PREVENTION PROGRAM AMONG TEENAGERS ATTENDING SECONDARY SCHOOL IN MONTÉRÉGIE

All of the Quebec experiments described so far have come out of local and regional initiatives that have been relatively independent of other community structures and organizations and have limited their activities to schools. One final example provides a useful illustration of the planning process in an HIV prevention program involving close links between the various school, social health, and community networks. Developed by the Public Health Department (DSP) of the Montérégie region, this process is consistent in every respect with the social planning model described by Rothman (1979) and is based on two models: the ecological model of Green et al. (1980), called PRECEDE (Predisposing, Reinforcing, and Enabling Causes in Educational Diagnosis and Evaluation) and the MATCH (Multi-Level Approach Toward Community Health) model (Simon-Morton et al., 1989).

First, the DSP played an advisory role in using its resources to identify the needs of teenagers recruited from both the schools (Otis et al., 1990) and the community (Otis et al., 1992). The results of these two studies, based on various social cognitive theories, made it possible to establish priorities and to target the program at predisposing, reinforcing, and enabling factors, as suggested in the PRECEDE model. Identification of these factors led to the formulation of multiple objectives, depending on the level of intervention—individual (the teenagers and interveners involved, whether teachers, parents, community workers, doctors, pharmacists, or others); organizational (schools, community bodies, pharmacies, local stores, the media); governmental (regional administration, Ministry of Education, Ministry of Health and Social Services, etc.)—and the settings selected: school, community, health network.

Second, the DSP had to serve as the liaison agent between the various settings so that, in keeping with the objectives that had been formulated, each one would take charge of the development and implementation of activities specifically designed for its culture. To facilitate this process, the DSP offered training courses for all the actors involved. The training courses varied with the tasks the actors were expected to perform, while suggesting certain activities for the young people, including pedagogical material. A list of other possible activities was presented to stimulate their creativity. Following the training courses, the DSP had to ensure that the activities planned were in keeping with the program's objectives (Longpré and Otis, 1994).

The value of this process was that it standardized the messages conveyed to the young people while orchestrating the actions of all the actors. On the other hand, its impact on individual young people depended on the ability of each setting to appropriate the principles of the program and put them into practice. The only deficiency in the Montérégie model was that funding was not available to provide regular and systematic support for the settings adopting the program, which had obvious repercussions for its effectiveness. In fact, the evaluation of this process has made it possible to illustrate the links between the depth of the implementation of educational actions in various settings and the achievement of the program's goals. Nevertheless, this experiment demonstrates how the health network can contribute to community empowerment in the area of preventing HIV infection.

EDUCATIONAL ACTIONS AMONG YOUTH IN HALFWAY HOUSES

A study carried out between 1991 and 1994 among youth in halfway houses reported a rate of prevalence of HIV infection of roughly 0.06 per cent (Frappier and Roy, 1995). Although this rate is relatively low, other studies underline the high vulnerability of these teenagers to infection. Compared to their peers recruited in the school setting, these young people are three to four times more likely to be sexually active and to have had more than five different partners since their first sexual experience, including several at risk. This group stands out even more when we consider the proportions of these young people who have engaged in prostitution (9 to 12 times more) or injection drug use (8 to 24 times more) (Otis, 1996). Furthermore, these risk factors are combined with a lower rate of condom use, precarious living conditions, and a social environment that is often dysfunctional.

The moment of admission to a halfway house can be a good opportunity to meet these young people and raise issues surrounding sex and prevention. Unfortunately, in Quebec, as in Canada as a whole, the frequency with which interventions are undertaken does not reflect the high priority that should be given to them. Halfway houses are closed settings, difficult to penetrate, especially since their responsibilities, centred on social rehabilitation, are so heavy that staff members find it difficult to see the relevance of including activities concerning prevention and promotion of sexual health.

In Quebec, two experiments with youth centres, including halfway houses for young people (CRJDAs), illustrate how it is possible to reach these young people and contribute to their sexual well-being.

INTERVENTION PROGRAM ON SEXUALITY AND PREVENTION OF STDs AND AIDS FOR YOUNG PEOPLE AND YOUNG MOTHERS IN HALFWAY HOUSES

The first experiment concerned all the CRJDAs (centres de réadaptation pour jeunes en difficulté d'adaptation) in eastern Quebec. After conducting a study of these young people aimed at better understanding the psychosocial factors related to their risk behaviours and safety practices (a study based on the theories of planned behaviour [Ajzen, 1985] and interpersonal behaviour [Triandis, 1979]), Godin et al. (1997) developed an intervention program targeting the factors that appeared to play a major role.

The program was developed in collaboration with representatives from the administration of each halfway house, which provided a more accurate picture of the dynamics of this population. One special characteristic of the program was its flexibility: a young person could enter it at any time. This feature acknowledged the reality of CRJDAs, since young people may be admitted to or leave them at any time during the year. In the 10 meetings offered, the following themes were raised: the reality of AIDS, knowledge about AIDS and STDs, the meaning of sexual relations, high- and low-risk sexual activities, the condom, advantages and disadvantages of condom use, values and sexuality, communication about sexuality, risk-free sex through negotiation of safety measures, assertiveness, initiating discussion and reasoning in the face of obstacles to the adoption of safe sex practices. These themes were raised through activities such as formal and informal presentations, exchanges of ideas, discussions, debates, personal reflection, teamwork, quiz games, role-playing, problem resolution, handling condoms, improvisation games, songs, and audiovisual materials. What made the program original was that it took into account not only knowledge but both cognitive and relational aspects.

The results of evaluative research on this program confirm the importance of developing interventions in a planned way and strongly refute the argument that the educational approach based on social cognitive theories (Fishbein, 1979; Ajzen, 1985, 1991; Triandis, 1979; Bandura, 1977, 1986, 1990, 1992) is not an effective guide for program development. In fact, at the end of the program the young people in the experimental group had a higher personal moral norm with respect to condom use than did the control group; their beliefs and attitudes concerning condom use were more favourable; and they had a greater perception of control and belief in their self-efficacy, as well as a stronger intention to use condoms in the following months (Godin et al., 1997).

Furthermore, for the educators, the experience of organizing this program had an impact on their practice of intervention itself, on the ways they looked at the problems of STDs and AIDS and approached sexuality with their clients. Changes that seem attributable to the discussions generated by the interventions were also observed at the institutional level. These exchanges forced the halfway houses to take a stand on the availability of condoms and HIV testing in their respective settings. In addition, because educators participated in this intervention, they consequently revealed a willingness to take responsibility for the prevention activities and services to be offered to their clients in the medium and long term (Michaud et al., 1997).

COMMUNITY ACTION PROGRAM TO PREVENT STDs/HIV AMONG YOUNG PEOPLE IN MONTREAL YOUTH CENTRES

If the program in halfway houses corresponds to a relatively classic model of social planning, the experiment currently being carried out under the direction of the Department of Public Health (DSP) of Montreal-Centre more closely reflects the locality development model (Bastien et al., 1996). The community action program proposed by the DSP takes a 'goal-free' perspective on planning, in which the evaluative research-action undertaken will encourage the Montreal youth centres and community bodies to take responsibility for HIV-prevention educational action among youth in care. Instead of defining objectives a priori and developing the same activities for all settings, the DSP acts as facilitator and liaison, leading the youth centres, first, to define their own priorities and develop educational activities around sexuality and drug addiction; second, to develop intersectoral links combining the efforts and expertise of community and institutional bodies; and, finally, to develop intersectoral projects promoting the mobilization and involvement of young people. This process has several advantages: it respects the culture of each organization, the youth centres bringing together other players (group homes, supervised housing, foster families, etc.); it gives them the support required at every stage in the development and implementation of their actions; and it creates close intra- and intersectoral links. On the other hand, it also accepts the absence of control over the various settings' adherence to the process and teenagers' involvement with their own sexual health.

In fact, the last two experiments are highly complementary. The DSP's Montreal-Centre community action program works more towards creating a macro-structure encouraging the various settings, and teenagers themselves, to take charge, while the program of Godin et al. could be a specific action that one of the settings within that macro-structure might decide to undertake because it is consistent with its priorities and the needs of its clientele. In the first case, the emphasis is on tackling the community and organizational environment, a necessary condition for the development of collective responsibility and the repetition of educational action; in the second, the accent is on teenagers themselves and the development of their abilities in the face of risk—conditions promoting the development of individual responsibility and self-protection.

EDUCATIONAL ACTIONS AMONG STREET YOUTH

Some studies undertaken at the national level and in Quebec illustrate the degree to which, among marginalized young people, street youth are a primary target. The Toronto study conducted by Read et al. (1993) reported a prevalence rate for HIV infection of 2.2 per cent (0.8 per cent in the 14–20 age group and

5.8 per cent among those aged 21–5), rates comparable to those obtained by Roy et al. (1996) in Montreal (0.4 per cent in those 20 and under, 3.6 per cent in those over 20). In the latter example, roughly one-third of the young people were characterized by high-risk activities: same-sex relations among boys, prostitution, or injection drug use (35.7 per cent). Unfortunately, preventive intervention and, even more, sexual-health education and promotion aimed specifically at them is almost a Utopian dream, at least from an individual perspective. On the one hand, we do not understand the culture of these young people; on the other, they are difficult to reach and mobilize except through street work and outreach, which limits the scope for educational action. In fact, to counter HIV infection among these young people we would have to tackle their living conditions as a whole, which would require serious reflection on current social and political structures and the place they leave for young people.

In Canada, efforts among street youth are at an embryonic stage. More often than not, they consist in making condoms and clean syringes available in the locations they frequent and offering them someone to talk to, in the person of a street worker.

INTERVENTION BY PEER HELPERS AMONG STREET YOUTH

On the Island of Montreal, a peer intervention program sought to bring together street youth in the downtown core. This program had three goals: to inform young people about how to protect themselves against STDs and HIV, and about the social and health services available to them; to effect change in their behaviour and the norms of their environment regarding safer behaviours (sexuality and injection drug use); and to encourage them to use the services and resources available.

This intervention, eight months in length, was carried out with the support and involvement of a youth clinic, a Community Health Centre (CLSC), and four community bodies working with downtown street youth. The liaison agents, the peer helpers, were young people operating in the field while receiving parallel training (27 four-hour meetings) consisting of two parts: the first dealing with knowledge, attitudes, and behaviour concerning STDs and HIV and the second aimed at developing the skills required to serve as liaison agents (communication, listening, mutual aid, information distribution, etc.). The latter involved a tour of the setting's resources and observation outings with a street worker. The peer helpers had two distinct mandates: work on the street or in a setting supervised by a professional sponsor and production of a special event designed for the street youth. Work in the street or supervised setting consisted of three successive stages, each lasting three weeks (four hours per week). The first stage was an observation period in which the peer helpers accompanied their sponsor-interveners at work; the second consisted in attempting, under supervision, to make contact with street youth; and the third, called 'personalized intervention', allowed the young peer helpers to use their skills to transmit a prevention message.

Evaluation of this intervention (essentially based on qualitative data) yielded the following effects: among the peer helpers, an increase in self-esteem was observed; among the street youth, there was no significant change in behaviour;

the norm of the setting did not seem to have altered. As for the partner organizations, the goal of referring young people to these services was achieved and the various services became aware of their deficiencies with respect to prevention of STDs and AIDS among these young people.

No doubt the main obstacle to success for this program was related to the reality within which street youth live and the situations they confront every day, which make it more difficult to effect change in behaviour and the environmental norm. In the implementation of this program, the lack of time to prepare the peer helpers, the lack of explanation of their role, and the insufficient time spent in the field compared to the time spent in training were all drawbacks, preventing them from appropriating the project in such a way as to make them effective (Mercier et al., 1996).

Despite these limitations, the program demonstrated its capacity to mobilize young people as agents of education and prevention; it promoted access to the appropriate resources for the street youth; and it allowed agencies to become aware of the needs of that clientele. A similar project should be attempted in a context where the trained peer helpers would spend enough time in the field to have a significant impact among the street youth.

EDUCATIONAL ACTIVITIES WITH WOMEN

The specific vulnerability of women to HIV infection is a growing reality that Canadian policies have taken into account only recently (Hankins, 1994). From 1990 to 1996, the proportion of declared AIDS cases in Canada among women rose from 6.2 per cent to 10 per cent of the total population of reported people with AIDS, with Quebec alone accounting for 50 per cent of them. The fact that, along with injection drug use, heterosexual transmission is the principal risk category identified among these known cases underlines women's dependence on their ability to negotiate protection and satisfaction with their sexual partners. According to Hankins (1994), this ability is closely related to women's position in society, a position that for many is still characterized by economic dependence and a state of subordination deriving from the powers exercised by men. Thus she suggests that, until there is an effective, acceptable method of protection—other than the condom—that depends exclusively on the woman, the various programs addressing women should emphasize the ability to communicate with sexual partners in order to improve the capacity for negotiation.

Until now, it has been possible to reach teenagers through activities in the schools or through media campaigns (most of them aimed specifically at heterosexuals under the age of 30), but adult women have been a neglected target. Yet they take just as many risks as their teenaged sisters, and they do not always have the skills required to manage these risks safely (Otis et al., 1997d). For them, however, the challenge of prevention is complex because not all women can be reached through the usual channels, and this is likely especially true of the most vulnerable. This complexity explains why so few interventions have been directed at adult women in Canada generally and in Quebec, as well as the lack of specificity and intensity of those that have been tried.

CONDOMANIA

The Condomania program, implemented in the Vancouver region, was one of the rare experiments targeted specifically at women in the general population (Wagman, 1993). Taking the form of a multimedia campaign, this program was intended to influence the behaviour of women aged 19 to 30 by making condoms more acceptable to them. The campaign was developed following the principles of social marketing. First, various small focus groups were formed among women in the larger target group to identify their beliefs and values concerning prevention, particularly condom use. The information gathered was then used as a guide in the development and production of the campaign materials. Promotion and publicity activities spread the message in various forms and locations (posters in public places, buses, bus shelters, etc.). In addition, the staffs of bars and discothèques were involved so that various short-term activities might be held there. To facilitate the implementation of these activities, volunteers were recruited and trained. In addition, stories and advertisements within both electronic and print media were used to reinforce these actions. This intensive two-month campaign was repeated every six months for three years, running into funding problems in the third year. Evaluation of the campaign (based on pre-test/post-test telephone surveys among random cross-sections and a series of in-depth interviews) produced inconclusive results as to achievement of the objective. In fact, few people could remember having seen the campaign material, and only 25 per cent of these had retained the message. The in-depth interviews suggested that this indifference reflected the women's entrenched beliefs that risk groups exist (and that they did not belong to such a group) and that their partners were trustworthy. In other words, even though they were the targets of the campaign, these women did not feel that the message to which they were exposed was directed at them personally.

NEVER ONE WITHOUT THE OTHER

In Quebec, the *Jamais l'un sans l'autre* campaign for women using oral contraceptives was another example of a strategy aimed at women, but this time through a specific channel: their pharmacists. Financed by the Quebec AIDS Coordination Centre (CQCS), this experiment was the result of collaboration between the health network and social services of the Lanaudière, Laurentides, and Outaouais regions and the Order of Pharmacists of Quebec. Throughout the month of November 1994, 159 pharmacists distributed an awareness package containing a condom to every customer asking to refill her prescription for birth-control pills. A poster repeating the campaign slogan indicated to customers that their pharmacist was taking part in the program. To support this endeavour, a broad public awareness campaign was carried out at the same time, in which the objectives and relevance of the *Jamais l'un sans l'autre* project were taken up by the regional print and electronic media.

Evaluation of this project focused on finding out whether the women saw their pharmacists as credible sources with respect to preventing HIV infection, whether the pharmacists themselves accepted this role, and whether involving them was a good way of reaching women at higher risk or those difficult to reach in other ways. During the campaign, 25,281 women aged 14 to 51 were contacted directly through the involvement of their pharmacists. Two months after the campaign, the women in the experimental group had a stronger perception of their risk of contracting HIV than did the control group; they said they were more aware than they had been and were more strongly motivated to protect themselves. The great majority recognized the usefulness, relevance, and effectiveness of such a campaign and even wanted to see it repeated. They also recognized the legitimacy and credibility of their pharmacist as an actor in the area of prevention and sexual health. Furthermore, analysis of the behavioural profile of these women indicated that the pharmacists were able to reach high-risk women: 9.4 per cent of them had had a partner at risk, and 0.5 per cent were injection drug users (Otis et al., 1996). This experiment thus demonstrated that pharmacists can be important actors in planning future educational activities with women.

WITHOUT A CONDOM, THE ANSWER IS NO

Another example in Quebec, the *Sans condom c'est non* project (Haïek and Brochu, 1996), but one addressed specifically to teenaged girls attending the youth service of a Community Health Clinic, was conducted with the specific aim of raising the rate of condom use among young girls. This intervention, based on Ajzen's (1985) theory of planned behaviour, Bandura's (1977) learning theory, and Triandis's (1979) theory of interpersonal behaviour, had five objectives: increasing knowledge; developing a positive attitude towards condom use; raising awareness of the internal factors (moral norm) and external factors (subjective norm) influencing this behaviour; and acquisition of technical skills in using condoms. This intervention, lasting three months, had two parts. The first worked as follows. After the teenager's appointment at the clinic, the intervener (doctor or nurse) gave her a package of educational material relating to the program's objectives (games similar to Monopoly, Boggle, and Quiz; role-playing games, such as how to visit the drug store). The contents of the package were explained to the teenager, who then was supposed to play the role of tutor with two student friends, covering all the suggested activities with them in the course of three meetings. After each meeting, the tutor visited the intervener again to discuss the results of this experiment. This constituted the second, more individualized part of the program.

The impact of this intervention with teenager-tutors was rigorously evaluated (quasi-experimental design, pre-test, post-tests, with a non-random control group). Immediately following the intervention, the teenager-tutors in the experimental group had a significantly higher rate of condom use for both vaginal and oral sex than did those in the control group (>14.6 per cent). Unfortunately, by the time of the follow-up visit, three months later, these significant differences had faded (Haïek and Brochu, 1996). Following this evaluation, the program was modified and reinforcement activities were added. The revised program will be re-evaluated, this time with respect to the group tutored as well as the tutors themselves.

Preventive education for women requires the use of multiple channels to reach them. Clearly, doctors and pharmacists play an important role. Nevertheless, preventive efforts must look beyond clinics and the work setting to less traditional channels (beauty salons, women's groups, local stores, shelters for battered women, etc.), settings that so far have been largely neglected by formal prevention interventions.

EDUCATIONAL ACTIONS AMONG MEN WHO HAVE SEX WITH MEN

In May 1997, in Canada, men who have sex with men accounted for 78.7 per cent of all declared cases of AIDS among men (LCDC, 1997), while in March 1997 this figure was 73.6 per cent in Quebec (CQCS, 1997). Yet it was not until the early 1990s that systematic studies were undertaken (Myers et al., 1993; Godin et al., 1993) and formal policy commitments were made to support prevention efforts among these men—a sign of unease about working with a community judged to be marginal. However, the gay community itself did not wait for such support to arrive before taking responsibility; the most severely affected community, it was the first to mobilize itself.

In general, intervention programs among gay and bisexual men have tried to understand the environmental and collective dimensions that help to reinforce the community and motivate it to take action (Vassal and Morrison, 1997). Action-research has also been developed in various forms, bringing together actors from various sectors around a common goal. Evaluations of interventions, which have been rarely undertaken, show that community work appears to be the most effective approach, especially on-site intervention and work using peers (Kelly et al., 1992).

THE TALKING SEX PROJECT

In Toronto, the Talking Sex Project (Tudiver et al., 1992) demonstrated its effectiveness in changing the risk practices of the men who took part in it. This program offered two types of intervention. The first, undertaken by community volunteers, consisted of one three-hour session with 8–12 participants in which the following themes were addressed: the impact of AIDS on individuals and the community, clarification of risks and guidelines for safer sex, obstacles to safer sex, and ways of incorporating fantasies into sexual scenarios to promote safer sex practices. The second intervention, organized by a trained male-female team who were paid for their work, consisted of four two-hour sessions emphasizing the construction of sexual and affective relations and the expression of emotions. Participants in these sessions had specific tasks to fulfil and discussed safer sex. Sharing personal experiences with risk-management strategies was encouraged. In addition, skills for negotiating safe sex were developed through role-playing. In these two forms, the program made it possible to improve knowledge and develop a feeling of competence about condom use. The single-session intervention, because it was organized by peers, was the most successful. This project is only one of many examples in which the gay community has taken on the responsibility for preventing HIV infection.

MEN'S ACTION SURVEY PLAN

There is now a structure that allows the gay community to take a critical look at its efforts. The Men's Action Survey Plan (MASP) provides the expertise required to various teams, notably in Sudbury, Winnipeg, and Toronto, to help gay and bisexual educators in the area of AIDS prevention to develop the skills they need to evaluate their programs. This structure assists them in their work, reviews and supervises what they do, and supplies the relevant material and documentation. An early assessment of the MASP team underlines the many difficulties encountered by gay community groups both in programming actions and in evaluating those actions. In fact, work within the gay community is constantly in question because, from year to year, that work depends on government funding, which is not always consistent. In this context it is impossible to make long-term plans or maintain stability in the resources invested.

The situation in Quebec is no different, but since 1985 the gay community has persisted in developing prevention programs. In Montreal, the Comité Sida Aide Montréal (C-SAM), a local community organization, in collaboration with the community health department of the Montreal General Hospital, coordinated the Jouez sûr-Play safe campaign, launched in 1986 (Adrien et al., 1987). Other interventions have been initiated by C-SAM and other groups such as ACT-UP. The gay press has published a constant stream of articles and advertisements about safe sex, while the gay and lesbian film festival, 'Image et Nation', has presented productions on the same subject. In 1990 community groups and social service and health agencies joined forces to launch Action Séro-Zéro, a project aimed at preventing HIV transmission among Montreal's gay and bisexual men. Its work in the city's bars and bathhouses demonstrates an important and productive partnership with business. In addition, it helps to promote positive images of homosexuality, notably through workshops on self-assertion and self-esteem and communication campaigns such as *Le Droit d'aimer sans peur et sans reproche* (The right to love without fear and without reproach). A number of these actions have been, or are currently, the subject of evaluation through a partnership between university and public health researchers and Action Séro-Zéro, which itself commissioned and ran these evaluations.

BAR-TO-BAR

After three years of involvement in Montreal's gay bars (eight in 1994 and 16 in 1996), Séro-Zéro wanted to assess the relevance of its work in these settings. This involvement consisted in making condoms and lubricant available to patrons for an amount left to the discretion of the beneficiary. In addition to condoms, the project offered pamphlets on safe sex and AIDS and took advantage of special events to present humorous shows on the risks of HIV transmission and how to prevent it. Twice every week, the head of the program visited each of the participating bars to refill the condom boxes and pamphlet containers and talk to managers and employees. This regular contact proved to be an important reinforcing factor in prevention efforts in these settings.

The evaluation of this intervention indicates that, over a period of 18 months, 155,000 condoms and 33,000 pamphlets were distributed. The program reached a diverse group of men who have sex with men—diverse in terms of both age and socio-economic resources. In fact, six of every 10 patrons of the participating bars took Séro-Zéro condoms. For these men, the Séro-Zéro box was the second most common source of condoms, just after drug stores. They took the Séro-Zéro condoms because they were easily available, inexpensive, accompanied by lubricant, and useful for last-minute encounters. Almost 95 per cent of the customers questioned found Séro-Zéro's prevention efforts in gay bars useful and necessary, and 61 per cent said they would like to see more such efforts. Moreover, the bar owners and managers were unanimous in saying that Séro-Zéro's work was completely satisfactory. The testimony of one of them illustrates how receptive they were to this intervention: 'To have had a Séro-Zéro condom from one of those famous boxes—there's no telling how many people they've saved.' According to several of them, considering tips and how little effort was required, the program benefited not only their patrons but the establishments themselves. In other words, although they would not be prepared to take responsibility for the program themselves, they were very favourable to Séro-Zéro's presence in their businesses (Dupont et al., 1997).

BATHHOUSE PROJECT

At the same time Action Séro-Zéro undertook an evaluation of *Au sauna . . . on s'emballe*, the bathhouse project it had launched in January 1992. Along the same lines as the bar project, this consisted in giving out a free condom with every admission (between 36,000 and 72,000 condoms per year at each bathhouse), offering additional condoms and lubricant at a reduced price, handing out pamphlets, and distributing other kinds of educational material: posters, postcards, key chains, condom cases, etc. The results of the evaluation showed the receptivity and openness of the bathhouse managers and employees and their desire to see the program continued and reinforced, as well as their customers' appreciation and perception of the program's impact on their knowledge, attitudes, and feelings of competence with respect to safer sex (Morrison et al., 1996). At present this program is continuing, with one additional feature: Séro-Zéro's presence in the bathhouses is so credible, and the houses themselves are so receptive, that an intervener now spends several hours a week in a room at one or another of the houses, offering information and advice to clients who wish it.

Séro-Zéro's work in the bars and bathhouses has stimulated the creation of environments favourable to the adoption and maintenance of a healthy and safety-conscious sex life; has promoted safer sex as a social norm; and, above all, has involved in the battle against AIDS the managers of commercial establishments—people whose mandate has nothing to do with prevention—by appealing to their sense of social responsibility and the image they present to their clients.

Séro-Zéro's persuasion and mobilization efforts among commercial establishments appear to have turned resistance and indifference into a kind of moral obligation to become involved.

TWO WORKSHOPS: 'I'M DIFFERENT' AND 'I'M HERE, AND I'M STAYING'

To provide a place where gay and bisexual men can talk and discuss the factors linked to risk-taking in relation to HIV/AIDS transmission, in April 1995 Action Séro-Zéro took on the mandate of increasing these men's negotiation and self-assertion skills by inviting them to participate in two workshops that are similar in form but different in content. The first, *Le sens d'une différence*, focuses on self-esteem; the second, *J'y suis, j'y reste*, on self-assertion. Taking the form of a small group (8–12 people), each of these workshops consists of five three-hour meetings. Two facilitators lead each group, and the meetings address the following themes: sexuality, body image, risk, eroticism, stereotypes and prejudices, communication and the condom, life assessment, the family, relations with others, and generally accepted messages about homosexuality. These themes are addressed through discussion, brainstorming, mental imaging, and role-playing. The workshops are currently undergoing evaluation (process and impact).

In these workshops Séro-Zéro has shown its willingness to confront HIV infection through the factors related to the social vulnerability of some of these men. For Séro-Zéro, the difficulty of affirming oneself as gay, on both the individual and the social levels, interferes with the capacity to negotiate life, emotional relationships, and sexual health.

PROJECT 10

Complementing the actions of Séro-Zéro, the Batshaw Youth and Family Centre in Montreal has launched several services for young people aged 14–25 who are questioning their sexual orientation or having difficulty being gay or bisexual in a society with little tolerance. The services of Project 10 take various forms: a telephone help line, individual counselling, separate support groups for those aged 14–18 and 19–25, and weekly 'drop-in' nights, informal gatherings where everyone can participate. In addition to promoting the adoption and maintenance of safe practices through improvement of knowledge, attitudes, and feelings of competence, the goals of Project 10 include heightened self-esteem and acceptance of one's sexual orientation, as well as development of adequate social support. The framework for intervention is based on the process of behavioural change (initiation, consolidation, and maintenance) discussed by Peterson et al. (1991) and on Harter's (1993) work on developing self-esteem. Each week, between three and five young people join Project 10, and on average they take part in 10 of the project's meetings. The evaluation now under way, to last three years, will show to what extent Project 10 has achieved its objectives. Nevertheless, the preliminary results point to the diversity of the needs of these young people who seek, above all, to break their isolation and take their place in society, which is the goal of the project.

PROVINCIAL INTERVENTION PROGRAM IN PARKS

In Quebec, Action Séro-Zéro is not the only body taking responsibility for preventing HIV infection, especially in locations where sexual activity takes place, such as parks. In the fall of 1996, ten Quebec community organizations met to share their experiences, draw up an overview assessing interventions in the parks, and adopt a plan for short- and medium-term action. Currently engaged in a process of evaluative action-research, they want to understand the profile of the men they contact and assess the relevance of their activities in the parks. Respecting the needs of each location, thanks to paid staff or volunteers, the men frequenting the park have access not only to condoms and lubricant but to someone who will listen and can also provide information and, if necessary, refer them to other resources (Otis et al., 1997e; Pelletier et al., 1997). For the organizations involved, intervention in the parks seems to be the only way to reach some men having sex with other men and expose them to a specific prevention message because they do not frequent gay businesses. This on-site work is thus essential.

These experiments in Quebec, which reflect the mobilization of gay communities across Canada, demonstrate the ability of these communities to take responsibility, linking communication strategies specifically oriented towards men having sex with other men to the mobilization of business people, the formation of support and discussion groups, and fieldwork in the locations where sex takes place. These concerted actions reinforce one another and work together towards the creation of a favourable environment for the promotion of safer sex.

TRAINING EDUCATORS

In most of the experiments described above, the program planners have made some reference to the training of interveners, regardless of their discipline or the intensity of the role they will have to play. In fact, training is a key factor determining the extent to which an intervention can be implemented and its eventual effects. The values, attitudes, knowledge, and abilities of the actors involved are essential to the design of the program. In the 1980s sex education was the preserve of a few specialists, but the emergence of the AIDS epidemic has forced an entire network of actors to become involved and learn on the spot how to do their jobs. Today education, promotion of sexual health, and prevention are everyone's responsibility: doctors, nurses, teachers, street workers, volunteers, peer helpers, parents. This diversity of expertise and knowledge is at once the strength and the weakness of current efforts at preventive education (Gaudreau, 1989). If some have benefited from a structure that allows them to acquire the skills necessary to fulfil their role, others have been thrown into action without those skills.

In Quebec, an extensive study by Gaudreau, Dupont, and Séguin (1994) examined the evolution of the training given to interveners working with young people in the area of AIDS prevention since the beginning of the 1980s. Based on analysis of 21 training programs offered in 13 different regions, mainly by the DSPs, this study indicates that the majority of interveners, both within and outside the school setting, had already received some training, whether through conferences or seminars, university courses, or systematic programs. On the whole, their knowledge of AIDS and AIDS prevention was good, although their understanding of sexuality was somewhat weaker; their attitudes towards their role were quite positive.

Beyond these forms of training, since 1990 the Quebec AIDS Coordination Centre (CQCS) has been responsible for the training of interveners at the provincial level. Having started with values education teachers, it later offered various interveners working with youth in care a training course entitled *Sortir des sentiers battus* (Getting off the beaten tracks). Since 1994 it has offered interveners at youth centres, community organizations, and Community Health Clinics a course on homosexuality entitled *Pour une nouvelle vision de l'homosexualité: intervenir dans le respect de la diversité des orientations sexuelles* (A New Look at Homosexuality). This course was introduced and evaluated as a pilot project in the context of a more general program established by the Public Health Department in Montérégie, and is described in the following section.

PLANNING A SERVICE IN MONTÉRÉGIE FOR YOUNG MEN AGED 15–24

To encourage the establishment, within the health network and community and institutional bodies, of assistance and support services for young gay and bisexual men, the Montérégie project consisted of four stages: raising awareness and mobilizing the target settings; participation of interveners in the provincial training programs on homosexuality; then, six weeks later, participation in a complementary workshop entitled 'Working at respecting diversity in sexual orientation'; and, finally, presentation of support activities in the settings through on-site visits. The provincial training program sought to increase interveners' knowledge of homosexuality and bisexuality, to develop favourable attitudes among them, and to enhance their feelings of competence in providing assistance and support to young gay and bisexual men. For its part, the Montérégie workshop sought to give the interveners the skills necessary to ensure better psychosexual follow-up with these young people and to plan outreach activities for them. Each session lasted one day. Evaluation of the training course and the workshop (quasi-experimental, pre-test/post-test design with non-random control group) indicates that, eight months after participating in these sessions, the interveners in the experimental group had a better knowledge of homosexuality than those in the control group. They believed they were better equipped to work with gay and bisexual youth, their attitudes towards homosexuality and their support role were more favourable, and their feelings of competence in terms of counselling and preventive education were higher (Otis and Chouinard, 1994, 1995; Vassal et al., 1996). Later on-site visits showed that this training had an impact on the establishment of certain services for young gay men. This experiment underlines the value of these training sessions and the importance of incorporating them in a more comprehensive process, including support and reinforcement activities.

Given the current challenges in the area of preventing HIV infection, government support for training is an important asset. It is certainly commendable that such support is available to interveners belonging to a formal structure, who have already received some professional training for work in this area; however, efforts should also be made to support the training of interveners for whom prevention is not the principal mandate and who lack the skills required to take on this task. Parents, managers of commercial establishments, volunteers—the actors involved in several of the experiments described above—should be targeted in this way.

FOSTER PARENTS AND PREVENTION OF STDS AND AIDS

The *Parents d'accueil et prévention des MTS et du sida* program was carried out with the goal of reaching young people in foster families through foster parents. Starting from the premise that young people are vulnerable to STDs and HIV infection, especially when they display behavioural difficulties, the program was aimed at preparing foster parents to serve as guides with respect to preventing STDs and HIV among the young people entrusted to them. Its objectives were as follows: 'to improve their knowledge so that they can intervene adequately with respect to the prevention of STDs-AIDS in the context of the love lives of young people in care, encourage them to think about attitudes favourable to communication, and help them to adopt strategies capable of reinforcing their interventions depending on the young people's requests and needs' (Berlinguet and Trottier, 1996). Achievement of these objectives was furthered by various activities (role-playing, self-assessment exercises, discussion periods, audiovisual presentations) over the course of five weekly group meetings, each lasting three hours.

Evaluation of this prevention program demonstrated that foster parents were interested in serving as educators in the area of STD and HIV prevention. In addition, they were interested in and comfortable with talking about sexuality and the emotional lives of the young people living with them. Finally, they thought the program met the expectations they had expressed, and emphasized the relevance of offering the program to all parents, as well as to young people themselves.

These two experiments testify to the importance of training the actors involved in the field of education and prevention of HIV infection. When a particular program is developed, it should include specific training about its objectives and prepare the interveners to organize the activities they offer. Training of interveners is also part of any process of empowerment.

CONCLUSION: THE BURDEN AND CHALLENGES OF PREVENTING HIV INFECTION

The state of research on all the factors surrounding HIV transmission and self-protection is sufficiently advanced to sustain the development of educational and preventive actions among most target groups. We know what we have to work on, individually and interpersonally, as well as at the social level (Otis et al., 1997a), but we have trouble knowing *how to do it*—how to transform what we have learned into actions that are relevant, effective, and tailored to the needs of each individual and community. Beyond the knowledge acquired through epidemiological, behavioural, and psychosocial research, we have to accept that educational and preventive action itself has been and will continue to be a source of lessons through its failures, and of new knowledge through its successes and creativity. The experiments described above are only a pale suggestion of the richness and diversity of the response to the threat of AIDS in Canada.

Thus the present chapter, while reporting on the current state of sexual-health education and promotion from the perspective of preventing HIV infection, has allowed us to draw certain conclusions and has stimulated reflection on the current reality: we must do *more*, do it *better*, and do it *differently*, for with the advent of new treatments and new hopes, the image of the epidemic has, rightly or wrongly, become destabilized and is in the process of redefinition.

DOING MORE

The conclusion that we must do more is based on several arguments. On the level of both research and intervention, a significant gap exists in the efforts directed at different groups, notably teenagers in secondary schools and others who in many cases are more vulnerable. Educational actions with elementary-school children are extremely rare, while actions in the college and university environments reach very few young adults. Youth in care, especially those outside institutional settings, are hard to reach, and initiatives on their behalf are still limited and superficial. Will we have the courage to address the sources of their precarious life conditions and the social and political structures capable of remedying them? Adults in general, especially women, receive too little attention, even though heterosexual transmission of HIV is increasing. Reaching them will mean exploiting new channels and moving into less traditional, more specific settings. Action on behalf of gay and bisexual men is continuing to develop; however, it is under constant threat because it is held at arm's length by community bodies whose annual survival depends on the goodwill of governments granting funds. Moreover, young gays are still a neglected group. The various ethnocultural communities represent a challenge; a recent cross-Canada study of some of these communities should assist in the development of new educational actions (Cappon et al., 1995). Finally, people living with physical or intellectual disabilities remain equally neglected in terms of both research and intervention. Yet some American efforts have clearly shown the relevance and feasibility of work on preventive education among people suffering from mental illness (McKinnon, Carey, and Cournos, 1997; Kelly et al., 1997).

Doing more also means being prepared to take the time required to bring about the desired changes. In fact, a number of experiments have been too brief to achieve any change at all (Drolet, 1996; Mercier et al., 1996). To modify behaviour or change a community's norms, multiple strategies must be deployed over the long term. Some programs, once implemented, call for follow-up and reinforcement activities if the gains achieved are to be maintained (Longpré and Otis, 1994; Haïek and Brochu, 1996; Warren et al., 1994; Otis and Chouinard, 1994, 1995; Vassal et al., 1996). In addition, linkage and complementarity, horizontal as well as vertical, are required between various structures, services, and resources to create synergy between actions (Longpré and Otis, 1994; Bastien et al., 1996). Thus, we must do more.

DOING BETTER

In a way, doing better means addressing the totality of the factors that may influence the depth of implementation of an intervention and its effectiveness. Although Lamptey et al. (1993) have attributed the failure of prevention not to preventive education itself but to the absence of the political will to make it available to everyone, in Canada this statement must be qualified. In fact, Canadian political will does exist and is manifested in various strategies, structures, resources, and services. The real problem is the absence of co-ordination and consultation between these various structures, which means there is no overall perspective on HIV/AIDS prevention and education efforts as a whole: their strengths and weaknesses, the needs that have and have not been met. This lack of co-ordination is even more flagrant when these structures must be linked with other structures (e.g., legal, community-based) whose first mandate is not prevention of HIV infection. Better co-ordination between the various ministries (health, education, justice, etc.) or other political or administrative levels is essential, especially since a reform at one or another of these levels can have a major impact on the quality of actions. The Quebec experience in the school setting (cutbacks in values education, the withdrawal of school nurses) is an excellent example of the fragility of the gains that are made and the problems that arise when consultation is lacking.

In addition, reflection is needed on the allocation of funds and the repetition of actions. At present, pilot projects are favoured, and interveners are constantly asked to submit new, original, innovative projects, which in the end means that everyone is obliged to reinvent the wheel each time. On the other hand, actions that have proved to be effective lose their grants, which means that their continuation, or their trial in other settings, is threatened (Warren et al., 1994; Wagman, 1993). If innovative experiments should be encouraged, does this have to be at the expense of those that have proved their worth? To make a return on their investments in the evaluation of educational actions, the granting bodies should arrange for sources of financing that are stable. Agencies alone cannot be expected to take full responsibility for these actions, especially when many of them rely on grants to survive. Beyond these funding problems, the repetition of educational actions also depends on the quality of the transfer of knowledge and experience. Due to the lack of time, resources, or knowledge as to how to make known the work that is done, too many relevant experiments remain in obscurity. Thus, government structures should take more responsibility for making these efforts known and reinvesting them in the various communities.

Doing better also means taking into account, in planning educational activities, the knowledge gained from previous experiments with respect to effectiveness criteria (see Chapter 1, Table 4). In addition, interveners must be capable of entering and becoming integrated into the target settings to reach those clients who are less accessible, and of taking into account their culture and characteristics. It is also important to anticipate the many constraints that can hamper the intervention. The prevailing values of the setting and the gap between these and the values conveyed by the intervention have been and remain major obstacles to implementation of prevention programs (Fafard et al., 1996; Djandji, 1996).

The question of interveners is of primary importance. On the one hand, their diversity and heterogeneity should be a strength in preventive efforts, not a drawback. Thus the training designed for them should take into account their specific needs and the roles they are expected to play. This training will be all the more crucial in the future, when the emphasis placed on empowerment will demand major readjustments in the educational and organizational styles adopted by prevention agents. In this context, the whole notion of partnership between educator and educatee, as described by Bouchard (1997) in his reflection on the social pedagogy of intervention, becomes more relevant than ever. Thus we must do better.

. . . AND DIFFERENTLY

A major shift in the paradigms on which educational actions are based underlines the fact that we must do things differently. Since public health authorities have taken responsibility for preventive education and the promotion of sexual health, sexuality has been reduced to risk behaviours and condom use has become equivalent to sexual health (Otis, 1996). To the extent that the knowledge we have gained now leads us to simultaneous consideration of individual, interpersonal, and social dimensions, integrating prevention of HIV infection into the larger context of sexual-health education and promotion, a shift is necessary from the perspective of health through education to one of education for health. Gaudreau (1994) maintains that from the point of view of public health, the definition of education used to refer to the notion of 'social system' education (the totality of structural components serving the development of persons and societies [Legendre, 1983]), and especially to 'process' education (the succession of interdependent stages aimed at the achievement of particular ends and goals [Legendre, 1983]).

In fact, the various political and social structures were established for prevention, while the programs planned primarily sought the modification of risk practices and the adoption of safety measures. Now, the experience of the last few years reinforces the importance of developing educational activities that are more experiential and of leaving more room for the actors involved to define the objects of change (Baillargeon et al., 1996; Schoonbroodt and Gélinas, 1997; Bastien et al., 1996; Bouchard, 1997), orientations that favour empowerment. These new perspectives permit the actualization of education defined in terms of finality: 'the harmonious development of the potentialities of the human being with a view to a superior ultimate state of perfection conferring autonomy of belief, thought, and action' (Legendre, 1983: 230).

In the future, education and prevention will no doubt have to combine all three definitions of education ('social system', 'process', and 'finality'), accept the coexistence of positivist and constructivist paradigms, and take more inspiration from other disciplines, notably sexology and theories of education. They will also have to accord a little more importance to the learning process itself and the involvement of the actors in this process, instead of focusing exclusively on the objectives to be achieved and the expected health effects. This will have a major impact on how evaluation of educational actions will be conceived and the indicators that will be selected for judging their effectiveness. To give education the whole responsibility for reducing the incidence of HIV infection and changing the risk behaviours of an entire population, to impose on it the heavy burden of controlling an epidemic, was a Utopian fantasy. On the other hand, it is entirely within the capacity of education to promote empowerment of individuals and communities. Thus, evaluators should revise their methods and select indicators that will make it possible to appreciate and to measure this process of appropriation, which is the only realistic effect that activities in the area of sexual-health education and promotion can be expected to achieve. And even there, things must be done *differently*.

REFERENCES

Abrahamson, L., M. Seligman, and J. Teasdale. 1978. 'Learned Helplessness in Humans: Critique and Reformulation', *Journal of Abnormal Psychology* 87: 49–74.

Adelman, M.B. 1992. 'Healthy Passions: Safer Sex as Play', in T. Edgar, M.A. Fitzpatrick, and V. Freimuth, eds, *AIDS: A Communication Perspective*. Hillsdale, NJ: Lawrence Erlbaum Associates, 69–90.

Adrien, A., J. Carsley, and S. Ioannou. 1987. 'Promotion de pratiques sexuelles sûres chez la population homosexuelle de Montréal-Québec', *Rapport hebdomadaire des maladies au Canada* 13, 3: 9–12.

Ajzen, I. 1985. 'From Intentions to Actions: A Theory of Planned Behavior', in J. Kuhl and J. Beckman, eds, *Action-Control: From Cognition to Behavior*. Heidelberg: Springer, 11–39.

———. 1991. 'The Theory of Planned Behavior', *Organizational Behavior and Human Decision Processes* 50: 179–211.

———, and M. Fishbein. 1980. 'Theoretical Implications', in Ajzen and Fishbein, eds, *Understanding Attitudes and Predicting Social Behavior*. Englewood Cliffs, NJ: Prentice-Hall, 79–91.

Amaro, H. 1995. 'Love, Sex and Power: Considering Women's Realities in HIV Prevention', *American Psychologist* 50: 437–49.

Arroyo, J., J.J. Lévy, J. Otis, and F. Pilote. 1997. 'Déterminants de l'usage du préservatif en milieu latino-américain', in N. Chevalier, J. Otis, and M.-P. Desaulniers, eds, *Sida et prévention*. Montréal: Les Éditions Logiques, 363–74.

Averill, J.R. 1987. 'The Role of Emotion and Psychological Defense in Self-protective Behavior', in N.D. Weinstein, ed., *Taking Care: Understanding and Encouraging Self-protective Behavior*. Cambridge: Cambridge University Press.

Baillargeon, L., S. Séguin, D. Veilleux, J. Otis, R. Burelle, R. Côté, and G. Godin. 1996. 'Approche expérientielle appliquée au bien-être sexuel et à la prévention auprès de jeunes en difficulté d'adaptation', 64e congrès de l'ACFAS, Montreal.

Bandura, A. 1977. 'Self-efficacy: Toward a Unifying Theory of Behavioral Change', *Psychology Review* 84: 191–215.

———. 1986. 'Self-efficacy Mechanism in Human Agency', *American Psychologist* 40: 359–73.

———. 1990. 'Perceived Self-efficacy in the Exercise of Control over AIDS Infection', *Evaluation and Program Planning* 13: 9–17.

———. 1992. 'A Social Cognitive Approach to the Exercise of Control over AIDS Infection', in R. DiClemente, ed., *Adolescents and AIDS: A Generation in Jeopardy*. Newbury Park, Calif.: Sage, 89–116.

Barrett, M. 1994. 'Sexuality Education in Canada Schools: An Overview in 1994', *Canadian Journal of Human Sexuality* 3: 199–208.

Bastien, R., E. Roy, et al. 1996. 'Programme d'action communautaire en prévention des MTS/VIH chez les jeunes des deux Centres jeunesse de Montréal'. Montréal: Direction de la santé publique Montréal-centre.

Berlinguet, M., and G. Trottier. 1996. 'Famille d'accueil et prévention des MTS et du VIH-sida auprès de jeunes: épilogue d'un programme à succès', *Service social* 45, 1: 137–45.

Botvin, G.D., S. Schinke, and M.A. Orlandi. 1995. 'School-based Health Promotion: Substance Use and Sexual Behavior', *Applied and Prevention Psychology* 4: 167–84.

Bouchard, J.M. 1997. 'Partenariat et pédagogie sociale de l'intervention', in N. Chevalier, J. Otis, and M.-P. Desaulniers, eds, *Sida et prévention*. Montréal: Les Éditions Logiques, 39–56.

Cappon, P., et al. 1995. 'HIV/AIDS in the Context of Culture: Selection of Ethnocultural Communities for Study in Canada', *Canadian Journal of Public Health* (May–June): 511–14.

Caron, F. 1996. *Évaluation d'un programme d'éducation à la sexualité orientée sur la prévention du sida présenté par des jeunes dans une école secondaire multi-ethnique de la Montérégie.* Rapport d'activité, Université du Québec à Montréal.

———, J. Otis, and F. Pilote. 1998. 'Evaluation of an AIDS Peer Education Program on Multiethnic Adolescents Attending an Urban High School in Quebec, Canada', *Journal of HIV/AIDS Prevention and Education for Adolescents and Children* 2, 1: 31–53.

Catania, J.A., S.M. Kegeles, and T.J. Coates. 1990. 'Towards an Understanding of Risk Behavior: An AIDS Risk Reduction Model (ARRM)', *Health Education Quarterly* 17, 1: 53–72.

Centers for Disease Control, Division of Adolescent and School Health. 1997. 'School-based HIV-Prevention Education—United States, 1994', *Journal of School Health* 67: 103–5.

Chandarana, P.C., P. Conlon, S. Noh, and V.A. Field. 1990. 'The Impact of AIDS Education among Elementary School Students', *Canadian Journal of Public Health* 81: 285–9.

Côté, R.L. 1990. *Processus expérientiel de changement et d'apprentissage: principes d'apprentissage, processus de changement et interventions pédagogiques facilitantes*. Québec, Département de psychopédagogie, Université Laval.

CQCS. 1997. *Rapport de consultation concernant la prévention des MTS et de l'infection au VIH pour les années 1992–1995*. Ministère de la Santé et des Services sociaux du Québec.

Denis, J.L., and F. Champagne. 1990. 'L'analyse de l'implantation: modèles et méthodes', *Canadian Journal of Program Evaluation* 5, 2: 47–67.

Desaulniers, M.-P. 1994. 'L'éducation sexuelle préventive du VIH-sida et les représentations sociales du corps et de la sexualité', in N. Chevalier, J. Otis, and M.-P. Desaulniers, eds, *Éduquer pour prévenir le sida*. Beauport, Que.: Publications MNH, 251–62.

———. 1996. 'Pour une approche globale de la sexualité adolescente', *Revue sexologique* 4, 1: 190–4.

Djandji, H. 1996. 'Le programme d'éducation à la sexualité "remettre à plus tard les relations sexuelles"', *Revue sexologique* 4, 1: 181–4.

Drolet, M. 1996. 'L'évaluation d'une intervention préventive auprès d'adolescents et d'adolescentes ou Quand les garçons nous font nous interroger', *Service Social* 45, 1: 31–60.

Dupont, M., J. Otis, and Action Séro-Zéro. 1997. 'Évaluation de "Bar en bar": un programme de prévention du VIH dans les bars gais de Montréal'. Montréal: Action Séro-Zéro.

Edgar, T. 1992. 'A Compliance-based Approach to the Study of Condom Use', in T. Edgar, M.A. Fitzpatrick, and V. Freimuth, eds, *AIDS: A Communication Perspective*. Hillsdale, NJ: Lawrence Erlbaum, 47–68.

———, M.A. Fitzpatrick, and V. Freimuth, eds. 1992. *AIDS: A Communication Perspective*. Hillsdale, NJ: Lawrence Erlbaum.

Evans, G., and S. Cohen. 1987. 'Environmental Stress', in D. Stokols and I. Altman, eds, *Handbook of Environmental Psychology*, vol. 1. New York: Wiley.

Fafard, A., G. Vermette, F. Letarte, and L. Roy. 1996. *La collégialité dans l'action. Le recours au pair aidant chez les jeunes: une méthode d'intervention pour la prévention des MTS et du sida*. Évaluation de l'implantation d'un projet. Lévis, Que.: DSP, Région Chaudière-Appalaches.

Festinger, L. 1950. 'Informal Social Communication', *Psychological Review* 57: 217–82.

Fishbein, M. 1979. 'A Theory of Reasoned Action: Some Applications and Implications', in H.E. Howe, ed., *Nebraska Symposium on Motivation*. Lincoln: University of Nebraska Press.

Fisher, J.D., and W.A. Fisher. 1992. 'Changing AIDS-Risk Behavior', *Psychological Bulletin* 111: 454–74.

Fisher, W.A., and J.D. Fisher. 1993. 'A General Social-Psychological Model for Changing AIDS Risk Behavior', in J.B. Pryor and G.D. Reeder, eds, *The Social Psychology of HIV Infection*. Hillsdale, NJ: Lawrence Erlbaum, 127–54.

Fournier, K. 1997. *L'accessibilité au condom en milieu scolaire québécois. Enquête auprès des CLSC et des directions d'école secondaire*. Québec: Ministère de la Santé et des Services sociaux, Direction générale de la santé publique.

Frappier, J.Y., and É. Roy. 1995. *HIV Seroprevalence and Risk Behaviors Study among Adolescents with Maladaptive and Social Problems in Montréal*. Montréal: Unité de maladies infectieuses, rapport de recherche—projet #5505–3744–AIDS, PNRDS.

Freire, P. 1973. *Pedagogy of the Oppressed*. New York: Seabury Press.

Gaudreau, L. 1989. 'La diversité des intervenants et intervenantes en éducation sexuelle', in A. Dupras, ed., *La sexologie au Québec*. Longueuil: Éditions Iris, 237–74.

———. 1997. 'Le sida et l'éducation', in J.J. Lévy and H. Cohen, eds, *Le Sida: aspects psychosociaux, culturels et éthiques*. Montreal: Éditions du Méridien, 299–331.

———, N. Chevalier, M. Dupont, and A. Caron. 1994. 'Les représentations sociales pour inspirer l'éducation en matière de prévention du sida', in N. Chevalier, J. Otis, and M.-P. Desaulniers, eds, *Éduquer pour prévenir le sida*. Beauport, Que.: Publications MNH, 291–308.

———, M. Dupont, and S. Séguin. 1994. *La formation québécoise d'intervenants en prévention du sida auprès des jeunes: Rapport de recherche*. Montréal: Centre de Recherches en éducation.

Gélinas, A., R. Fortin, C. Schoonbrodt, and A. Vanasse. 1995. 'Éducation pour la santé: vers une gestion appropriative de la santé', paper presented at IVe Congrès des Sciences de l'Éducation sous l'égide de l'Association Francophone des Doyennes, Doyens et Directrices, Directeurs d'éducation du Canada, Québec, Université de Montréal.

Gillis, P.A. 1994. 'Sex Education and HIV/AIDS Prevention', *Sexual and Marital Therapy* 9, 2: 159–70.

Glanz, K. 1991. 'Perspectives on Group, Organization, and Community Interventions', in K. Glanz, F.M. Lewis, and B.K. Rimer, eds, *Health Behavior and Health Education: Theory, Research and Practice*. San Francisco: Jossey-Bass, 387–402.

Godin, G. 1991. 'L'éducation pour la santé: les fondements psychosociaux de la définition des messages éducatifs', *Sciences sociales et santé* 9, 1: 121–39.

———, and F. Michaud. 1996. 'La prévention des MTS-sida chez les jeunes', in *La santé et ses déterminants*. Ottawa: Forum national sur la santé.

———, J. Carsley, K. Morrison, and R. Bradet. 1993. *Enquête québécoise Entre hommes*, Coalition des organismes communautaires québécois de lutte contre le sida et Université Laval.

———, F. Michaud, M. Alary, J. Otis, C. Fortin, and B. Masse. 1997. 'Évaluation d'un programme d'intervention sur la sexualité et la prévention des MTS et du sida chez les jeunes en centre de réadaptation', paper presented at 65e Congrès de l'ACFAS, Trois-Rivières, abstract 2078–R.

Green, L.W., and M.W. Kreuter. 1991. *Health Promotion Planning, an Educational and Environmental Approach*, 2nd edn. Toronto and London: Mayfield.

———, ———, S.G. Deeds, and K.B. Partridge. 1980. *Health Education Planning: A Diagnostic Approach*. Palo Alto, Calif.: Mayfield.

Haïek, L.N., and S. Brochu. 1996. ' "Sans condom c'est non": Intervention auprès d'adolescentes fréquentant une clinique de jeunes', *Revue sexologique* 4, 1: 7–22.

Hamel, J.-G., L. St-Onge, and M.-P. Desaulniers. 1994. 'L'éducation et la prévention du VIH-sida en milieu scolaire', in N. Chevalier, J. Otis, and M.-P. Desaulniers, eds, *Éduquer pour prévenir le sida*. Beauport, Que.: Publications MNH, 149–60.

Hankins, C.A. 1994. 'La femme et l'infection par le VIH', in N. Chevalier, J. Otis, and M.-P. Desaulniers, eds, *Éduquer pour prévenir le sida*. Beauport, Que.: Publications MNH, 76–84.

Harter, S. 1993. 'Causes and Consequences of Low Self-esteem in Children and Adolescents', in R.F. Baumeister, ed., *Self-esteem: The Puzzle of Low Self-regard*. New York: Plenum Press, 86–116.

Health Canada. 1994. *National Guidelines for Sexual Health Education*. Ottawa.

Heider, F. 1958. *The Psychology of Interpersonal Relations*. New York: Wiley.

Holland, J., C. Ramazanoglu, S. Scott, S. Sharpe, and R. Thomson. 1992. 'Risk, Power and the Possibility of Pleasure: Young Women and Safer Sex', *AIDS Care* 4, 3: 273–83.

Janis, I.L. 1967. 'Effects of Fear Arousal on Attitude Change: Recent Developments in Theory and Experimental Research', in L. Berkowitz, ed., *Advances in Experimental Social Psychology*, vol. 3. New York: Academic Press.

Joos, S.K., and D.H. Hickam. 1991. 'How Health Professionals Influence Health Behavior: Patient-Provider Interaction and Health Care Outcomes', in K. Glanz, F.M. Lewis, and B.K. Rimer, eds, *Health Behavior and Health Education: Theory, Research and Practice*. San Francisco: Jossey-Bass, 216–41.

Kelly, J.A., J.S. St Lawrence, L.Y. Stevenson, et al. 1992. 'Community AIDS/HIV Risk Reduction: The Effects of Endorsements by Popular People in Three Cities', *American Journal of Public Health* 82: 1483–9.

———, T.L. McAuliffe, K.J. Sikkema, D.A. Murphy, A.M. Somlai, G. Mulry, J.G. Miller, L.Y. Stevenson, and M.I. Fernandez. 1997. 'Reduction in Risk Behavior among Adults with Severe Mental Illness Who Learned to Advocate for HIV Prevention', *Psychiatric Service* 48, 10: 1283–8.

Kirby, D., L. Short, J. Collins, D. Rugg, L. Kolbe, M. Howard, B. Miller, F. Sonenstein, and L.S. Zaben. 1994. 'School-based Programs to Reduce Sexual Risk Behaviors: A Review of Effectiveness', *Public Health Reports* 109, 3: 339–60.

Kleinman, A. 1980. *Patients and Healers in the Context of Culture: An Exploration of the Borderland between Anthropology, Medicine, and Psychiatry*. Berkeley: University of California Press.

Kotler, P. 1982. *Marketing for Nonprofit Organizations*. Englewood Cliffs, NJ.: Prentice-Hall.

Laboratory Centre for Disease Control (LCDC). 1997. *Inventory of HIV Incidence and Prevalence Studies in Canada*. Ottawa: Health Canada, Division of HIV Epidemiology, Bureau of HIV/AIDS and STD.

Lamptey, P., T. Coates, P. Piot, and G. Slutkin. 1993. 'Prevention: Is It Working?', paper presented at IXth International Conference on AIDS, abstract PS–01–2.

Lazarus, R. 1966. *Psychological Stress and the Coping Process*. New York: McGraw-Hill.

Lazes, P., L.H. Kaplan, and K.A. Gordon. 1987. *The Handbook of Health Education*. Rockville, Md: Aspen Publications.

Legendre, R. 1983. *L'éducation totale*. Paris, Montréal: Nathan/Ville-Marie.

Leventhal, H. 1985. 'The Role of Theory in the Study of Adherence to Treatment and Doctor-Patient Interactions', *Medical Care* 23: 556–63.

———, M.A. Safer, and D.M. Panagis. 1983. 'The Impact of Communications on the Self-regulation of Health Beliefs, Decisions and Behavior', *Health Education Quarterly* 10: 3–29.

Lewis, F.M. 1991. 'Perspectives on Models of Interpersonal Health', in K. Glanz, F.M. Lewis, and B.K. Rimer, eds, *Health Behavior and Health Education: Theory, Research and Practice*. San Francisco: Jossey-Bass, 242–52.

Longpré, D., and J. Otis. 1994. 'Le processus de planification d'un programme de prévention du VIH chez les jeunes: L'exemple de l'Unité de santé publique de l'Hôpital Charles-Lemoyne', in N. Chevalier, J. Otis, and M.-P. Desaulniers, eds, *Éduquer pour prévenir le sida*. Beauport, Que.: Publications MNH, 179–90.

Lovelock, C.H., and C.B. Weinberg. 1984. *Marketing: For Public and Nonprofit Managers*. New York: John Wiley & Sons.

McCreary Centre Society. 1993. *Adolescents Health Survey*. Vancouver: Greater Vancouver Region.

McGuire, W.J. 1968. 'Personality and Attitude Change: An Information-processing Theory', in A.G. Greenwalt, T.C. Brock, and T.M. Ostrom, eds, *Psychological Foundations of Attitudes*. New York: Academic Press.

———. 1985. 'Attitudes and Attitude Change', in G. Lindzey and E. Aronson, eds, *Handbook of Social Psychology*. New York: Random House.

McKinnon, K., M.P. Carey, and F. Cournos. 1997. 'Research on HIV, AIDS, and Severe Mental Illness: Recommendations from the NIMH National Conference', *Clinical Psychology Review* 17, 3: 327–31.

Marlatt, G.A., and W. George. 1984. 'Relapse Prevention: An Introduction and Overview of the Model', *British Journal of Addiction* 79, 3: 261–73.

Maticka-Tyndale, E. 1997. 'Prévenir la transmission sexuelle du VIH, en sommes-nous capables? Avons-nous fait suffisamment d'efforts?', in J.J. Lévy and H. Cohen, eds, *Le Sida: aspects psychosociaux, culturels et éthiques*. Montréal: Éditions du Méridien, 333–65.

Mercier, C., J. Fortier, and J. Cordova. 1996. 'L'intervention par les pairs auprès des jeunes de la rue du centre-ville de Montréal'. Rapport de recherche remis à la RRSSSM-C, Régie régionale de la Santé et des Services sociaux de Montréal-Centre.

Metz, S., and M.A. Fitzpatrick. 1992. 'Thinking about Safer Sex: The Risky Business of "Know Your Partner" Advice', in T. Edgar, M.A. Fitzpatrick, and V. Freimuth, eds, *AIDS: A Communication Perspective*. Hillsdale, NJ: Lawrence Erlbaum, 1–20.

Michaud, F., R. Morin, and G. Godin. 1997. 'De la formation à l'implantation d'un programme sur la sexualité et la prévention des MTS et du sida chez les jeunes en centre de réadaptation', paper presented at the 65e Congrès de l'ACFAS, Trois-Rivières, abstract 2078–R.

Miller, L.C., B.A. Bettencourt, S.C. DeBro, and V. Hoffman. 1993. 'Negotiating Safer Sex: Interpersonal Dynamics', in J.B. Pryor and G.D. Reeder, eds, *The Social Psychology of HIV Infection*. Hillsdale, NJ: Lawrence Erlbaum, 85–126.

Ministry of Education. 1996. *Selecting Indicators to Report on Progress in School-based HIV Prevention and Sexual Health Promotion*. Ottawa: Health Canada.

Morrison, K., J. Otis, and R. Bernèche. 1996. *Au sauna . . . on s'adapte. Évaluation du programme Au sauna . . . on s'emballe*. Montréal: Séro-Zéro.

Moscovici, S. 1985. *Psychologie sociale*. Paris: Presses Universitaires de France.

Myers, T., G. Godin, L. Calzavara, J. Lambert, and D. Locker. 1993. *The Canadian Survey of Gay and Bisexual Men and HIV Infection: Men's Survey*. Ottawa: Canadian AIDS Society.

Nutbeam, D. 1986. 'Health Promotion Glossary', *Health Promotion* 1, 1: 113–27.

Otis, J. 1996. *Santé sexuelle et prévention des MTS et de l'infection au VIH: Bilan d'une décennie de recherche au Québec auprès des adolescents et adolescentes et des jeunes adultes*. Québec: Ministère de la Santé et des Services sociaux.

———, D. Charest, F. Pilote, et al. 1996. 'Jamais l'un sans l'autre'. Évaluation d'une campagne de prévention des MTS et du VIH à l'intention des utilisatrices de contraceptifs oraux. Montréal: Département de sexologie, Université du Québec à Montréal.

———, and N. Chouinard. 1994, 1995. *Évaluation du projet: 'Planification d'une structure d'accueil en Montérégie destinée aux jeunes hommes de 15 à 24 ans ayant des comportements homosexuels'*, 2 vols. Unité de santé publique de l'Hôpital Charles LeMoyne. Régie régionale de la Santé et des Services sociaux de la Montérégie.

———, G. Godin, J. Lambert, and R. Pronovost. 1990. *Étude des déterminants psychosociaux de l'utilisation du condom chez les adolescents et adolescentes de cinquième secondaire. Rapport de recherche.* Dépôt légal: Bibliothèque nationale du Québec, Bibliothèque nationale du Canada, 4e trimestre.

———, B. Gomez, D. Longpré, and R. Thomas. 1992. *Étude des déterminants psychosociaux de l'utilisation du condom chez les adolescents et adolescentes fréquentant les organismes communautaires du Département de santé communautaire de l'Hôpital Charles LeMoyne*. Rapport de recherche. Dépôt légal: Bibliothèque nationale du Québec, Bibliothèque nationale du Canada, 4e trimestre.

———, E. Roy, R. Burelle, and C. Thabet. 1997a. 'Le sida et ses répercussions chez les adolescents', in J.J. Lévy and H. Cohen, eds, *Le Sida: aspects psychosociaux, culturels et éthiques*. Montréal: Éditions du Méridien, 195–236.

———, J.J. Lévy, J.M. Samson, F. Pilote, and A. Fugère. 1997b. 'Différences de genre et usage du préservatif', in N. Chevalier, J. Otis, and M.-P. Desaulniers, eds, *Sida et prévention*. Montréal: Les Éditions Logiques, 375–92.

———, R. Burelle, L. Baillargeon, R. Côté, et al. 1997c. 'L'approche expérientielle ou l'autre façon d'aborder la promotion de la santé et du bien-être sexuel chez les adolescents', paper presented at 65e Congrès de l'ACFAS, Trois-Rivières, abstract 1093–R.

———, S. Cummings, D. Charest, F. Pilote, R. Tremblay, and J. Boissinot. 1997d. 'Vulnérabilité des adolescentes et des femmes adultes', in N. Chevalier, J. Otis, and M.-P. Desaulniers, eds, *Sida et prévention*. Montréal: Les Éditions Logiques, 191–222.

———, et al. 1997e. *L'évaluation des interventions dans les parcs auprès des hommes ayant des relations sexuelles avec d'autres hommes: un projet de recherche-action*. Québec: Ministère de la Santé et des Services sociaux.

Ouellet, F., and J. Lindsay. 1991. *Évaluation de l'implantation d'une activité d'animation théâtrale, comme moyen de prévention du sida, auprès des jeunes de niveau secondaire.* Projet subventionné par le Conseil québécois de la recherche sociale (Projet EA–233 A89).

Paicheler, G. 1997. 'Communication publique et gestion du risque de sida par le public', in N. Chevalier, J. Otis, and M.-P. Desaulniers, eds, *Sida et prévention*. Montréal: Les Éditions Logiques, 21–38.

Pelletier, R., J. Otis, R. Bastien, A. Beaudry, R. Leroux, K. Lournier, and K. Morrison. 1998. 'Implanter efficacement des interventions préventives dans les parcs auprès des HARASAH: resultats d'une expérience québécoise', *Journal Canadien des Maladies Infectieuses* 9 (supp. A), 15A (résumé no. 132).

Peterson, L., D.G. Ostrow, and D.J. McKirman. 1991. 'Behavioral Interventions for the Primary Prevention of HIV Infection among Homosexual and Bisexual Men', *Journal of Primary Prevention* 12: 19–34.

Petty, R.E., F. Gleincher, and B.G. Jarvis. 1993. 'Persuasion Theory and AIDS Prevention', in J.B. Pryor and G.D. Reeder, eds, *The Social Psychology of HIV Infection*. Hillsdale, NJ: Lawrence Erlbaum, 155–82.

Prochaska, J.O., C.A. Reeding, L.L. Harlow, J.S. Rossi, and W.F. Velicer. 1994. 'The Transtheoretical Model of Change and HIV Prevention: A Review', *Health Education Quarterly* 21: 471–86.

Read, S., D. DeMalleo, and B. Bock. 1993. *HIV Prevalence in Toronto Street Youths*. Toronto: Hospital for Sick Children.

Régie Régionale de la Santé et des Services sociaux. 1997a. *Surveillance des cas de syndrome d'immunodéficience acquise (sida), Québec cas cumulatifs 1979–1997. Province de Québec.* Direction de la santé publique, mise à jour no. 97–1.

———. 1997b. *Surveillance des cas de syndrome d'immunodéficience acquise (sida), Québec cas cumulatifs 1979–1997. Montréal-Centre.* Direction de la santé publique, mise à jour no. 97–1.

Rimer, B.K. 1991. 'Perspectives on Interpersonal Theories in Health Education and Health Behavior', in K. Glanz, F.M. Lewis, and B.K. Rimer, eds, *Health Behavior and Health Education: Theory, Research and Practice*. San Francisco: Jossey-Bass, 140–58.

Rogers, E.M., and F.F. Shoemaker. 1971. *Communication of Innovations: A Cross-Cultural Approach*, 2nd edn. New York: Free Press.

Rogers, R.W. 1983. 'Cognitive and Physiologicial Processes in Fear Appeals and Attitude Change: A Revised Theory of Protection Motivation', in J. Petty, ed., *Social Psychophysiology*. New York: Guilford Press, 153–76.

———, and C.R. Mewhorn. 1976. 'Fear Appeals and Attitude Change: Effects of a Threat's Noxiousness, Probability of Occurrence and the Efficacy of Coping Responses', *Journal of Personality and Social Psychology* 34: 54–61.

Rosenstock, I.M., V.J. Strecher, and M.H. Becker. 1994. 'The Health Belief Model and HIV Risk Behavior Change', in R.J. DiClemente and J.L. Peterson, eds, *AIDS Prevention and Mental Health*. New York: Plenum Press, 5–24.

Rothman, J. 1979. 'Three Models of Community Organization Practice', in F.M. Fox, J.L. Erlich, J. Rotherman, and H.E. Tropman, eds, *Strategies of Community Organization*. Chicago: Peacock, 20–36.

Roy, E. 1993. 'L'épidémiologie du VIH-SIDA chez les adolescents', *Journal Canadien des Maladies Infectieuses* 4, supp. D: 13D.

———, D. Haley, J.-F. Boivere, J.-Y. Frappier, C. Claesseris, and L. Lemire. 1996. *L'infection au VIH chez les jeunes de la rue de Montréal*. Rapport final. Montréal: Unité de Santé Publique, Division des maladies infectieuses.

Samson, J.-M. 1995. 'Les objectifs de l'éducation sexuelle préventive du sida', *Sexologies* 4, 18: 45–53.

Schoonbroodt, C., and A. Gélinas. 1996. 'La prévention par le changement émergent: apprendre à gérer les problèmes!', *Éducation santé* 108.

———, and ———. 1997. 'Gestion appropriative et méthodologie du changement émergent', in N. Chevalier, J. Otis, and M.-P. Desaulniers, eds, *Sida et prévention*. Montréal: Les Éditions Logiques, 83–104.

Scott, F., L.W. Chambers, J. Underwood, S. Walter, and L. Pickard. 1990. 'AIDS Seminars for Senior Grades in Secondary Schools', *Canadian Journal of Public Health* 81: 290–4.

Simon, W., and J.H. Gagnon. 1986. 'Sexual Scripts: Permanence and Change', *Archives of Sexual Behavior* 15: 97–120.

Simon-Morton, B.G., et al. 1989. 'An Ecological Approach to the Prevention of Injuries due to Drinking and Driving', *Health Education Quarterly* 16, 3: 397–411.

Skinner, B.F. 1969. *Contingencies of Reinforcement: A Theoretical Analysis*. New York: Appleton-Century-Crofts.

Steinaker, N.W., and M.R. Bell. 1979. *The Experiential Taxonomy: A New Approach to Teaching and Learning*. New York: Academic Press.

Sutton, S.R. 1982. 'Fear-arousing Communications: A Critical Examination of Theory and Research', in J.R. Eiser, ed., *Social Psychology and Behavioral Medicine*. New York: Wiley.

Triandis, H.C. 1979. 'Attitudes and Interpersonal Behavior', in H.E. Howe, ed., *Nebraska Symposium on Motivation*. Lincoln: University of Nebraska Press.

Tudiver, F., T. Myers, R.G. Kurtz, K. Orr, C. Rowe, E. Jackson, and S.L. Bullock. 1992. 'The Talking Sex Project: Results of a Randomized Controlled Trial of Small-Group AIDS Education for 612 Gay and Bisexual Men', *Evaluation and the Health Professions* 15, 4: 26–42.

Valdiserri, R.O., D.W. Lyter, L.C. Leviton, et al. 1989. 'AIDS Prevention in Homosexual and Bisexual Men: Results of a Randomized Trial Evaluating Two Risk Reduction Interventions', *AIDS* 3: 21–6.

Vassal, A., and K. Morrison. 1997. 'Les hommes gais, le sida et la science', in J.J. Lévy and H. Cohen, eds, *Le sida: aspects psychosociaux, culturels et éthiques*. Montréal: Éditions du Méridien, 143–70.

———, J. Otis, N. Chouinard, and F. Pilote. 1996. 'Long term effects of training addressed to health care personnel working with young gays and bisexuals', paper presented at XIth International Conference on AIDS, Vancouver, 10 July, abstract #LB045.

Wagman, L.M. 1993. 'Condomania: A Public Education Intervention', *Canadian Journal of Public Health* 84, supp. 1: S62–5.

Wallston, K.A., and B.S. Wallston. 1978. 'Locus of Control and Health: A Review of the Literature', *Health Education Monographs* 6: 107–17.

Warren, W.K., and A.J.C. King. 1994. Development and Evaluation of an AIDS/STD/Sexuality Program for Grade 9 Students. Final research report. Kingston: Queen's University.

———, ———, R.P. Beazley, and M.A. King. 1994. 'Les effets d'un programme d'enseignement au sujet du sida et des MTS auprès d'élèves de 14 et 15 ans', in N. Chevalier, J. Otis, and M.-P. Desaulniers, eds, *Éduquer pour prévenir le sida*. Beauport, Que.: Publications MNH, 161–78.

Weiner, B. 1993. 'AIDS from an Attributional Perspective', in J.B. Pryor and G.D. Reeder, eds, *The Social Psychology of HIV Infection*. Hillsdale, NJ: Lawrence Erlbaum, 287–302.

Chapter 3

Social Workers and HIV Prevention

A Neglected Dyad

LYNNE LEONARD

The human immunodeficiency virus is silent, slipping unfairly and unheralded into its host.

Unfairly, because effective transmission takes place through those activities generally considered, at least by some of the people some of the time, to be pleasurable.

Unfairly, because in contrast to other health risk behaviours such as smoking, or eating a high fat diet or failing to exercise, just one instance of this risk-taking behaviour can result in an immediate health-altering condition.

Unfairly, because the antibodies, developed by the body within weeks or months following infection, do not have the protective properties of those formed in the more common viral infections.

Unheralded, because the immediate post-infection symptoms parallel the early signs of flu and in the absence of visible discrete markers of infection, the virus settles, largely undetected, to lie dormant for many years.

> But then, like a quietly malevolent guest, the human immunodeficiency virus gradually activates; and once roused from its dormancy it inexorably subverts both immune and nervous system functions, resulting in a dreadful array of infections and tumours, fevers and dementia, and a wasting of both body and spirit over months of clinical decline. (Osborne, 1989: 25)

In the quiet of its initial stage and in the tumult of its final stage, the pathogenesis of the infection can be seen as a metaphor of social work's own dominant response to the epidemic: relatively silent over the circumstances of infection with the virus, but full of activity once the consequences of infection are manifest; emphasis on clients living with the disease, scant attention to enabling clients to live disease-free.

From where does this unbalanced perspective on the priorities of social work practice in the HIV field emanate? Its origins can be seen in the policy and practice documents originating from our own professional association, the Canadian Association of Social Workers (CASW). In its 1989 statement on HIV/AIDS, the CASW recognized that 'as a national organization for social workers and as a member of the international social work community, CASW must address the human and professional concerns which relate to the prevention of HIV infection, the control of its transmission and the care and support needed by individuals, groups, communities and, perhaps, entire societies in coping with AIDS' (CASW, 1989: 1). The CASW has certainly addressed the latter issue with excellent results, including the recent compilation of the advanced social work practice manual, the *Comprehensive Guide for the Care of Persons with HIV Disease: Module 6—Psychosocial Care.*

The first two issues—prevention and control of transmission—have largely been ignored, however. As an example, in 1990, the CASW, in partnership with the Federal Centre for AIDS, developed and distributed to social workers throughout Canada a resource kit to enable social workers to extend their skills in responding to the HIV/AIDS epidemic. In the context of the emphasis in its statement of just a year earlier, of the need for a social work focus on both HIV prevention and AIDS care, and given the title of this kit—*Preparing for HIV and AIDS*—it is reasonable for social workers to expect attention to be given to HIV transmission as well as to the disease of AIDS. This expectation was not to be fulfilled. The objectives identified in the introductory pages of the report (Blue, 1990: 2, 7) speak of only one priority:

> This resource kit has been developed on the premise that all social workers will have contact with people living with AIDS (PLWAs), their families, friends and care-givers, regardless of the agency they are employed in, the tasks they are involved in and the type of social work they do, including counselling, policy development or community work. . . .
>
> The challenges of caring for PLWAs, their friends and families means relying on existing skills and being open to change and possibly the development of new skills. This kit aims to provide practical information and guidance for intervention in this area.

While this comprehensive manual does indeed address the complex issues of responding to the need for care and support for people living with AIDS—the end-stage consequence of HIV infection—it gives little more than passing mention to the issue of prevention of HIV infection. Already we see the development of the priorities of the social work intervention in this field, of the narrowing of the broader perspective contained in the original 1989 statement, to an emphasis on care and support for people living with AIDS.

Some five years later, the CASW's most recent publication in this area, *Social Work Practice and Practice Wisdom in the Field of HIV/AIDS* (Clarke, 1995), continues to focus on practice with people infected with or affected by the virus. This CASW research paper, like the earlier publication, risks fostering two inappropriate messages for social workers. First, it suggests that the only social work contribution in the area of HIV/AIDS is with clients who are aware of and have disclosed their positive status, with their lovers, family of choice, and friends. Second, and equally as limiting for social work practice, is the notion that a discrete number of social workers are working in the area of HIV/AIDS, thus implying that only 'specialist' social workers can respond to the challenges this crisis has thrust upon us.

The first message is illustrated in the recruitment methodology. While the first goal of the project and the corresponding recruitment objective was to 'identify and survey Canadian social workers in the field of HIV/AIDS' (Clarke, 1995: 1), participation in the study was circumscribed by focusing on the end-stage of HIV transmission. By relying chiefly on participant referrals from agencies and committees whose mandate is towards those people living with HIV infection, a more inclusive description of the lives and work, challenges and successes of those social workers practising in the field of HIV prevention is lost.

I am sure there are many social workers like myself, committed to practise in the HIV/AIDS battlefield but primarily concerned with prevention activities, who feel excluded by the research author's concluding remarks: 'Social work is in an optimal position to respond to the suffering of [persons living with] HIV/AIDS and thereby make a huge difference in the course of this epidemic' (Clarke, 1995: 32). Amen to that, but how about the recognition that if social work incorporated a primary prevention perspective, it would be in 'an optimal position to make a huge difference in the course of the epidemic' by actively working towards lowering the incidence of HIV, of diminishing new infections by promoting prevention activities?

The second message of exclusivity, of specialism, is also demonstrated by recruiting into the project only those social workers involved with people actively fighting the disease. The research instrument used to survey the 299 participants was based on a series of six questions, the first of which was: 'Who are the social workers in this field?' I would suggest that by widening the definition of the social worker's response to the epidemic to include interventions that may enable clients to lower the HIV risk created by some activities—often the essence of their existence—the answer to this question would be a resounding 'All of us!'

The potential harm to our profession in maintaining this perception of exclusivity is discussed by Alcock (1996: 150), who describes the challenges to establishing HIV/AIDS as a 'presence' in social work: 'many professional social workers seem to regard HIV/AIDS as a "special" topic and despite the information distributed by CASW, are unprepared for the day when some aspect of HIV/AIDS will arise in their practices.'

I would state the issue more strongly. The consequences for clients of this mystification of expertise and the distancing that it must produce in social workers who see themselves as 'outside' the HIV field are profound. When they eventually meet clients who need their help on risk-reduction decisions, on prevention, these social workers will deliver a diminished standard of service. The result of a failure to respond effectively to a client's need for skilled support in reducing the risk of HIV infection is potentially catastrophic and ethically indefensible.

Perhaps, and this is certainly true for the earlier resource kit, the CASW focus has primarily reflected the paradigm of care and understanding prevalent at the time. Indeed, until the mid-1980s the main focus of epidemiological understanding, research initiatives, and clinical management was focused on AIDS itself. However, since then there has been a significant paradigm shift, described by Kelly (1995: 2) as 'a reconceptualization of HIV illness as a continuum ranging from initial HIV infection and a period of asymptomatic infection without clinical illness, through the initial onset of illnesses and to the diagnosis of major life threatening illnesses.' In conceptualizing HIV as a 'continuum of infection stages and clinical illnesses varying in severity rather than as an AIDS/not AIDS dichotomy', Kelly remarks, 'de-emphasis on the AIDS label in favour of HIV also reminds us that the true disease culprit—and thus the true focus of prevention efforts—is infection with HIV.'

In this second decade of the epidemic, it is now critical for social workers to explore their responsibilities and contributions in working with people to ensure that they do not enter this continuum at all—or if they do, that it is with a true understanding of the level of HIV risk they wish to tolerate. A shift from exclusive attention to the end-stage of the illness continuum to a focus on social work interventions that address the key issue of risk reduction in the wider context of health behaviour change is urgently needed. Within such a preventive perspective, therefore, this chapter will highlight policy frameworks and behavioural change theories that could inform social work in the HIV/AIDS field. First, I will place social work interventions in the context of current, primarily structural, paradigms of Canadian public health policy. Second, I will draw on some recent developments in behavioural science to identify a model of risk-reducing interventions that might be used by social workers concerned with prevention at both the individual and community levels. The theme of this chapter is therefore health, not disease.

THE CONTEXT OF PUBLIC HEALTH POLICY

Emphasizing health rather than disease is the essence of a public health perspective, a field with a long tradition in promoting and implementing prevention activities to control communicable disease. Given this pedigree, what has been the public health response to HIV infection and AIDS? Are there lessons for social work in this profession's framework of preventive responses to the epidemic?

Perhaps the most fundamental and appropriate lesson for social work, certainly at this stage in the profession's unbalanced focus of its intervention objectives to address HIV infection and AIDS, is the principle outlined by Albee (1989: 18), who asserts that 'the field of public health has traditionally taught us much of what we need to know to prevent plagues effectively. First of all, it is well established that no mass disorder afflicting humankind has ever been eliminated by attempts at treating only infected individuals.'

If social work is to build on the idea that we must go further than the treatment and support of infected individuals and those living with them, crucial as these activities are, then on which conceptions of prevention might we draw? Two major paradigms of prevention currently permeate thinking and action in the Canadian public health arena: health promotion theory and population health theory. These conceptual frameworks have something to offer social work because they both draw attention to how health and risks to health are socially constituted as well as how they are determined by individual biological and behavioural factors. These approaches resonate with the social work perspective, which situates the individual within a determining or constraining economic, social, and cultural environment. This environment constructs the possibilities of conscious choice—the limits of client self-determination. On this basis, these two dominant approaches to prevention and the current attempt to amalgamate them into a single new framework, as described by Wong (1997) in *Paradigms Lost*, merit further consideration.

The fundamental feature of the health promotion approach has been to encourage a process whereby people are empowered to increase control over their health and to improve it. It is an approach that identifies the 'prerequisites' of health—peace, shelter, education, food, income, stable ecosystems, sustainable resources, social justice, and equity (WHO, 1986). At least in theory, this approach demands that we cannot expect people to improve their own health and reduce risks when many of their illnesses and disabilities are the outcome of wider economic and social forces—poverty, injustice, and other forms of oppression—over which they have no control.

Within the health promotion framework, Health Canada, working in partnership with the communities concerned with HIV/AIDS, developed the National AIDS Strategy based on a community action approach in setting priorities and planning and implementing programs. The strategy included a focus on prevention through the achievement of behavioural changes that would reduce risks of HIV infection. There is, however, a problem with this approach as it applies to HIV/AIDS. As a single-issue, community-specific focus of intervention, it does not have the necessary theoretical and political resources to tackle the social context of populations most at risk of infection, a context that includes inequality, social injustice, poverty, homophobia, and racism. This problem, among others, has made public health professionals receptive to another model of prevention.

The population health perspective places central emphasis on the determinants of health and disease. This approach has the effect of diminishing the focus on individual lifestyles and emphasizing the importance of the economic and social environment in constructing health and the incidence of disease. The population health framework has been the basis of an argument that there should be less public expenditure on health care and more (equivalent to that cut from health expenditures) on the social determinants—welfare payments, education, employment, housing, etc. Although this approach to resource allocation has been criticized, rightly in my view, as providing an ideological justification for cost-cutting operations, the overall model of population health has attractions for social work. It is a framework within which socio-economic inequality could be placed as a central determinant of health, illness, and risk, especially if buttressed by an explicit theory of the origins of inequality and how it is reproduced in society.

In the face of the competing biomedical models of health and disease, it is perhaps unrealistic to expect government to adopt such a radical, critical version of the population health perspective to guide resource allocation, because it would challenge major economic and ideological elements of the existing social structure. However, a more cautious, consensual population health promotion framework is gaining influence in informing the strategic direction of government policies (Hamilton and Bhatti, 1996). What emerges from this framework is a distinction between risk factors or risk behaviours personal to the individual (personal risk perception, physiological attributes, self-efficacy, and, due to the biological sexism of the virus, sex) and risk conditions that play a determining role in constructing the decisions and choices of individuals and communities about behaviours that may place them at risk of HIV infection.

The importance of the application of this paradigm shift to conceptualizing and positioning HIV prevention activities is gaining credibility (Aggleton et al., 1994; Piot and Aggleton, 1998; Hankins, 1998). Specifically, this development in the discourse on risk involves moving from the much maligned and distracting concept of risk groups to the concept of risk factors and risk behaviour and to the concept of risk conditions or risk situations. While Hankins (1998: S150) asserts that 'the paradigm of individual risk has clearly been superseded by a discourse of vulnerability or risk situation', Aggleton et al. (1994: 343) argue for a more balanced approach with a dual emphasis on individual factors and social and community factors: 'a number of factors are now known to influence risk behaviour. These can be divided into two main types: those that are linked to attributes of the individual (including risk perception, outcome expectations, and self-efficacy) and those that derive from the community or society of which the individual is part.'

It is in the context of this discussion of the development of conceptualizations of prevention in the health field that I turn to an exposition of a particular preventive model. It is a model with the potential to synthesize the two patterns of risk discussed by Aggleton et al., and can be applied to work with clients to help them consider the personal relevance of changing health risk behaviours and adopting protective behaviours in the wider context of the risk conditions experienced in their daily lives. It is a model that, though individualistic in its origins in a behavioural paradigm and more usually applied in clinical practice as a clear individual behaviouralist approach to intervention, is capable of development into a more socially contextualized model well suited to use by social workers.

KNOWLEDGE AND BEHAVIOUR CHANGE

Early on in the HIV epidemic, many studies carried out in diverse populations attested to the increase in HIV/AIDS knowledge as the outcome of awareness training, education, and sensitization programs (Bandura, 1992; Mayes et al., 1992; Jemmott and Jemmott, 1991; MacDonald et al., 1990; Goodman and Cohall, 1989; Richard and Van De Pligt, 1991). As discrete interventions, these programs were based on two premises. First, behaviours conferring high risk of HIV infection are engaged in out of ignorance of both the risk created and the changes needed to lower that risk. Second, increasing awareness of behaviours that confer risk would result in a reduction in HIV risk behaviours—that finite number of HIV risk-related sexual and drug injection practices. Indeed, in the CASW's own manual, prevention of HIV infection appears to be synonymous with education: 'The importance of education in an attempt to prevent HIV transmission is paramount. To date, in the absence of a cure or vaccine, education designed to affect activities and attitudes is the most effective strategy to prevent HIV transmission' (Blue, 1990: 114). While brief educational interventions can increase an individual's HIV-related knowledge by between 6 and 21 per cent (Alteneder et al., 1992), interventions relying on health information alone to promote changes in behaviour have yielded inconsistent, often disappointing results (Eisen, Zellman, and McAlister, 1990; Silvestre et al., 1989; Becker and Joseph, 1988). It is now clear that knowledge is a necessary but insufficient determinant of change, that is, behavioural changes to prevent or lower the risk of HIV infection or transmission are not consistently produced by increased knowledge alone.

What makes knowledge something a person can act on? One answer is to suggest that the ability to act on knowledge is determined by a person's readiness to engage in behaviour change. Understanding the factors that determine readiness is thus central to risk reduction efforts. The more we can understand why people engage in risk behaviours, despite having the requisite knowledge of disease transmission and protective behaviours, the more appropriate our interventions are likely to become. As Fishbein and Guinau (1996: 6) write in their overview of the relationship between behavioural science and public health in the field of HIV prevention, 'Clearly, the more one understands the factors influencing (or underlying) a person's decision to perform (or not perform) a given behaviour, the more likely one is to develop interventions that can effectively change that behaviour.' Thus, in the same way that conceptualizing HIV illness as a continuum helps us to develop a deeper understanding of the differing manifestations of the disease, viewing the process of changing behaviour and adopting new behaviours as representing a continuum of readiness to change enables us to tailor social work responses to each individual based on his/her degree of readiness to change.

Most current theories of behaviour change (Becker and Joseph, 1998; Bandura, 1977, 1994b; Fishbein, 1980) generally include elements of an acknowledgement by the individual that he/she is at risk; that he/she is committed to change and is capable of making that change and has the skills to do so; that others are also changing and that the individual is able to identify reinforcing consequences of change. Unique in their differing emphasis on the above factors, these theories converge in their basic premise that individuals have potential control over their own behaviour and are nominally free to make decisions to engage in protective or risk behaviours.

While integrating key concepts from these individualistic theories of human behaviour to explain why and how behaviour change occurs, the transtheoretical model (TTM), discussed here, pushes our understanding of the dynamics of individual behaviour change in terms of the actual process of initiating and maintaining change and, I will suggest, has the potential to ground the mechanics of that change in the social context or risk condition in which the risk behaviours take place. Our understanding of the process of change, of the work of change, is enhanced by the model's conceptualization of the relative importance of components of individualistic models of behaviour change at different times or stages in the change process. In addition, the TTM may be flexible enough to take into account the context of the relations of gender, class, and culture within which individual behaviour is embedded.

THE TRANSTHEORETICAL MODEL OF BEHAVIOUR CHANGE

The transtheoretical model was developed in the early 1980s by James Prochaska and Carlo DiClemente. With its origins in psychotherapy research and smoking cessation, the model conceptualizes behaviour change as a continuous process in which people move through a sequence conceptualized as five successive stages as depicted in the following figure (Prochaska, DiClemente, and Norcross, 1992).

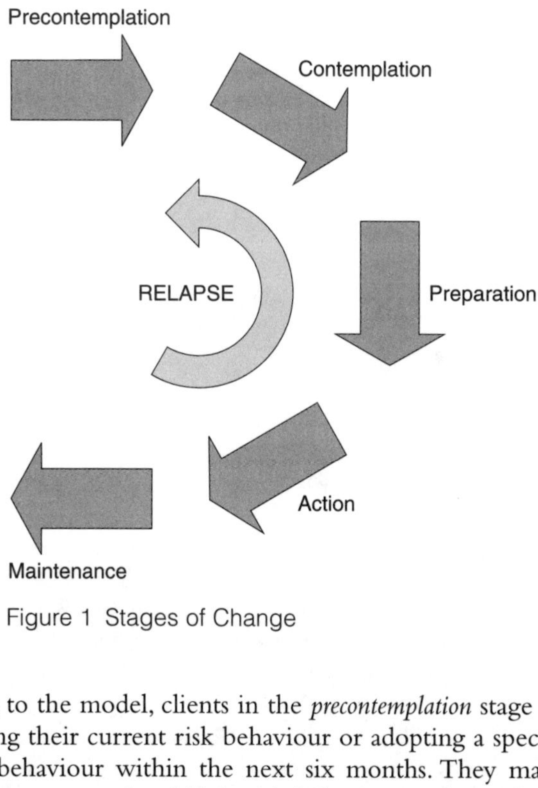

Figure 1 Stages of Change

According to the model, clients in the *precontemplation* stage have no intention of changing their current risk behaviour or adopting a specified protective or preventive behaviour within the next six months. They may be defensive about their present HIV-related high-risk behaviour and may lack awareness of the personal consequences and the consequences for others of such behaviour. In addition, the behaviour may be perceived either as positively functional or as a rational response to their individual circumstances. Whatever the cause, little time is spent in thinking about their present HIV-related high-risk behaviour. Examples of clients in this precontemplation stage would be injection drug users who share needles as a consequence of sharing a hit of drug or adolescents who do not use condoms as they do not perceive themselves to be susceptible to HIV.

In contrast, clients in the *contemplation* stage are seriously considering changing their current risk behaviour and have formed an intention to adopt the preventive behaviour within the foreseeable future—generally defined as within the next six months. The consequences of their current behaviour for themselves and others have become apparent, yet there remains ambivalence regarding the relative benefits of longer-term gains against the short-term costs of change. An example of a client in the contemplation stage would be a woman who realizes the risks for herself in allowing her partner to determine her sexual protective behaviour but who feels that the potential conflict with her partner if she insisted on condom use would be too difficult to experience.

This ambivalence resolves in the *preparation* stage as the personal relevance of change increases and clients seriously plan to change their risk behaviour and adopt the new preventive behaviour within the immediate future—usually defined as within the next 30 days. An injection drug user is actively seeking out sources of clean needles, adolescent girls may be actively seeking assistance in asserting their need for protection with their sexual partners, and gay men may be actively considering alternate recreation locations less conducive to casual sexual encounters.

In the *action* stage, clients have changed their HIV-related high-risk behaviour, have adopted the new preventive behaviour, and are actively engaged in strategies to lower their HIV risk. Condoms are used every time for intercourse and clean, unused needles are used every time for injection drug use. The lower-risk behaviour is still relatively new at this most challenging stage but the client is using specific strategies to support the new behaviours and avoid relapse.

As the low-risk behaviour becomes more routine and with accumulated experience in using coping strategies in high-risk situations, clients move into the *maintenance* stage. This stage is characterized by having sustained their HIV-related low-risk behaviour for a substantial period, usually thought of as six months or more.

The TTM acknowledges that initiating and sustaining a new behaviour is challenging and recognizes *relapse* as a normative event occurring at any stage and requiring a repetition of movement through the stages. In fact, particularly with addictive behaviours, most people who change will cycle through the five stages several times before they reach the end of maintenance.

WHAT DETERMINES A CLIENT'S STAGE OF READINESS TO CHANGE?

Three other key concepts of this model, *decisional balance*, *processes of change*, and *self-efficacy*, are the variables that influence the transition from one stage of behaviour change to another.

In a recent study our research team investigated the salience of competing theories of health behaviour change to understand the determinants of condom use for HIV prevention among heterosexually active youth and young adults (Leonard et al., 1998). The constructs of the TTM were an integral part of this exploratory study. To illustrate these three stage-defining concepts, the definitions of each of the concepts are presented followed by examples of the ques-

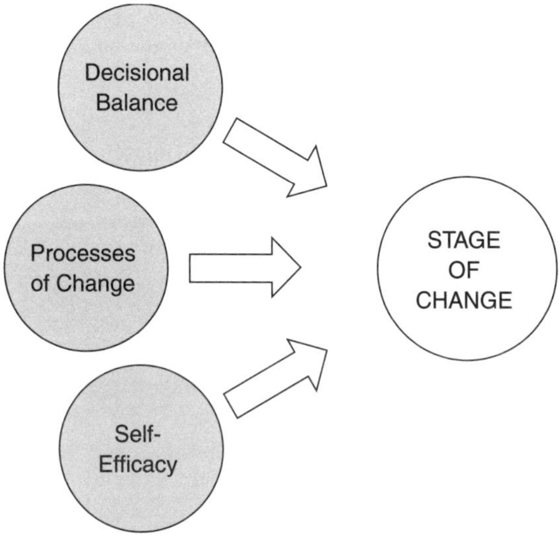

Figure 2 The Transtheoretical Model

tions used in this study to measure the constructs. The examples are therefore specific to the use of condoms for HIV prevention.

DECISIONAL BALANCE

Drawing on Janis and Mann's (1977) decision-making theory, the TTM conceptualizes how clients consider changes in their health behaviour in terms of a balance of comparative gains and losses. The motivation for change, the development of intention to change, is strongly determined by how people view the gains and losses (or the pros and cons) of their current behaviour *vis-à-vis* the pros and cons of adopting a new behaviour.

How clients view the relative importance of the pros, the benefits of adopting the new behaviour, in relation to the cons, the costs of adopting the new behaviour, varies across the stages of readiness to change. In virtually all behaviours studied to date, the pattern of decisional balance at each stage has been consistent (Prochaska et al., 1994). Thus, knowing the characteristics of a client's decisional balance, of his/her ranking of the benefits and costs of adopting a new behaviour at each stage of readiness to adopt that new behaviour, is of central importance. This understanding enables the social worker to tailor counselling interventions to address that balance in order to initiate, with the client, a shift in the decisional balance congruent with that of the next stage of change.

In *precontemplation*, the cons, the costs of changing the risk behaviour, exceed the pros, the benefits. Clients perceive that for their own personal circumstances, there are more negative outcomes about adopting HIV-related lower-risk behaviours than there are positive outcomes. There is therefore little motivation to change. Concerning adopting consistent condom use for HIV prevention, examples of statements reflecting the negatives of behaviour change would be clients saying introducing condoms would cause stress in their relationships, that using condoms when having sex would feel unnatural, that condoms would be too much trouble, or that their partners would get upset.

During *contemplation* the pros—the benefits of behaviour change—increase significantly. Clients now see about as many personally salient reasons for changing as they do for maintaining the HIV-related high-risk behaviours. In the *preparation* stage, the pros that support reducing risk behaviours outweigh the cons, thereby providing motivation for change. For example, clients might believe that by using condoms every time they would be safe from diseases and would feel more responsible in terms of their own protective behaviour.

During *action* and *maintenance*, the cons of change decrease somewhat while the pros remain relatively constant and decisional balance becomes less of a mediator of change or exerts less influence on the change process.

PROCESSES OF CHANGE

The strategies that clients use as they progress through the varying stages of readiness to change risk behaviour are termed the processes of change. In the TTM there are 10 processes of change (DiClemente and Prochaska, 1985). Five are related to experiential or cognitive strategies that modify thoughts, feelings, and emotions to promote change, while five processes are related to behavioural strategies to promote change.

Again, drawing on examples of scales used to investigate the utility of the TTM to understand the prevalence of condom use for HIV prevention, the *experiential or cognitive processes* are the following:

- *Consciousness-raising* relates to activities or strategies clients use to increase their awareness of their risk behaviours. A client might begin thinking about things he/she has seen or heard about how one can become infected with HIV through unprotected sex, or about things seen or heard about how condoms help to provide protection from contracting HIV during sex.
- *Dramatic relief* occurs when a client experiences a strong emotional reaction to a situation linked to risk behaviours—for example, feeling upset when seeing pictures of people dying of AIDS or on hearing warnings about sex without a condom.
- *Social liberation* is characterized by the client becoming increasingly aware of changes in the environment that provide alternatives to risk behaviours. Becoming aware that more and more people are choosing to use condoms during sex and recognizing that condoms are now easier to find in stores and health-care clinics are social liberation strategies.
- *Self re-evaluation* occurs when a client reappraises the consequences associated with modifying behaviour as being personally salient. For example, one may feel bad about oneself having sex without a condom because it increases the risk for HIV infection or feel better about oneself using condoms to reduce the risk of infection with HIV.

- *Environmental re-evaluation* occurs as clients become aware of the impact of their behaviour on others. For example, clients stop to think that if everyone used a condom every time during sex, HIV would not be spreading so fast in their community, or they think about the fact that they are helping to stop the spread of HIV in their community by using a condom every time they have sex.

The *behavioural processes* follow:

- *Self-liberation* reflects activities that support the client's commitment to reducing HIV-related risk. An example would be when clients are with partners who don't want to use a condom and they tell themselves that their health is too important to risk getting infected with HIV.
- *Counter-conditioning* involves strategies that replace risk behaviours with incompatible substitute behaviours, such as finding alternatives to unprotected sex to provide fun and satisfaction when condoms are not available.
- *Stimulus control* strategies involve changing the environment to avoid high-risk situations, such as maintaining a readily available supply of condoms at home and carrying condoms at all times.
- *Reinforcement management* refers to those strategies employed by clients to reward themselves for change efforts, for example, using positive self-statements or tangible rewards when condoms have been used to reduce their risk of HIV infection.
- *Helping relationships* refers to the efforts clients make to gain the professional or social support they need to maintain their change efforts. Examples include identifying people in their social circle who encourage and support their use of condoms during sex, or on whom they can count for encouragement when they are having a hard time using condoms every time they have sex.

Understanding which processes of change or which strategies clients generally engage in to make positive transitions between stages gives social workers a framework for tailoring interventions with their clients to enable movement to the next stage. For most health behaviours the experiential processes—those strategies related to modifying feelings, thoughts, and emotions to change behaviour—are generally used in the early stages of behaviour change, that is, in the precontemplation and contemplation stages. The behavioural processes are used later to increase and maintain the new behaviours. Table 1, from Prochaska et al. (1992), provides a schema for detailing the stage-specific processes.

SELF-EFFICACY

Successfully changing health-impairing behaviours has been consistently linked to people's confidence in their ability to do the work of change—to a strong personal belief in their capability to engage in the specific health-promoting behaviour in a varying range of risk situations. Bandura (1994a: 26) posits that this fac-

Table 1 Matching Process to Stage

Precontemplation	*Contemplation*	*Preparation*	*Action*	*Maintenance*
Consciousness-raising Dramatic relief Environmental re-evaluation				
	Self re-evaluation			
	Social liberation			
		Self-liberation		
			Reinforcement management Helping relationships Counter-conditioning Stimulus control	

tor, self-efficacy, is a major determinant or causal influence on whether a person both initiates engagement and continues engagement in adaptive behaviour:

> Perceived self-efficacy is concerned with people's beliefs that they can exert control over their own motivation, thought processes, emotional states, and patterns of behaviour. People's beliefs about their capabilities affect what they choose to do, how much effort they mobilize, how long they will persevere in the face of difficulties.

As Bandura explains, the consequence of a lack of this sense of self-efficacy, this belief that the recommended behaviour can be performed under a variety of circumstances, results in poor behavioural outcomes even when the required skill set and knowledge base are in place. 'Self-doubts over-ride knowledge and self-protective action' (Bandura, 1994a: 26). Self-efficacy is an integral feature of the TTM. In the same way that processes of change and decisional balance vary across stages, so does self-efficacy (DiClemente, 1986). It is lowest in precontemplation and reaches its highest levels in maintenance. To assess a client's self-efficacy in consistently using condoms for each act of sexual intercourse, for example, a social worker might ask a client how confident or sure he is that he would use condoms every time when he thinks his partner might get angry or when he has been using alcohol. Similarly, for assessing self-efficacy in terms of stopping sharing needles for injection drug use, social workers could ask how confident the client is that he or she would not share a needle when a friend has a hit of a drug and only one needle.

USING THE MODEL IN SOCIAL WORK PRACTICE: STAGE-MATCHED INTERVENTIONS

The transtheoretical model challenges the view that populations engaging in high risk-related behaviours, such as injection drug users sharing injection equipment or adolescents having unprotected sex with many partners, are homogeneous in respect to their risk behaviour.

The essence of the TTM is that people engaging in health risk behaviours are heterogeneous with respect to their intentions to engage in or maintain health-protective behaviours. The TTM shows us that clients need to be seen as constituting discrete groups defined not only by their specific risk situations, but by their readiness to change risk behaviours and by their stage of change, and therefore as requiring different stage-matched interventions.

Practitioners using the TTM will be able to initiate an effective tailored approach to intervention based on 'stage-matching'. Knowing an individual client's stage allows a social worker to intervene by encouraging the use of stage-appropriate processes of change, that is, activating the processes that will help the client progress to the next stage. Furthermore, the model brings into focus the need to address motivation directly among those in the pre-action stages by shifting decisional balance, and at all stages to embed intervention in the context of enhancing a client's self-efficacy with respect to the new adaptive preventive behaviour.

With few exceptions, outside the parameters of the Centers For Disease Control (CDC) demonstration projects in the US that operationalized stage-matched assessments and interventions based on Prochaska's work, little empirical or evaluative evidence exists of applying the core elements of the TTM to HIV-related risk behaviours. Similarly, work on developing the model to encompass the two concepts necessary to any effective prevention strategy—a focus on how the individual client might be helped to progressively adopt new behaviours that constitute a lessening of risk and prime emphasis on the social and cultural determinants of those behaviours—is in its infancy.

Extending the very valid principles of stage assessment and stage-matched interventions from the original, individualistic perspective to a new perspective that respects, highlights, integrates, and makes visible to the client the risk conditions mediating his/her own HIV-related risk behaviours is therefore a challenge and an opportunity. It is a challenge that can be uniquely and effectively met by social work, with its historical theoretical underpinning of understanding the determining nature of the social environment in which behaviour unfolds. It is an opportunity to use a model, which has typically demonstrated such great promise in relation to effecting change in other health-impairing behaviours, to inform a sense of direction in the formulation of vital prevention protocols demanded of social workers within the urgency of the Canadian HIV epidemic.

The following section delineates that challenge and opportunity by generalizing the traditional TTM principles to a new domain of health behaviours and by expanding the TTM individualistic determinants of behaviour to an inclusive paradigm that synthesizes individual and societal or structural determinants of risk, as well as risk behaviours and risk conditions.

THE SOCIAL WORKERS' RESPONSE

ASSESSMENT

To formulate appropriate interventions, the first step, using the model, is to assess with the client his/her stage of change or readiness to change activities that confer high HIV risk and to adopt lower-risk behaviours. As the activities that currently confer greatest risk for HIV infection are sexual and injection drug use practices, the challenge for social workers is to establish the context in which such issues can be freely discussed. Achieving a comfort level in talking about these issues may require some additional preparation on the social worker's part. Learning about the diversity that exists in the social expression of human sexuality is a necessary foundation for understanding healthy sexuality in the context of the risk conditions that many clients experience.

Aside from this issue, social workers using a client-centred approach are well positioned in terms of their ability to engage in reflective listening, use a questioning style based on open-ended questions, and express empathy to determine with the client his or her stage of change without increasing resistance to the work of change. Essentially, using the skills specified above and the use of open-ended questions such as 'How do you see the situation with condom use in your relationship?' or 'How does injecting drugs fit into your life right now?', practitioners can begin to understand the determinants of a client's stage in relation to those behaviours that confer or transmit the risk of HIV infection.

Having ascertained the client's readiness to change risk behaviour, having placed him/her in a 'pre-action stage' of precontemplation (sees *no need* to use condoms consistently), contemplation (sees *need* to use condoms consistently *but*), or preparation (*ready* to start using condoms consistently) or in the 'action stages' of action (*using* condoms consistently for less than six months) and maintenance (*using* condoms consistently for more than six months), the social worker and client can jointly consider interventions tailored to the client's stage (Levenkron et al., 1995). These stage-matched interventions are then implemented with the intent to facilitate movement to the next stage.

PRECONTEMPLATION INTERVENTIONS

As we have seen, clients in the precontemplation stage perceive no problems with their current behaviours and are not seriously thinking of changing their HIV-related risk behaviour during the next six months. They may feel resigned ('Look, I figure if I've got it, I've got it, so what's the point of using condoms?'), may rationalize the problem away ('Everyone I know shares and they're not positive.'), may be reluctant to adopt protective behaviour ('But you know, really, I don't think it's worth the hassle of trying to use condoms every time we have sex.'), or may become defensive or rebellious when presented with advice ('It's easy for you to say, you've never had to deal with this stuff.') (Miller and Rollnick, 1991).

The goal of the social worker's intervention in the precontemplation stage is to work with the client to shift the energy invested in the problem towards contemplation, towards considering changing in the foreseeable future. The focus of intervention here is to ease the client into thinking about current high-risk HIV-related behaviour, and the consequences of continuing it, in a manner that is personally relevant. Clients need to talk about risk behaviour from their own perspective, to have acknowledged the risk conditions contributing to their risk behaviour, and to be supported in starting work on re-evaluating the costs and benefits of change in order to achieve a more balanced view of their situation. This is achieved by addressing the client's decisional balance, which in precontemplation is strongly weighted to the cons of changing the behaviour exceeding the pros, the benefits of changing behaviour. Enhancing the pros of changing ('What would be some of the benefits for you if you used condoms all the time?') and the cons of not changing through emphasizing the personal relevance of risk ('Think about all the people you know who have got infected through dirty needles and imagine what it would be like for you.') and raising doubts concerning the advantages of risk behaviour ('What do you think will happen to you if you keep on sharing needles?') are techniques to shift decisional balance in this stage (Hotz and Leonard, 1998).

One of Prochaska's earliest empirical integrations was the discovery of systematic relationships between the stage people were in and the processes they were applying. Table 1 details the latest empirical integration of the 10 processes and the five stages across such behaviours as smoking, diet, cocaine use, exercise use, condom use, and sun exposure. The practical application of this integration schema for clients in the precontemplation stage is to target the processes specific to precontemplation to encourage movement to the next stage, contemplation (Prochaska and Velicer, 1997). In precontemplation, consciousness-raising ('What do you do to minimize your worry about not using condoms?'), eliciting dramatic relief ('How do you feel when you hear that someone you know has got AIDS?'), and initiating environmental re-evaluation ('What is the effect of your needle-sharing on your girlfriend?') are the cognitive processes to be enhanced. In addition, to the extent that clients can be helped to identify alternative means of achieving change goals and to see choices in how they might go about doing so, they are likely to begin seeing change as being possible or even desirable.

CONTEMPLATION INTERVENTIONS

Moving from the precontemplator's firm conviction of maintaining the status quo by never changing, we find that clients in the contemplation stage are seriously considering changing their current risk behaviour 'someday' within the next six months. Although the consequences of their current behaviour are understood, doubts regarding the relative balance of long-term benefits and short-term costs of change prevent a firm commitment to change. Clients in this stage frequently suffer a motivational paralysis because they can perceive almost as many reasons for changing as they do for continuing their risky behaviour: 'I know that sharing is not the way to go, but that's the way me and my buddies do it and I don't want them mad at me.' Thus, despite having meaningful reasons for change, the individual experiences anxiety over its consequences and the stresses inherent in adopting new ways of behaving, particularly when those behaviours involve others such as in sexual decision-making. These factors serve as profound sources of ambivalence: 'I don't want to get sick, but he's told me he's out of that door if I make him wear a safe.'

For clients in contemplation, therefore, enabling them to resolve their ambivalence about change and to tip the decisional balance in favour of change is the primary focus of the social worker's intervention. This is accomplished by working with the client to disclose all the pros and cons concerning the issue: 'What would be some of the good things for you in making a change to using condoms?', 'What would be some of the problems for you in using condoms?', 'What are some of the good things for you in continuing to not use condoms?', 'What are some of the not so good things for you in continuing to not use condoms?' At this stage on the change continuum, the social worker's goals are to use these personally relevant perceptions to increase the client's awareness of the risk behaviour as a problem (the cons of not changing) and to enhance his/her own perception of the value of changing (the pros of change) by helping the individual attend to and explore his/her own reasons for change. To deepen awareness of the cons of staying the same, social workers can use open-ended questions to elicit problem recognition, for example, 'What problems could occur in the future if you didn't address the issue of condom use in your relationship?' Similarly, to deepen awareness of the pros of changing, open-ended questions can be used to elicit the intention to change, 'How would you feel if you were able to always protect yourself from infection during sex?', 'How would your life be more positive if you were able to achieve this?' (Miller and Rollnick, 1991).

Reflecting back to the client his or her own areas of concern (the cons of not changing) and highlighting the discrepancy between current behaviour and personal goals (the pros for changing) are strongly related to the self re-evaluation process of change. Reappraising the consequences associated with modifying behaviour as being personally relevant is considered to be the process of change to be targeted to enable clients to move from precontemplation to contemplation: 'On the one hand it is important to you to have a relationship with your boyfriend and on the other you want to remain healthy and disease free'; 'Keeping in with your buddies is important to you, yet keeping on sharing needles actually causes you more worries.'

PREPARATION INTERVENTIONS

The contemplator's intention to change 'someday' becomes an intention to change 'soon' (within the next month) as he/she moves into the preparation stage. The ambivalence characteristic of the contemplation stage resolves as the pros of changing outweigh the cons of changing previous high-risk behaviour. Clients in the preparation stage are now getting ready to change by planning the specific steps to be undertaken to protect themselves from risk.

During this stage clients need the kind of support from social workers that helps them feel more confident about changing. At this point on the stage continuum, the focus of intervention needs to be on the positive dimensions of engaging in risk-reducing behaviours and of making change a priority. Consequently, strategies that enhance commitment and help clients to define the very specific change goals in behavioural terms are indicated here.

Enhancing commitment to change involves helping clients learn the coping strategies that will be required to make change happen. First steps include identifying with clients the personal risk situations that will make risk behaviour likely for them and establishing and practising the basic coping skills to use in response to those risk situations, for example, role playing with the client assertive responses in sexual encounters with a partner who doesn't want to use condoms, establishing the means to ensure a ready supply of clean needles at all times, and discussing best condom practices as well as local sources of free or maximally accessible condoms. Identifying with the client the time at which the new behaviours will be implemented and supporting the client in communicating his/her goal to significant others (which will at least convey clear limits or expectations and at best generate support) also help to strengthen commitment.

As clients prepare to move towards the action stages, a behavioural process of self-liberation is key to target in order to facilitate movement to the first action stage. Self-liberation can be initiated by social workers suggesting to their clients that they review together the reasons for wanting to change and why these reasons are important, by establishing what they will use to chart their progress and by posing such questions as, 'What do you need to keep this goal as your priority?' (Miller and Rollnick, 1991).

ACTION INTERVENTIONS

Intention becomes reality, 'soon' transforms to 'now', as clients move, at their own pace, into the action stage. Action is the stage at which clients have made specific overt modifications in their HIV-related risk behaviour within the past six months. As the new lower-risk behaviour has only recently been adopted, clients are most vulnerable to the risk of relapse at this stage. Relapse is the return from the action stages of action and maintenance to one of the earlier pre-action stages of precontemplation, contemplation, or preparation, although most people usually relapse to preparation or contemplation. 'The bad news is that relapse tends to be the rule when action is taken for most health behaviour problems' (Prochaska and Velicer, 1997).

The immediate goal of the social worker for work with clients in the action stage is to support, by acknowledging, praising, and celebrating, the clients' continuous efforts to maintain the new behaviour. Self-efficacy is greatly increased at this stage in the recognition of the achievement of short-term, targeted goals such as the consistent use of condoms for one month, or injecting alone with clean needles, outside of all social interactions, for one month. The behavioural processes of change are those that clients make the most use of in this stage to move towards maintenance. To assist with this first goal, concentrating on the process of reinforcement management will be helpful. This can be achieved initially by planning reinforcement ('How would rewarding your successes help your confidence and motivation?'), and then by helping the client decide on the nature of those rewards in terms of positive self-statements or perhaps something more tangible, such as a trip to the movies or dinner at a favourite restaurant or with friends.

The second, concurrent, goal is to strategize with the client personal coping strategies to identify and deal with situations that may cause relapse to the previous risk behaviour. Specifically, the social worker needs to work with the client to anticipate and to prepare to survive relapse crisis situations, those situations that will challenge the new position and tempt the individual to go back to his/her previous behaviour. In working with clients to anticipate relapse crisis situations, social workers can focus on stimulus control, a behavioural process found to be helpful in this stage. Stimulus control involves assisting the client in identifying those personally relevant cues that may lead to the risk behaviours and explore ways to avoid or counter these stimuli: 'What kind of things might tempt you to have sex without a condom again?' or 'What kind of situations will make you feel like sharing needles again?'

In preparing to survive relapse crisis situations, identifying alternatives to risk behaviour aligned with the needs that were being met for the client by the previous risk behaviour is a further key process to initiate at this stage. Counter-conditioning strategies can be worked on with the client through such questions as, 'What could you do when you feel yourself under pressure to share a needle with your friend?' or 'What could you do when you really want to have sex but neither you nor your partner has a condom?'

Finally, as the lower-risk behaviour is still new at this stage and not necessarily well integrated to respond to a range of risk situations, it is important for the client to identify needed supports or helping relationships to maintain the unfamiliar behaviour. The social worker will therefore need to explore with the client what kind of support is personally needed ('What kind of support from others will help you put your plans into action?'), to explore the source of such support ('Who do you think will be able to give you this sort of support?'), and to plan to initiate such support from among the client's identified sources in his/her social circle and from community agencies and organizations.

MAINTENANCE INTERVENTIONS

Maintenance is the stage in which clients have sustained their lower-risk behaviour for more than six months. While still making strenuous efforts to avoid relapse, they do not use the change processes to prevent relapse as frequently as do those in the first six months of action because they are increasingly more confident that they can continue with their adaptive preventive behaviours, which are becoming more routinized. Nevertheless, the behavioural strategies initiated in the action stage need to be reinforced with the client with particular emphasis on helping the client identify risk situations ('What signs would warn that you are at risk for a slip?') and working with the client to rehearse coping strategies to deal with those situations ('Okay, the needle exchange van has not turned up, you're joneseying, desperate for a hit and have no clean needles. What could you do to make sure you don't end up sharing needles again?').

ASSESSING RISK CONDITIONS

Integrated into the process of stage-matching is the social worker's involvement of the client in assessing the conditions that may be associated with high-risk behaviour. The descriptions of these risk conditions should be made accessible to the client and clearly relevant to the individual's experiences and, perhaps, should avoid or move beyond the abstractions of class, gender, culture, or racism. The language for describing typical risk conditions might be in terms of obstacles to a client being able to exercise choice over risk-related behaviours. Such obstacles may be both external or structural and also internalizations of ideologies and identities that severely restrict the client's agency—that is, the ability to make choices in one's own self-defined interests.

At this preliminary stage in developing the TTM in a more structural way, we might begin to work on descriptors of structural obstacles that could be refined, reformulated, and expanded as social workers begin to use the model. The following overlapping categories of risk conditions as obstacles to reducing risk-related behaviour might be used as a starting point.

- Inadequate material resources, ranging from the lack of free or inexpensive items such as clean needles or condoms, to the depressing and invalidating experiences of living at a poverty level that not only leads to paralysing feelings of worthlessness but also saps the energy needed to make changes in behaviour.
- Relative powerlessness in relation to significant others (friends, lovers) that prevents the client from acting on a decision believed to be in the interests of his/her protective health. The internalization of this powerlessness may lead to fatalism about the possibilities of change and a reluctance to mount resistance to the exercise of power by others.
- Cultural norms that act to inhibit, or at least delegitimate, lower-risk practices. Such cultural norms may be associated with religious beliefs, such as prohibitions on the use of condoms, or with subcultural practices that act as a source of identity, such as needle-sharing.

Other categories could be added to this initial identification of risk conditions that affect risk-related behaviour. The challenge here, of course, is for the social worker and client to attempt to move from the identification of obstacles to the means by which they might be overcome. Within the process of stage-matching, therefore, the social worker and the client try to identify resources and activities that might be used to assert the client's demand for greater autonomy and security. These resources and activities might include, for example, the client joining a sex trade worker's support group; the social worker arguing for the development of more needle exchanges; the client seeking support within a group committed to the empowerment of its gay and lesbian members; or the social worker contributing to a piece of action research on the effects of poverty on HIV risk.

CONCLUSION

> The role of the behavioural sciences is to assist in the promotion of changes in behaviour that most effectively reduce the rate of spread of HIV infection, and thus reduce the scale of the pandemic. (Aggleton et al., 1994: 342)

The attraction of this statement lies in the notion of behavioural scientists, although it could just as easily apply to social workers, *assisting* in the promotion of changes in behaviour—working with the client, at the client's pace, grounded in the client's lived experience of HIV-related risk. The statement is also attractive because, by not specifying individual or societal or political behaviour change, Aggleton et al. neatly sidestep the unnecessary distraction of defending reductionist arguments if only individual behaviour change was emphasized. At the same time, it is implicitly suggested that changes in behaviour need to happen at every level. Change is required not only by the actor but on the stage on which he/she acts, and the director and producer must also engage in behaviour change if the scale of the pandemic is to be reduced.

Does adopting the TTM both as an assessment tool and as an intervention model to guide our work with clients suggest that we are only concerned with changing the actors? Would we, as a profession, be contributing to Rhodes's view (1996: 4) that focus on individual change has not been adequately matched by interventions at other levels:

> Contemporary HIV prevention responses have been overwhelmingly focused on targeting individuals with the aim of encouraging individual behavior change. . . . The over-reliance on targeting individuals and individual behavior changes alone restricts both the possibilities and parameters of change to individuals.

I have suggested that the assessment and intervention techniques specific to the transtheoretical model of behaviour change have the potential to be developed and applied by social workers in their preventive work with individual clients in an intervention that exposes, respects, and integrates the social construction of a client's risk behaviour. Exposing, understanding, and integrating structural determinants of health risk in clinical practice interventions are essential to providing a meaningful and tailored social work response to the HIV preventive needs of clients—essential but not sufficient.

What is required, at a different time and in a different place, is for the determinants of risk conditions to be addressed by individual social workers and by our profession working collectively. Ensuring a constant supply of free condoms and lubricants in washrooms used by clients, entering into partnerships with HIV prevention programs to become satellite needle exchange programs and sites for anonymous HIV counselling and testing, and creating, posting, and supplying generic HIV prevention posters and brochures to create awareness and to give information in waiting areas and in the offices of workers in all social service agencies and welfare offices are attainable goals to ameliorate risk conditions at a local level. On a collective level, as a profession, through the auspices of the CASW, we must assume a prominent public role in supporting Canadian strategies to address the structural determinants of HIV-related risk behaviour. For example, public endorsement of the recommendations detailed in *HIV, AIDS and Injection Drug Use: A Nation Action Plan* (CPHA and CCSA, 1997) and their adoption and integration into the university curricula of professional social work courses would be a major contribution to the massive prevention effort that is required.

This chapter commenced with a critical review of the social work profession's unbalanced response to the challenges of the disease; it seems only fitting to end with a sense of optimism that perhaps the dichotomy between care, treatment, and support and prevention activities is slowly being eroded. The CASW, in its latest publication, *Comprehensive Guide for the Care of Persons with HIV Disease*, includes a chapter on prevention that emphasizes the prevention potential of social work: 'With its focus on both the psycho (personal skills and abilities) and the social (the broader environment where people must use these skills), social work practice has great potential to influence the root causes of this illness and a responsibility to help prevent the spread of HIV' (CASW, 1997: 139). The model described in this chapter can be used to direct and inform preventive social work practice to address risk behaviour change in the context of constraining risk conditions, and perhaps with the help of this model the sentiments expressed by one social worker (CASW, 1997: 139) will be echoed far and wide:

> One of the most important contributions that I can make as a social worker is to help prevent the spread of HIV. In my ability to start where the client is, foster self-esteem and help people get the resources they need to enjoy better quality of life and avoid other factors, such as poverty and drug use, that make them more vulnerable to social and health problems like HIV, I believe I am doing something to stop this virus.

Dedication and Acknowledgements

This chapter is dedicated to the memory of Dr Maurice Moreau, past professor of social work at Carleton University and l'Université de Montréal. Dear friend and colleague, Maurice led the development of the structural approach in Canadian social work practice and exemplified why HIV prevention is so vital.

Portions of this chapter were initially published in L. Leonard and S. Hotz, 'Social Workers and HIV Prevention: A Model for Preventive Practice', *The Social Worker* 64, 4 (1996): 108–21. The author thanks Stephen Hotz and Janice Hansen for their comments on an earlier draft of this chapter and gives special thanks to

Peter Leonard for his encouraging scepticism, which pushed my thinking to the beat of a different drum.

REFERENCES

Aggleton, P., K. O'Reilly, G. Slutkin, and P. Davies. 1994. 'Risking Everything? Risk Behavior, Behavior Change, and AIDS', *Science* 265: 341–5.

Albee, G. 1989. 'Primary Prevention in Public Health: Problems and Challenges of Behaviour Change as Prevention', in V. Mays, G. Albee, and S. Schneider, eds, *Primary Prevention of AIDS: Psychological Approaches*. Newbury Park, Calif.: Sage.

Alcock, S. 1996. 'Visible and Connected: The BCASW Committee on HIV/AIDS', *The Social Worker* 64, 4: 149–51.

Alteneder, R., J. Price, S. Telljohann, J. Didion, and A. Locher. 1992. 'Using the PRECEDE Model to Determine Junior High School Students' Knowledge, Attitudes, and Beliefs about AIDS', *Journal of School Health* 62, 10: 464–70.

Bandura, A. 1977. *Social Learning Theory*. Englewood Cliffs, NJ: Prentice-Hall.

———. 1992. 'A Social Cognitive Approach to the Exercise of Control over AIDS Infection', in R. DiClemente, *Adolescents and AIDS: A Generation in Jeopardy*. Newbury Park, Calif.: Sage.

———. 1994a. *Social Foundations of Thought and Action: A Social Cognitive Theory*. Englewood Cliffs, NJ: Prentice-Hall.

———. 1994b. 'Social Cognitive Theory and Exercise of Control over HIV Infection', in R. DiClemente and J. Peterson, *Preventing AIDS: Theories and Methods of Behavioural Interventions*. New York: Plenum Press.

Becker, M., and J. Joseph. 1988. 'AIDS and Behavioural Change to Reduce Risk: A Review', *American Journal of Public Health* 78: 394–410.

Blue, L. 1990. *Preparing for HIV and AIDS: A Resource Kit for Social Workers*. Ottawa: CASW.

Canadian Association of Social Workers (CASW). 1989. CASW Statement on HIV/AIDS. Ottawa: CASW.

———. 1997. *Comprehensive Guide for the Care of Persons with HIV Disease*. Ottawa: CASW.

Canadian Centre on Substance Abuse (CCSA) and Canadian Public Health Association (CPHA). 1997. *HIV/AIDS and Injection Drug Use: A National Action Plan*. Ottawa: Health Canada.

Canadian Public Health Association (CPHA). 1993. *HIV/AIDS: A Public Health Perspective*. Ottawa: CPHA.

Clarke, R. 1995. *Social Work Practice and Practice Wisdom in the Field of HIV/AIDS: A Research Report*. Ottawa: CASW.

DiClemente, C. 1986. 'Self-efficacy and the Addictive Behaviours', *Journal of Social and Clinical Psychology* 4: 302–15.

———, and J. Prochaska. 1985. 'Processes and Stages of Change: Coping and Competence in Smoking Behaviour Change', in S. Shiffman and T. Wills, eds, *Coping and Substance Use*. New York: Academic Press, 319–43.

Eisen, M., G. Zellman, and A. McAlister. 1990. 'Evaluating the Impact of a Theory-based Sexuality and Contraceptive Education Programme', *Family Planning Perspectives* 22, 6: 261–71.

Fishbein, M. 1980. 'A Theory of Reasoned Action: Some Applications and Implications', in H. Howe and M. Page, eds, *Nebraska Symposium on Motivation, 1979*. Lincoln: University of Nebraska, 65–116.

———, and M. Guinam. 1996. 'Behavioural Science and Public Health: A Necessary Partnership for HIV Prevention', *Public Health Reports* 111, 1: 5–10.

Goodman, E., and A. Cohall. 1989. 'Acquired Immunodeficiency Syndrome and Adolescents: Knowledge, Attitudes and Beliefs, and Behaviours in a New York City Adolescent Minority Population', *Paediatrics* 84: 36–42.

Hamilton, N., and T. Bhatti. 1996. *Population Health Promotion: An Integrated Model of Population Health and Health Promotion*. Ottawa.

Hankins, C. 1998. 'Changes in Patterns of Risk', *AIDS Care* 10, 2: S147–53.

Hotz, S. 1996. 'Modifying Risk Behaviours: A Practical Approach for Helping Patients to Change', *Issues in Lipidology* 5, 1: 10–15.

———, and L. Leonard. 1998. 'Beyond Knowledge and Willpower: New Ways to Work Together to Change HIV-Related Risk Behaviour', workshop presented at the Canadian HIV/AIDS Skills Building Symposium, Toronto.

———, ———, R. Plotnikoff, C. Redding, and J. Hansen. 1997. 'The Stages of Condom Use among Heterosexual 15–29 Year Olds', paper presented at annual meeting of the Society for Behavioral Medicine, San Francisco.

Janis, I., and I. Mann. 1977. *Decision Making: A Psychological Analysis of Conflict, Choice, and Commitment*. New York: Free Press.

Jemmott, L., and J. Jemmott. 1991. 'Applying the Theory of Reasoned Action to AIDS Risk Behaviour', *Nursing Research* 40, 4: 228–34.

Kelly, J. 1995. *Changing HIV Risk Behaviour: Practical Strategies*. New York: Guilford Press.

Leonard, L., S. Hotz, J. Hansen, and R. Plotnikoff. 1998. *A Critical and Comparative Examination of Four Theories of Health Behaviour Change Applied to HIV Preventive Behaviour*. Ottawa: Community Health Research Unit, University of Ottawa.

Levenkron, J., P. Coury-Doniger, and S. Cowell. 1995. *Overview of Behavioral Counseling for STD/HIV Risk Reduction*. Rochester, NY: University of Rochester and Monroe County Health Department.

Macdonald, N., G. Wells, W. Fisher, et al. 1990. 'High-risk STD/HIV Behaviour among College Students', *Journal of the American Medical Association* 263: 3155–9.

Mayes, S., V. Elsesser, J. Schaefer, H. Handford, and L. Michaelgood. 1992. 'Sexual Practices and AIDS Knowledge among Women Partners of HIV-infected Hemophiliacs', *Public Health Reports* 107, 5: 504–13.

Miller, W., and S. Rollnick. 1991. *Motivational Interviewing: Preparing People to Change Addictive Behaviour*. New York: Guilford Press.

Osborne, J. 1989. 'A Risk Assessment of the AIDS Epidemic', in V. Mays, G. Albee, and S. Schneider, eds, *Primary Prevention of AIDS: Psychological Approaches*. Newbury Park, Calif.: Sage.

Piot, P., and P. Aggleton. 1998. 'AIDS, Inequality and Prevention', *International AIDS Society Newsletter* 10: 8–10.

Prochaska, J., C. DiClemente, and J. Norcross. 1992. 'In Search of How People Change: Applications to Addictive Behaviors', *American Psychologist* 47: 1102–14.

———, J. Rossi, and N. Wilcox. 1991. 'Change Processes and Psychotherapy Outcome in Integrative Case Research', *Journal of Psychotherapy and Integration* 1: 103–20.

———, and W. Velicer. 1997. 'The Transtheoretical Model of Health Behavior Change', *American Journal of Health Promotion* 12, 1: 38–48.

———, ———, J. Rossi, M. Goldstein, B. Marcus, W. Rakowski, C. Fiore, L. Harlow, C. Redding, D. Rosenbloom, and S. Rossi. 1994. 'Stages of Change and Decisional Balance for Twelve Problem Behaviors', *Health Psychology* 13: 39–46.

Rhodes, T. 1996. 'Individual and Community Action in HIV Prevention', in T. Rhodes and R. Hartnoll, eds, *AIDS, Drugs and Prevention: Perspectives on Individual and Community Action*. New York: Routledge.

Richard, R., and J. Van De Pligt. 1991. 'Factors Affecting Condom Use among Adolescents', *Journal of Community and Applied Social Psychology* 1: 105–16.

Silvestre, A., D. Lyter, R. Valdisseri, J. Huggins, and R. Rinaldo Jr. 1989. 'Factors Related to Seroconversion among Homo- and Bi-sexual Men after Attending a Risk-reduction Educational Session', *AIDS* 3, 10: 647–50.

WHO (World Health Organization) and Canadian Public Health Association. 1986. 'Ottawa Charter for Health Promotion', *Health Promotion* 1: iii–v.

Wong. C. 1997. *Paradigms Lost: Examining the Impact of a Shift from Health Promotion to Population Health on HIV/AIDS Policy and Programs in Canada*. Ottawa: Health Canada.

Chapter 4

The Challenge of Risk Reduction Practices

WILLIAM ROWE AND GLENN MARCOTTE

BACKGROUND

The 1993 *Founding Document* of the Harm Reduction Coalition (1993: 7) defines harm reduction as:

> a set of strategies and tactics that encourage [drug] users to reduce harm done to themselves and communities by their licit and illicit substance use. In allowing users access to the tools with which to become healthier, we recognize the competency of their efforts to protect themselves, their loved ones and their communities.

Evolving from a community-based approach to drug use as a health issue, harm reduction challenges the traditional models of disease and criminalization in addictions. Rather than being guided by a rigid abstinence-based model of chemical dependency, harm reduction stresses the '*complexity, fluidity and individuality of the user's life*' (Harm Reduction Coalition, 1993: 3). Instead of stressing the linear 'all or nothing' disease model of addiction where both the drug and the drug user are objectified, harm reduction adheres to the competing adaptive model (Alexander and Hadaway, 1982; Alexander, 1987) where the drug user is a subject involved in his/her own healing and treatment. This circular person-centred approach can therefore be applied to any individual at any given stage of drug use.

Harm reduction addresses people's relationships to drugs, as opposed to vilifying the individual drug user or the drug itself. Positive change is the operating principle in harm reduction; it aims to enhance self-esteem and self-efficacy. Harm reduction does not support all behaviours; rather, it recognizes that people are not defined by behaviour alone. A global approach to the person is therefore favoured, with the intervener starting where the drug user is at. Risk is accepted as a natural part of all lives, with harm viewed on a continuum within the context of the individual's life. Understanding the entire person is therefore inseparable from the context of that person. The isolation, survival needs, and the drug use of the user are addressed within this context.

NEW APPROACHES TO RELATIONSHIPS

The Harm Reduction Coalition outlines new, redefined relationships espoused by the adherents of the model. These redefined relationships span the spheres of influence relevant to intravenous drug users (IDUs), including their relationship to themselves and the drug, rapport to the community, and interaction with society at large. The intrinsic non-judgemental value of the IDU as a unique person who interacts with the drug and who is competent in decision-making serve as a backdrop for empowerment of the user. 'The users have power in their willingness to take risk' (Harm Reduction Coalition, 1993: 5). As trust and change develop, user participation and ownership in decision-making evolve. This empowering process occurs in a structure where egalitarian relationships are fostered. A less hierarchical structure of mutual exchange moulds a consultative rapport between the user and the health-care provider; the provider gives the user tools to reduce risk. This is done in a non-coercive way, with the user seen as an expert who actualizes his/her ability to function with his/her own drug use.

Community-based interventions are at the core of the model. Communities of users and of those affected by drug use must become involved in the organization of harm reduction interventions. There must be means of receiving feedback from communities of users and ways in which the programs can be modified to reflect this feedback. The empowerment of the user can occur only when the communities affected accept, protect, and incorporate them. This can be a significant challenge where drug use is considered to be offensive or criminal. Community input is therefore essential not only in decreasing harm but in increasing acceptance. The scope of intervention must therefore be wide enough for agents of change to manoeuvre at both the micro and the macro levels. Harm reduction introduces changes in individual risky behaviour, in injection drug cultures where risky behaviours are normalized, and in the community at large.

RATIONALE

UNDERSTANDING BEHAVIOUR

The dominant abstinence approach to addiction focuses on the chemical acting on the object-oriented and powerless user. Mere exposure to alcohol and other addicting substances can lead to chemical dependency—the drug causes the addiction. As a unique, diagnosable, and irreversible disease, alcoholism is seen to entail a predictable progression of symptoms through which the drinker loses control. The 'exposure perspective' of alcohol and other drugs leads to a linear, causal understanding of why people consume drugs. It holds a very simplistic deterministic view of human nature (Alexander and Hadaway, 1982; Alexander, 1987).

A richer way of understanding human behaviour views 'opiate addiction as an attempt to adapt to chronic distress of any sort through habitual use of opiate drugs' (Alexander and Hadaway, 1982: 367). This 'adaptive perspective' to addiction focuses not on the symptom, being addicted, but on the problem, chronic distress. The drug is used as a coping strategy and addiction occurs only when there is a stressful situation. 'The role of drugs in their lives is often that of a coping tool, without which they might commit homicide or suicide' (Springer, 1991: 144). The adaptive orientation seeks to reduce the demand for drugs as a coping strategy for stress, as opposed to limiting the supply of the drug to the user. Stressors, which can lead to anxiety and depression, are adapted to in ways that reduce the demand for the drug. This richer understanding follows a subjective and humanistic orientation, with a purposive, not deterministic and linear, view of human nature.

HEALTH PROMOTION

In 1986, the World Health Organization presented the *Ottawa Charter for Health Promotion*, which included a recognition of the importance of environmental factors to health: 'To reach a state of complete physical, mental and social well-being, an individual must be able to identify and to realize aspirations to satisfy . . . needs and to change the environment or adapt to it.' The Ottawa Charter, therefore, not only considers health to be the absence of disease but also integrates notions of increased quality of life and life expectancy. The social and physical environments become means by which health can be enhanced.

Health promotion confers on populations means of enhancing health and of assuring a greater control over health issues. Health promotion focuses on the development of individual attitudes regarding health and also underscores environmental interventions that reinforce the adoption of healthy lifestyles. Environmental factors can also stand in the way of healthy choices.

In 1994 the Federal, Provincial, and Territorial Consultative Committee on Health described individual determinants of health to include biological and genetic factors, lifestyle habits, and adaptive personal competencies. The committee included healthy childhood development, level of education, income and social situation, social support network, employment and work conditions, physical environment, and health services as population-based determinants of health (Boyer, 1995). Harm reduction practice understands health in a similar way. In 1987, the Canadian government adopted harm reduction as the framework for Canada's National Drug Strategy encompassing sickness, death, social misery, crime, violence, and economic costs to all levels of government (Riley, 1994).

Addiction is viewed as an adaptive response to a wide cross-section of individual and collective determinants. By retaining value-neutral views of the person and the activity, a spirit of non-judgementalism can pervade intervention. This not only allows for the users' greater control of health issues but also opens doors whereby users can enhance their health in ways appropriate for them. Harm reduction programs are user-centred, thereby impacting changes in lifestyle habits and enabling adaptive personal competencies. Previously used ways of enhancing health can be expanded on. By focusing on the problem of HIV transmission, the IDU can develop healthier individual attitudes and alternatives, even if these are not ideal. The problems of HIV transmission and addiction can be addressed separately, allaying intervention confusion between these two stigmatized issues. Social support networks, as a population-based determinant of health, will reflect these different degrees of stigma. These networks can be called on differently when the focus of the problem shifts from HIV transmission to addiction itself. Environmental factors, such as the legality of injection drug use, will impact on how successfully these healthier lifestyles can be adopted if the focus of the problem is clearly identified—addiction or HIV transmission. The extent to which total abstinence affects the individual determinants of health, including biological and genetic factors, can be crucial. This is particularly the case as the link between genetic predisposition and chemical dependency is further understood. Clearly, health promotion and harm reduction both borrow from the same vocabulary in understanding problems and creating strategies of intervention for these issues.

COST-BENEFIT ANALYSIS OR AN INDIVIDUALISTIC APPROACH?

The Harm Reduction Coalition (1993: 3) states that harm reduction 'moves away from cost-benefit analysis of public health, and towards a humanistic, individualistic approach.' This approach can be concordant with the use of the cost-benefit analysis tool when the costs and benefits are defined in both individual and public health terms. Cost-benefit analysis is a tool that describes in concrete terms the private or public harm being minimized and at the same time outlines the countervailing benefit (individual or collective) of keeping that harm reduced.

METHADONE TREATMENT

Methadone maintenance treatment programs (MMTPs) are a case in point. The harm reduced in taking methadone orally is that injection ceases. The countervailing benefits were initially defined only in the terms of public issues, namely perceived crime control. With the arrival of HIV, the countervailing benefits of MMTPs also include the slowing down of HIV contagion among opiate drug users. This new countervailing benefit, individually and collectively, supersedes the old public security reward of MMTPs.

NEEDLE EXCHANGES

Similar reasoning can be applied to needle exchange programs. Reduced costs do not include the elimination of injection but rather the *clean* injection of the drug. The perceived potential harm of injection drug use is reduced so that the countervailing benefit, slowing down HIV contagion, can be experienced by both the IDU and his/her community. 'The underlying theory and principles are applicable to any social welfare and/or public health issue, particularly those that largely affect marginalized individuals and communities. . . . [We] are dealing not solely with behaviours, but with whole people with complex needs' (Harm Reduction Coalition, 1993: 7).

SAFER SEX FOR GAY MEN

Harm reduction is an important vehicle in understanding behaviour change outside of addictions. Unprotected oral sex can be viewed as a safer-sex harm reduction strategy for gay men, particularly when practised as an alternative to unprotected anal sex. It is therefore important for public health authorities to distinguish nuances between the HIV risks of unprotected oral and unprotected anal sex for this harm reduction strategy to be available to gay men. Once accepted as a safer-sex alternative, the reduced costs of HIV transmission inherent to oral sex can be reinforced. The individual and social benefits of accepting oral sex as a safer-sex alternative include empowerment for gay men, where safer alternatives to unprotected anal intercourse can be exercised.

COMBINATION THERAPY AS A PANACEA

The understanding of behaviour change can be improved by harm reduction principles when applied to such issues as the administration of combination therapies. The benefit of such treatment regimes (better health outcomes) also carries another type of risk—that people will worry less about the seriousness of becoming infected and, consequently, will reduce safer-sex behaviours. Decisional empowerment can correct this faulty perception and reduce risk-taking behaviours.

COMPARING CANADIAN AND AMERICAN POLICY

As a neighbour to the United States, Canada has had some difficulty in focusing on injection drug use as primarily a health promotion issue, let alone where harm reduction interventions can be applied. The 'zero-tolerance' supply-side interventions, based on the 'Just Say No' campaign from the US, criminalize chemical dependency and lead to policies that try to limit the drug supply. Because this approach adheres to the linear disease model of addictions, the user is objectified and powerless. Interventions recognizing the competency of users to make choices are not considered realistic. Mere exposure to the chemical is defined as the problem. This is in opposition to the understanding of drug use as a mechanism of adaptation to the environment. Rather, demand for the drug is considered the problem and, thus, becomes the focus of intervention.

Canada's policy of health promotion includes five strategies that affect the demand for drugs. Health education shifts the locus of control from the substance to the user. Communication and social marketing bridge the 'private trouble' of addiction with the original 'public issue' of security and the unfolding public issue of the HIV epidemic. Community development creates networks where chemical dependency can be understood as a social problem. Social action can provide feedback to decision-makers and legislators, challenging the status quo of criminalization.

Physical proximity, the relatively fluid exchange of persons, services, and products across the shared Canada-US border, and the domination of Canadian culture by American interests mitigate against the application of health promotion and harm reduction in Canada. Dr Diane Riley (1994: 15) of the Canadian Centre for Substance Abuse concludes:

> Among barriers to acceptance of harm reduction in many countries is a widespread devotion to a limited definition of idealism. Harm reduction accepts that some harm is inevitable, whereas the 'ideal' of zero-tolerance excludes all compromise and sets impossible goals. In North America, total abstinence has long been seen as the only acceptable goal of treatment. . . .

Clearly, this American approach of zero-tolerance has not reduced drug use. If anything, it has made drug use more dangerous and has led to enormous costs in the criminal justice system. As Canadian social workers begin to advocate for the use of harm reduction strategies, it is important that they also recognize the powerful influence exerted by US policies.

TENETS AND PRINCIPLES OF HARM REDUCTION

A number of tenets and principles are important and necessary for workers in the area of harm reduction and HIV. The following tenets apply to harm reduction:

- intrinsic value and dignity of all human beings;
- maximizing social and health assistance, disease prevention, and education;
- minimizing repressive and punitive measures;
- comprehensive and non-judgemental medical and social services for all;
- holistic approach to drug use;
- non-judgemental understanding of user's relationship to drugs;
- emphasis on reduction of drug-related harm;
- competency of drug user in decision-making;
- interventions focused on non-coercive and non-judgemental presentation of options;
- involvement of affected persons and communities in strategy creation;
- uniqueness of every drug user;
- accessibility to non-judgemental drug treatment, including MMTPs;
- support of needle exchanges;
- challenge of current drug policy.

From these tenets, five principles of harm reduction regarding HIV can be identified.

1. *Retain a value-neutral view of the activity.* The worker must recognize that the activity is the experience and expression of the client and must be cautious not to stray from this neutrality in discussing the activity. Its inherent value to the client must be understood by the health-care provider.

2. *Retain a value-neutral view of the person.* The importance of a non-judgemental attitude cannot be overstated, as an evaluative attitude can bias the worker's approach to the client.

3. *Focus on the problem*—the reduction of HIV transmission.

4. *Understand the place of abstinence* in harm reduction. Abstinence is not the main issue in harm reduction; its focus can lead to frustration and interference in the reduction of HIV transmission.

5. *Recognize the client's role.* Harm reduction programs are user-centred, where the client must be an active part of the process.

Harm reduction is based on a hierarchy of change, where a series of steps can lead to safety. The first step towards safety for the IDU who shares needles is

Table 1 The Ladder Approach To Harm Reduction

Intravenous Drug Use	*High Number of Anonymous or Known Sexual Liaisons*	*Homeless Youth in Sex Trade*
alternative to harmful drugs	fewer sexual partners	reducing influence of alcohol and drugs
↑	↑	↑
not injecting	alternatives to penetrative sex	supplementary sources of income
↑	↑	↑
not sharing needles	reducing the influence of alcohol and drugs during sex	safer location for sex trade
↑	↑	↑
cleaning needles	use of condoms for penetrative sex	food and shelter
↑	↑	↑
sharing needles	unprotected penetrative sex	turning tricks on the street

the recognition and understanding of the importance of not sharing needles. A second step is the acquisition of information and the resources to clean needles. Later steps involve the exploration of alternatives to injecting, such as MMTPs. This step approach to harm reduction is outlined in Table 1.

In all examples it is critical to remember that many things influence risk behaviour and that relapse is common. Reinforcing self-esteem, providing support, and emphasizing choice are important aspects of the harm reduction approach.

CHEZ MA COUSINE EVELYNE (CMCE): A HARM REDUCTION MODEL

Chez Ma Cousine Evelyne was Montreal's first care facility for persons living with AIDS (PLWAs), serving the community between 1988 and 1991. As other organizations were established to meet the shelter needs of PLWAs, the original Chez Ma Cousine ceased operations in July of 1991.

Persons living with AIDS who continued to use street drugs were considered by the extant AIDS hospices and shelters to be too difficult to place. Mental health concerns, as well as addictions and HIV, were an issue. Often, street involvement, such as prostitution, was present, making service delivery very difficult. Finally, IDUs were uncomfortable when integrated into mainstream AIDS hospices where the majority of the clientele were gay. Fear of identification with gay men stymied IDUs' use of the rapidly evolving AIDS hospice network as the needs of the largest population impacted by the pandemic were addressed. Abstinent IDUs, let alone those unable or unwilling to stop consuming, became the doubly marginalized.

A new CMCE opened its doors on 1 October 1995 in an effort to respond to the needs of these marginalized 'twice removed'. With harm reduction as the *modus operandi* of the program, mutual respect and dignity became the cornerstones of service delivery. A global approach to the resident focuses on the person's life, as opposed to the life-defeating aspects of HIV disease. Residents are encouraged to assume a role in the ongoing activities of the centre and to reappropriate their lives by building a sense of belonging to the program.

During the first year of operations, 17 residents lived in the home, with stays ranging from 28 to 335 days. Of the 17 admissions, six were still present by the end of this period. The average stay at the centre was less than six months. Three resident deaths occurred, two at CMCE and one in hospital. All other departures from CMCE were voluntary, except for one resident who left the facility at the request of CMCE. This expulsion resulted from acts of physical violence on another resident. One resident was discharged into his own apartment, one into a detox centre, and one resident chose to return to the street, while the balance of discharged residents returned to families of origin, spouses, and/or friends.

ADMISSION

Three admission criteria existed: homelessness, chemical dependency, and an HIV/AIDS diagnosis. Admission to CMCE was generally sought in the absence of other solutions: refusal elsewhere or voluntary departure from other helping venues. Criteria *not* considered in admission included the type and length of chemical dependency and the health status and subsequent degree of physical autonomy. Issues of readmission to CMCE, where there could be perceived to be a 'revolving door' access to the home, have been a source of concern. CMCE has also questioned whether its mandate should be limited to hospice care, where the focus is on end-of-life issues. It has concluded that its mission is not limited to persons living with AIDS who are approaching the end of life.

By the end of the first year of operations, CMCE had concluded that admissions would exclude those who could 'manage on their own' (Rozier and Laberge, 1997: 97). Those persons who had a higher degree of autonomy and who were physically mobile would be admitted only in very special circumstances. As a result, the following admission parameters have now evolved: mental health condition, degree of psychosocial distress, and the capacity to use one's own resources.

SERVICES

The four problem areas encountered by residents—addictions, HIV/AIDS, homelessness, and mental health—are addressed by service delivery along four axes: basic services, such as food and shelter, medical services, social follow-up, and, finally, pyschorelational follow-up.

Operating 24 hours per day, CMCE provides food and shelter in a 30-room building in central Montreal, all in a family ambience. Nine individual rooms are available, with shared bathrooms, living-rooms, dining-rooms, and clothes washing facilities. Meals are served three times per day, and residents have access to the kitchen outside of these fixed times.

No single physician is allocated to CMCE, as residents are encouraged to develop and sustain a rapport with their own physicians. While this implies a continuity of care for the person after leaving CMCE, the problems of fragmented care from several unco-ordinated specialists are also present if the resident is not followed by a general practitioner.

CMCE has about 25 staff paid through government funding who work in three daily shifts. These people foster resident access to health care as intermediaries between the medical institutions and the residents. As liaison agents, they act as interpreters between worlds that are often perceived to be in opposition.

The services of a nurse are available during the week, so that the team of CMCE workers can manage the distribution of prescribed medications. Negotiation is generally necessary with the drug-using resident, where mediating and educating become important elements in harm reduction: eliminating or reducing the risks of resale of prescribed medication, the risks of overdose, and risks of concurrent and contraindicated consumption of other medications. Unbridled access to fresh syringes, disinfecting pads, and condoms continues to be an important means of HIV prevention. Information about safer injection sites on the body are also provided as a means of minimizing harm to the injection drug user. Palliative care and pain control are also available to those residents wishing to die at CMCE, which provides an environment for reconciliation both for the resident and for those close to him or her.

Staff are available particularly where support is sought in following procedures required by other caregiving or corrections institutions. This can entail accompanying the resident in interfacing with medical, social service delivery, judicial, or corrections-based institutions. CMCE also reaches out to residents through 'time management' coaching and recreational and educational programs. Opportunities for establishing a rapport and communication can be integrated into the ongoing social support available to each resident. Referrals are also made to community-based organizations, according to the needs expressed.

A cognitive behavioural approach serves as a theoretical guide where the relationship between the self and others is worked out within a social environment. Social integration is sought in all realms, including the economic and the social. Pet therapy also plays a role at CMCE. The presence of pets speaks to the importance of CMCE as a humane and family-based milieu as well as a professionally anchored program.

CHALLENGES AND RECOMMENDATIONS

Rozier and Laberge (1997), of the Collectif de recherche sur l'itinérance (the Homelessness Research Collective) at the Université du Québec à Montréal, posit that an important challenge for social workers is to act as a bridge between the traditional medical community, which is often abstinence-based, and those medical workers practising within the harm reduction framework. The empowerment of the drug user must be fostered within the social and professional networks that do not necessarily prize autonomy as highly as do adherents of the harm reduction model. For example, balancing mental health and autonomy issues becomes pertinent. Great flexibility is required in meeting the often changing needs of the user, particularly when the needs unfold *after* an initial needs assessment. Realistic objectives must be adhered to while service delivery adapts to the multiple needs of the user. These realistic objectives can include the acquisition of new skills or, more concretely, simple food and shelter for those for whom survival is a daily issue. From these concrete issues can unfold support, counselling, and biomedical needs.

Needs cannot be met in a social vacuum. The harm reduction model as a community-based approach implies some degree of structure. Balancing two cultures where individual and collective needs coexist is not easy to manage and remains a challenge. The advent of HIV disease has underscored the importance of community-based outreach initiatives in exploring the many-faceted cultures of the marginalized. This exploration, when implemented in the context of zero-tolerance, limits the degree to which the principles of harm reduction can be applied. For example, it is difficult to implement needle exchange programs when the possession of syringes remains criminalized. It is the challenge of social workers to determine whether they can be agents of social change at both the collective and individual levels. Important axes of intervention leading to individual and collective change can include harm reduction at three interrelated levels: individual harm, harm impacting the immediate surroundings, and broadly based social harm. A future challenge consists of prioritizing among the three (Rozier and Laberge, 1997).

CONCLUSION

The practical aspects of integrating harm reduction principles into agency practice can be difficult to resolve. While the previous program example is an illustration of some success, it has yet to be fully evaluated and followed over time. Agencies can use the following practical questions to assess an agency's or social worker's anxiety of working with injection drug users. They are not intended to shock or frighten, but to highlight issues that social workers must consider.

1. As a social worker, do you continue a counselling session if a client is high or stoned?
2. If the client is new to the area, do you help him or her find out where to make drug purchases?
3. Do you allow the residents or clients to make drug purchases on the premises? If not, how far away—one block, two blocks?
4. Would you allow residents whose only source of income is the sex trade to use their rooms to turn tricks?

5. What is your relationship to the police?
6. What is your relationship to the neighbours?
7. Does your organization allow clients to drop in even if it disrupts schedules and routines?
8. Does your organization provide a drop-in room for clients?
9. Are solid boundaries important to build structure in lives that have known little or no structure?

The questions become more ethically and morally challenging when the clients are minors or children. For example:

1. To what degree do we teach homeless minors how to do drugs safely?
2. Do we show adolescents involved in the sex trade the safest place to do business?
3. Should we facilitate the development of 'safe houses' so that street youth don't run the risks associated with parks and alleys?

These questions illustrate the complexity of the issues and highlight the social work value of client self-determination and the social work maxim to 'start where the client is'. In some cases, this will create a serious internal struggle for the social worker.

Most social workers embrace the values of client self-determination and the recognition of the dignity and worth of all individuals. Risk-reduction practices put these values to a greater test because they often call for the acceptance of behaviours or activities outside the comfort zones of most social workers. It is important that practitioners reframe these circumstances as learning zones if they are to be effective in working with clients who respond better to this approach. The use of risk-reduction strategies in HIV prevention is both challenging and changing the profession.

Our challenge is to dovetail service delivery with the marginalized using a traditional structure that is quite hierarchical and embedded with inequalities. This traditional structure uses a vocabulary that excludes the very concept of marginalization itself.

REFERENCES

Alexander, B. 1987. 'The Disease and Adaptive Models of Addiction: A Framework Evaluation', *Journal Of Drug Issues* 17, 1: 47–66.

———, and P. Hadaway. 1982. 'Opiate Addiction: The Case for an Adaptive Orientation', *Psychological Bulletin* 92, 2: 367–81.

Boyer, M. 1995. 'La promotion de la santé', lecture to the Colloque québécois sur la prévention du sida en milieu gai, Coalition des organismes communautaires québécois de lutte contre le sida (COCQ-Sida), Montréal, 8 Dec.

Harm Reduction Coalition. 1993. *Founding Document.* Oakland, Calif.: Harm Reduction Coalition.

Riley, D. 1994. *The Harm Reduction Model: Pragmatic Approaches to Drug Use from the Area between Tolerance and Neglect.* Ottawa: Canadian Centre on Substance Abuse.

Rozier, M., and D. Laberge. 1997. *Rapport d'évaluation: L'implantation de 'Chez Ma Cousine Evelyne'.* Montréal: Collectif de recherche sur l'itinérance, Département de Sociologie, Université du Québec à Montréal.

Springer, E. 1991. 'Effective AIDS Prevention with Active Drug Users: The Harm Reduction Model', in E. Springer, ed., *Counselling Chemically Dependent People with HIV Illness.* Binghamton, NY: Haworth Press.

World Health Organization. 1986. *The Ottawa Charter of Health Promotion.* Ottawa: WHO.

Part Two

Care

As hospitals and health professionals began to see their first cases of AIDS in the early 1980s, the evolution of the disease was easy to predict. The person with AIDS, named the 'AIDS victim' in those days, would be sick, require intensive interventions, find no respite from ever-developing symptoms, require hospice care, and, finally, die. Our role was to comfort, advocate for palliative services, try to keep the family involved, empower the loved one, and hang on as the roller-coaster of AIDS continued its course. No effective treatments existed to slow down the course of the illness.

Classical definitions of care sufficed in most cases—with one notable exception: the people with HIV were coming from populations previously invisible to us and that were unknown. They were marginalized and confronted enormous resistance from the health-care system, they did not elicit sympathy or empathy socially, and governments did not seem to care about their fate.

As the 1980s were a decade of despair and absence of treatments that saw an emphasis on the development of services for people with HIV who were inevitably going to be sick, and then sicker, so the 1990s have been a decade of some hope, much anguish, and some encouragement as new treatments became available. These treatments held much promise, and for some they continue to hold promise as viral loads plummet and CD4 cell counts rise . . . for some. For others the new therapies do not work at all, or their benefits do not last.

In the 1990s the definition of care is much more complex as community-based organizations have developed services and people with HIV have become articulate advocates for their own care and are living longer. The disease is not less complex, but more so. The role of health-care professionals has evolved enormously in the context of HIV. As 'AIDS victims' became 'people with AIDS' and then 'people with HIV', so, too, health-care 'professionals' became 'partners', 'collaborators', 'advisers', and sometimes 'people to fight against'. No longer were we the experts, all-knowing, able to tell the 'patient' what to do because it was good for him or her.

In this section on care, eight chapters offer stories, insights, experiences, and reflections on how care has evolved in the last decade and how emerging trends and needs might impact on the need for new services and new ways of seeing things.

In Chapter 5, Shirley Grosser writes of the experiences of caregivers who, like people with HIV, have experienced isolation and marginalization, and yet find tremendous meaning in their experience. This experience illuminates for social workers what clients' expectations of us are in an era of shrinking budgets and diminishing resources. In that context, social workers must increasingly play a liaison role, building networks, advocating for clients, and making connections between social service, medical, and legal bureaucracies.

Lois Jackson in Chapter 6 outlines the experiences of working with HIV-positive women, a little-known population that is becoming increasingly impacted by the disease. As she states, even though women, worldwide, have been the sex most affected by HIV, 'only 7 per cent of all publications on HIV' are concerned with women. Medically and psychosocially, women have specific needs and issues that merit an examination and a response.

Lillian Wells, Robyn Salter-Goldie, Dale D'Amatteo, and Susan King, in Chapter 7, report on the largest Canadian study to date of traditional families and HIV. This study, with 110 families participating and a total of 172 living children, is an important contribution to an understanding of the needs of the population affected by HIV. Because social workers and social service agencies are so often involved with these families because of their pre-existent client status, which adds to their vulnerability as families with HIV, the chapter is of particular interest in articulating their needs in the context of social work values.

Claude Olivier, in Chapter 8, provides a glimpse of the outreach experiences of a social worker in smaller cities and rural areas of New Brunswick. With other illnesses, being in a rural environment or living in a small city could be of benefit to the sick person, but the experience of having HIV evokes too often the opposite—isolation and rejection. Facing this, AIDS New Brunswick developed innovative ways to reach out to people with HIV and to bring them together.

On 1 December 1997 (World AIDS Day) the federal Minister of Health, Allan Rock, outlined the guiding principles of the Third Canadian Strategy on AIDS. In it he identified the serious and increasing impact of HIV on rural and urban Aboriginal communities across Canada. Although Aboriginal leaders had been warning for years that their communities were at particular risk, until recently there were few clear initiatives aimed at preventing HIV infection in Aboriginal communities. In Chapter 9, Judy Weiser, with Connie Fife, Albert McLeod, Kecia Larkin, Dolan Badger, and Tia Eagles-Claw, speaks about the Aboriginal experience and the particular challenges that confront Native peoples. Of particular interest in this chapter is the collaborative effort of dozens of Aboriginal leaders, street workers, counsellors, and health-care workers who were consulted. For those of us not experienced in the renewal of Aboriginal traditions across the country and in how these traditions can be applied to a phenomenon like HIV prevention, we acknowledge that we have much to learn about respecting and listening to our communities before undertaking action.

Perhaps the population that causes us the most difficulty in terms of understanding their experiences and needs is that of the injection drug user. Long considered a criminal, and only now beginning to be understood as someone who has a health problem, the injection drug user is confronted by a lack of services and a lack of understanding, and, more often than not, is caught up in the criminal justice system rather than in the health-care system. In Chapter 10, Anne Bowlby questions some of our society's basic assumptions about users and articulates responses to their needs that are all-too-often lacking, both in our professional training and in our service-responses to this population. Understanding them and their needs will necessarily be a crucial factor in our ability to slow down the progress of HIV in Canada. We will learn this lesson, sooner or later, but we will learn it.

In the late 1980s Health Canada funded two demonstration projects designed to better co-ordinate the various players offering care to persons with HIV. These projects, Caring Together in Edmonton and Projet Accès in Montreal, were meant to stimulate better articulation of the needs of people with HIV to care providers (both public and community-based), as well as to improve the co-ordination of the response these various players offered to persons with HIV. David Fitzgerald, who directed this effort, describes in Chapter 11 the Caring Together project in Edmonton, which excelled in a 'consumer empowerment' approach, giving an authoritative voice to people with HIV and developing services from that perspective.

In Chapter 12, Bill Ryan, Marc A. Hamel, and Cheh Cho address a phenomenon that affects the gay male community profoundly. First in urban settings and increasingly in rural areas, gay male communities have been devastated by HIV-related deaths. In some cities whole age cohorts have been decimitated by HIV. The social status of gay men, even though improved in the last 10 years, contributes to an overwhelming sense of grief, which is often left unexpressed and finds no legitimacy in mainstream society.

Chapter 5

The Management of Caregiving

Who Pays in Hidden Ways, or Pathways to Empowerment

SHIRLEY GROSSER

The observations presented here emerged as a result of a qualitative research study conducted in 1994. The study explored caregivers' perceptions of psychosocial services available to them while they were acting as primary caregivers to persons living with and dying of HIV disease. A number of assumptions were brought to the study. Because of the impression that the profession of social work had limited involvement in HIV/AIDS work, one could assume that caregivers might have little awareness of or understanding about the ways in which social workers might be helpful to them. It was anticipated that caregivers in cities such as Toronto and Vancouver, with larger HIV-affected populations and more visible social work services for HIV-affected persons, would be more aware of how social workers might offer assistance within many dimensions of caring.

Usually, social workers in hospital settings have been the profession's representatives in the HIV/AIDS field. Their experiences have ranged broadly, as is normally the case when acting with or on behalf of those living with a chronic, debilitating, and life-threatening condition. It was less likely that caregivers in the early stages of confronting HIV infection would have encountered social workers who might, for example, practice advocacy on their behalf within the social assistance system, or social workers who were open to exploring preparation of young persons for disability and death during a time of health. In other words, social workers likely entered the lives of caregivers late in the course of living with HIV disease. At the same time, it was hoped that some of the services available in the three cities under study could be seen as positive role models for all of us.

The study was conducted in three Canadian cities (Winnipeg, Vancouver, Toronto) with the clients of three different service delivery systems (a specialized HIV/AIDS-care hospital; a community-based health and social service clinic; and a voluntary community outreach program). The outcome and report of the study may be found elsewhere (Grosser, 1996). Today, as a result of the study, it is important to continue to pay attention to the stories people tell, to how they express and understand their experiences as caregivers, and to the consequences of their choices (or conscriptions by default) into the role of primary caregivers.

SCOPE OF THE STUDY AND ASSUMPTIONS ABOUT CAREGIVING: CAPTURING THE EXPERIENCE OF THE MARGINALIZED AND SILENT HELPERS

Not all caregivers may be willing or feel able to fulfil what is increasingly a presumptive societal expectation—that they provide a full range of complex caregiving acts. This presumption on the part of professionals, and the 'helping systems' they represent, frequently presents a socio-economic expectation for selflessness rather than a balanced assessment of the capacities of the caregiver within the size of the caregiving task. The tasks of caregiving to HIV-infected persons demand an escalating and unlimited output of human energy and monetary resources. What became patently clear as caregivers told their stories was how few opportunities they had to do just this, that is, to tell their stories, to be acknowledged in their commitment, to be recognized for their creativity in dealing with cumbersome, system-serving, and scarce resources (when these were available to them) or to 'make do' without help.

What also became clear were the ways in which the existing social resource systems (for which, parenthetically, caregivers were grateful, regardless of their miserly inadequacy) were of significantly variable and limited use to caregivers. These resources neither assumed necessary tasks nor supported the caregivers in tasks that were theirs alone. In essence, the caregiver to a person living and dying with HIV disease may find him or herself socially isolated and marginalized, fighting a solitary battle with diminishing personal energy and the inflexibility of various bureaucracies, whether lodged in formal services or in the voluntary sector. An unspoken but none the less real lament of many caregivers stated: 'It fell to me to go to work, and come home and do the laundry, and care for him, and cook, and shop, and do the rest of that stuff. To try to get a buddy . . . the hassle . . . it was so hideous . . . it was like going to the government.' Of course, this is *not* what the informants said *directly*. All were, as most of us are, socialized to accept and conform to the expectations of our culture. We care *for* the people we care *about*. And we'll take up the challenge to demonstrate that caring in the most intensive, long-term, complex, self-sacrificing, and intimate ways.

When one acknowledges and adds the social stigma of caring for a loved one living with HIV, the possibility of burden and the likelihood of significant psychological consequences are heightened. The words of the Canadian caregivers will provide the elaboration of these ideas throughout this chapter.

AFFECTED POPULATIONS

The caregivers involved in the study included eight men and four women. The relationships caregivers had with those under their care included connections by birth (a mother, a sister), chosen partners in life, spouse, friend, and volunteer care team veteran. Seven of these were partners in life. Caregivers ranged in age from 21 to 59, with the majority between the ages of 33 and 48. Most had held semi-professional or professional positions in the workforce, although most were unemployed at the time of the interviews. Most had at least high school education. Most were White. Two people were of Aboriginal background. All had been caregivers to men.

While the caregivers in the study reflected a reasonable range of individuals and brought their personal and relational commitments to the experience, they cannot be considered to represent the much more extensive efforts provided by a vast population of volunteers. So while this paper will highlight some of the experiences of caregivers in personal relationships, it cannot address the impacts or the work of that even larger sector of often hidden, unaccounted for, volunteer service provision.

THE EXPERIENCES OF CAREGIVING

Most of the literature on caregiving examines caregivers' *individual psychological capacity* to cope (i.e., coping styles). Models that address psychological capacities and skills of individuals are examined in such studies and often provide detailed and significant evidence of the psychological complexity inherent in caregiver coping. While this approach makes an important contribution to our assessment of individual resiliency and adaptability, the question of what factors support the development of personal resiliency remains.

Little of this information distinguishes between the differences in life experiences of one caregiver compared to another. The studies tend not to take into account such contextual factors as gender, the nature of the relationship, geographic location, community connections, economic viability, and so on (Green, 1993: 99). Whether, for example, a caregiver lives in a small town or in an urban setting, has responsibility for children or elders—these and other significant dimensions of personal lives impact the caregiving experience. It would perhaps be more appropriate to explore the relevance of particular services and resources for different people, in order to facilitate a match between styles and capacities and existing services and unfilled needs.

A second dimension that has received attention in the literature regarding the experiences of caregiving is the notion of *social support*, its presence or absence, its forms, its utility, its effectiveness (Kadushin, 1996; Wardlaw, 1994). This is particularly relevant when speaking of marginalized persons. For marginalized people and in marginalized communities (and both people infected and those affected by HIV may perceive themselves or be perceived as such), the notion of social support may take on unique meaning. For example, most people in this study, gay and straight, male and female, reported conflicts with families of origin, with both their own families and that of the person for whom they were giving care.

A third area of inquiry has examined the caregiver's perception of caregiver *burden* (Folkman et al., 1994; Packenham et al., 1994). More will be said about this point later.

ASSESSING COMPLEXITY IN TASKS AND CONSTRAINTS IN THEIR EXECUTION

The literature offers little attention to complexity in caregiving tasks or to the notions of *different dynamics of needs* and *different relevance of resources* for different caregivers. It is important for us to know what forms of service would make sense for different caregivers, and to have ways of discovering this information.

Several authors, when examining particular populations living with HIV, caution that findings regarding social support constellations or caregiver coping styles extracted from examining other populations do not necessarily fit for those dealing with HIV/AIDS (Britton et al., 1993; Green, 1993). Britton, Zarski, and Hobfoll state that 'One cannot ignore the lack of studies that have explored the often unique experience of this minority culture [the gay community], and as clinicians and researchers we again are reminded that generalization of findings from a majority culture to specific groups of people may be dangerously misleading' (Britton et al., 1993: 53). Green asserts that 'there is a substantial gap between the general social support literature in which social parameters such as gender, class and race are basic differentiators, and much of the HIV literature which emphasizes differences by transmission category' (Green, 1993: 99).

In contrast, one study (Delgado and Rose, 1994: 1) describes a model of caregiving, termed a 'caregiver constellation', that 'mobilized to help fill a void resulting from inadequate public and private insurance and services, and lack of family involvement'. This caregiver constellation provided all the societally expected functions of the (often mythologically and heroically idealized) well-oiled, extended family, caregiving machine to persons living with AIDS at late stages of illness. It is likely that such caregiver constellations are not uncommon but, rather, are considerably under-reported and, as such, provide another example of the hidden costs of caregiving activity.

It is important, too, that recognition be given to some of the built-in constraints we as professionals place on ourselves as we narrow our attention to how individuals cope. We might profitably explore how our selection of an assessment framework shapes what we notice. By focusing on individual coping styles, capacities, and attributes, we are in danger of minimizing the dynamics and the complexity of what each person deals with in his or her everyday life. We risk minimizing how they accomplish their 'taken-for-granted' tasks. Whether we focus our attention only on the caregiver's perceptions and definitions, or on the researcher's interpretation of these, or on the delivery system's procedures, or on the policy-maker's ideology, we are in danger of turning our attention away from a substantial dimension of the caregiving equation: the *complexities* and *constraints* to caregiving, most often represented by the *sociopolitical* contexts within which people attempt to do their coping and by the dynamic interplay of social, political, and economic factors.

BALANCING THE COSTS OF CAREGIVING WITH INDIVIDUAL CAREGIVER RESILIENCE

Caregiving work is generally hidden in our North American economic system and within our health-care system. Patients are encouraged to heal at home and die at home. Unaccounted for hours are spent by caregivers, at home, providing basic nursing care. Some quite complex nursing tasks, which were more commonly done in hospitals just a few years ago, are now accomplished at home. If no caregiver were available to do them, would they be done in hospital today or would the ill and dying be left to fend for themselves at home?

So what is the cost of caregiving? If we examine caregiver burden from the perspective of the caregiver, we may gain some sense of this. Yet even researchers who clearly identify that HIV-positive caregivers report greater burden than HIV-negative caregivers, and who indicate that 'Instrumental needs of the care recipient are a key factor in burden', state that 'health professionals [should] train caregivers in the skills that they need to care for individuals with advanced HIV infection.' Folkman and his colleagues cite an example of a 'necessary' form of caregiving, as described by a caregiver: 'It's a sublavian catheter that runs directly into his heart so you have to be careful for infection . . . so you don't want to kill some one. . . . this was the first time I've had to do this type of nurse care' (Folkman et al., 1994: 755). The authors seem to see no paradox in their report of burden, on the one hand, and the requirement for the training of lay persons to perform nursing functions, on the other.

Caregivers in the Canadian study found themselves providing similar services. As one explained:

> I made notes . . . for a couple of days, and tried to do it from my notes and found that my notes weren't too good. So we brushed up on the notes . . . I ended up with a 52-step procedure, 'cause with this type of IV you had to clean . . . there's this tubing . . . a cleaning solution you'd inject in to keep it sterile . . . I still have the procedure in case I ever need it.

This caregiver laughed as he considered the absurdity of his 52-step procedure. Another one described a similar quasi-professional expectation placed on his caregiving: 'He was . . . fed on a liquid diet through a portacath . . . and the TPN (total parenteral nutrition) was quite involved because it had to be completely sanitary . . . like I had to go on a course for three weeks to learn how to do this thing.'

The stigma of AIDS and the fear of the stigma of AIDS may compromise care and access to care regardless of gender or of relationships, i.e., whether the caregiver is a mother, sister, lover, friend, partner, wife, or team volunteer. Several female participants in the Canadian study reported incidents:

> I did feel very alone and needed someone to talk to about him. I didn't know who to talk to, and you don't want to burden people you don't know well . . . There was some phobia there (in the workplace) because it was AIDS connected.

> The ignorance, the stigma, . . . they had all this isolation stuff out on the table . . . a nurse come into his room, she had a gown, a mask, she had goggles, she had a cap on and her rubber gloves on and boots . . .

> Never once did they [shave] him [in hospital]. Why? Because they were afraid? Because he had AIDS?

Powell-Cope (1995), in a study of gay couples' experiences living with HIV, broadens the definition of family and reframes the traditional scholarly focus on the perceptions and tasks of caregiving. The study highlights caregiving in the context of a major life transition, with the particular meanings the participants of this transition attribute to the situation. This study cites stigma as one of several factors distinguishing the act of caregiving to persons with AIDS from other forms of caregiving: 'The social stigma surrounding AIDS and people with AIDS is well known, but the stigma of those people indirectly affected by AIDS, such as family caregivers, is less well documented' (Powell-Cope, 1995: 38).

Whether or not people are sophisticated about seeking or accessing help can play an important part in the maintenance or development of their capacity to provide caregiving. As one informant explained, 'As far as finding help, it's really up to the tenacity of the individual, and just how resourceful they really are. . . . The average person . . . would just have to pretty much luck into someone . . . otherwise they don't show up at your door.'

Our culture admires and praises independence and the person's capacity to 'do it alone', especially as a male. People are not generally acknowledged for their ability to tap into systems for helping. The studies that examine people's appraisal of stress and their capacities to cope may influence us towards an idealization of the 'courageous' sufferers of illness and their 'loyal' companions. We need to ask ourselves how people access social support services, if they do at all. We need to explore a variety of ways that formal social support is initiated. Currently, our efforts are minimal. We need to question whether those social support services available or accessible to caregivers differ from one caregiver to another, depending on such factors as the form of relationship, gender, and social and individual expectations. We need to question our agencies regarding their sharing of information, their accessibility, openness, innovation.

In the caregiver study, for example, it appeared as if gay men in urban settings usually had access to community supports and made a deliberate choice about using or avoiding these and seeking out professionals instead. There was evidence of a conscious use or non-use of community resources. But even this 'deliberateness' depended on availability of choice within resources, knowledge of resources, and the man's geographic location, at the least. As one said, 'You need to know, 'cause they aren't going to tell you unless you ask.' Women, on the other hand, seemed to have access to psychiatrists, mostly as an outcome of referral from other professionals, and used these in contrast to family, friends, or community supports. One wonders how these different uses of support services reflect such dimensions as the form of relationship caregivers had with their care receivers, their gender, and both social and individual socialization and expectations of help-seeking behaviour.

INTERVENTION IMPERATIVE 1: DEVELOPING A CONTEXTUAL MODEL FOR SOCIAL WORK ASSESSMENT OF CAREGIVING

Many of the issues of importance in a consideration of caregiving point to a need for an organizing framework that focuses our attention on the context in which the everyday acts of individual caregivers are performed. Social workers, like those in any field of practice, bring their own professional interpretations of which 'needs' are 'legitimate' within the helping encounter. The work of Nancy Fraser (1989) provides us with a comprehensive and extensive examination of just how complex the idea of identifying and defining 'needs' may be in our pluralistic society:

> Moralistic and scientific discourses about the needs of people with AIDS, and of people at risk with respect to AIDS, are well represented on government commissions; in contrast, gay and lesbian rights activists' interpretations of those needs are largely excluded. From this perspective, needs talk appears as a site for struggle. . . . Dominant groups articulate need interpretations intended to exclude, defuse, and/or co-opt counter-interpretations. Subordinate or oppositional groups . . . articulate need interpretations intended to challenge, displace, and/or modify dominant ones. In neither case are the interpretations simply 'representations'. In both cases, rather, they are acts and interventions. (Fraser, 1989: 165–6)

Fraser speaks of multiple ways of perceiving needs that may exist in a particular context and then identifies the 'politics of need interpretation' as a subject for discourse. She suggests that needs are open to the impacts of the environments/contexts in which they appear. They are influenced by whoever or whatever has the power to identify them, define them, and shape them. The purpose of discourse is directed to three dimensions. The first dimension addresses the question of whether the stated need is a political concern or a personal concern, that is, *either establishing or denying the political status* of a given need. (When one of the partners in the caregiver study challenged the pharmaceutical insurance system for disallowing coverage of the costs of an over-the-counter drug by threatening to have his partner admitted to an acute-care hospital, he was acting with social awareness of a way to transform his 'domestic' economic problem into a broader, 'political' economic one.) The second dimension represents the struggle over *interpreting or defining the need* (who gets to say what it is, to whom, and who hears the statement) and thus the determination of what will satisfy it. The third dimension represents the actual *act of satisfying the need*. These are the types of decisions that institutional practice (i.e., agency procedure) tries to homogenize—the same service for all. These are also the types of decisions that may make significant differences to the ongoing capacity of caregivers to maintain their unpaid and socially required functions.

NEEDS TALK: COMPETING MEANINGS IN THE DEFINITION OF NEEDS

There is considerable difference possible in meanings and interpretations, as well as impacts, when needs are defined as 'needs' or as 'interests' or as 'rights'. Fraser suggests that the range of acceptable social vocabularies for this discourse is quite extensive. For example, the interpretations of the words by those speaking about needs or interests or rights can come from a therapeutic perspective, an administrative perspective, a religious perspective, and so on (Fraser, 1989: 164–5). Caregivers in the study defined 'needs' in pragmatic ways—economic hardship balanced with non-responsive social and health resources, and both influenced by stigma, challenged the caregivers relentlessly. Most of the caregivers who identified as part of the gay community were sufficiently politicized to identify their caregiving tasks as other and more than 'needs'—to define them as rights. But both male and female caregivers, and a range of personal relationships, are represented in these words:

> You do learn that you have to question everything. For a lay person it's hard.
>
> The nurse said, unless the patient asks for certain things we don't do them unless they ask. He was so far out of it he couldn't ask for anything. . . . The family or the caregiver or whatever, they have to oversee these things.
>
> It scares me to wonder how many suffer needlessly because there isn't somebody to advocate for them.
>
> I truly believe that the only way a person gets good health care is to have someone advocating for them full time.

Fraser refers to the people controlling resource allocation decisions as 'the sociocultural means of interpretation and communication' (Fraser, 1989: 164) at the point that these powers speak with those in need. As professionals, we may consider ourselves one of the bridges in this process, one of the sources of power in the allocation of resources. The way in which the 'needy', that is, those seeking to have needs met, are perceived by us (whether as normal or deviant, victim or social activist, unique individuals or members of social groups) provides one sociocultural interpretation.

FRASER'S REINTERPRETATION OF STRUCTURAL ARRANGEMENTS AS CULTURAL/IDEOLOGICAL CLASSIFICATIONS

Fraser challenges the 'structural' separation of economic issues from political issues and both of these from domestic issues. She identifies their commonplace differentiation in our cultural context as a false separation:

> In male-dominated, capitalist societies, what is 'political' is normally defined contrastively over against what is 'economic' and what is 'domestic' or 'personal'. Here, then, we can identify two principal sets of institutions that depoliticize social discourses: they are, first, domestic institutions, especially the normative domestic form, namely, the modern restricted male-headed nuclear family; and, second, official economic capitalist system institutions, especially paid workplaces, markets, credit mechanisms and 'private' enterprises and corporations. Domestic institutions depoliticize certain matters by personalizing and/or familializing them; they cast these as private—domestic or personal—familial matters in contradistinction to public, political matters. Official economic capitalist system institutions, on the other

> hand, depoliticize certain matters by economizing them; the issues in question here are cast as impersonal market imperatives, or as 'private' ownership prerogatives, or as technical problems for managers and planners, all in contradistinction to political matters. (Fraser, 1989: 168)

Instead, what is proposed is that we encourage the persons experiencing the events to define their experience. This serves to challenge the false boundaries erected by external powers naming the experience and ascribing an economic or political or domestic label to the experience to suit the prevailing power agendas. In other words, 'needs' as defined by the ones who are experiencing the events or who are asking for help do not differentiate a clearly separable domestic, economic, or political dimension but instead are experienced as each permeating the other. Fraser calls this phenomenon 'leaky' or 'runaway' needs, and identifies them as 'markers of major social-structural shifts' (p. 171). She refers to the point at which these converge as 'the social' or 'switch point' (p. 170). This 'switch point' represents the key location for social work intervention.

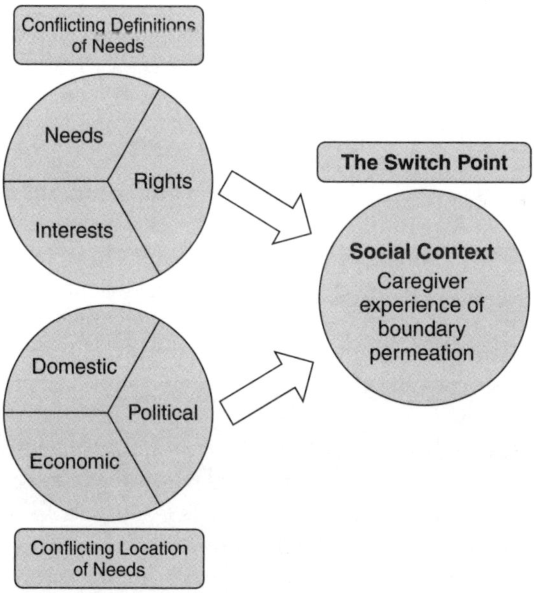

Figure 1 Markers of Major Social-Structural Shifts

Figure 1 provides a visual explanation of Fraser's reinterpretation of cultural/ideological classifications. 'Needs', 'interests', and 'rights' are dynamically interrelated under the notion of conflicting definitions of needs, or the several ways in which needs may be labelled. Similarly, the domestic, economic, and political arenas are joined in a dynamic interrelationship. Each dynamic feeds into the caregiver's experience, the social context, and Fraser's 'switch point'. By highlighting specific issues or various combinations of issues and feeding these into the caregiver's social context or Fraser's 'switch point', we can see how the definition of 'need' may be re-created several times and with different emphases, depending on the perceptions and proclivities of both the caregiver and the 'outsider'.

One caregiver, for example, spoke of the daily personal, intimate tasks involved in caring for his partner. 'How could I have done this [caregiving] if I was working full time? I wouldn't have.' Hearing this, an outsider (whether social worker, policy-maker, or administrator) might choose to define this caregiver's concern as located in an economic, or domestic, or political sphere and represent it as reflecting personal needs or interests or rights. He went on to say, 'I wouldn't have . . . it gets complicated. Because then spousal leave is necessary. You have to be recognized as a person's spouse if you're a gay couple. If you want to die at home it's going to cost.'

The dimensions of what this male partner demonstrates in his role as primary caregiver cross all classifications or locations of needs. The following interpretation is offered as an example of how this social worker chose to interpret what was heard. First, the speaker acknowledged the economic/domestic implications of remaining in the workforce or of removing himself ('if I was working full time . . . I wouldn't have [been able to provide the caregiving]'). He goes on to identify the political/domestic implications of acting in a partnership that is unacknowledged and ignored by the dominant culture ('you have to be recognized'). Finally, he identifies the political/economic/domestic implications of a societal expectation for 'hidden' caregiving ('if you want to die at home') along with its multiple costs (although the speaker may mean only monetary cost in this example).

So where would a social worker choose to intervene? Encourage the caregiver to work outside the home and find a substitute caregiver? What if his own health is uncertain? Encourage his social action regarding justice for persons in same-sex partnerships in the hope that the laws of the land, in a timely way, will provide for people in his situation, as well as for the many others currently unacknowledged? Pay attention to the psychological and social costs of isolation and abandonment? And to what degree does the agency dictate 'professional' perception and interpretation?

The example may bring home an important aspect of Fraser's argument, the notion that 'boundary permeation' extends to the lives of those giving and receiving care because of its impacts on *prescribed* social institutions such as 'the family', 'the official economy', and 'the state'. In contrast, societal arrangements that provide support for caregivers' and sufferers' interests, needs, and rights (such as those social services staffed by social workers) would be expected to notice and assess these with the intention of making a difference through selective intervention.

INTERVENTION IMPERATIVE 2: HEARING THE CLIENT AND LOCATING ASPECTS FOR INTERVENTION

Caregivers in the study were open in expressing their ideas about how systems might have been helpful to them.

One dimension of the work, valued by professionals—privacy, secrecy, confidentiality—was expressed as working against the best interests of caregivers, who need to know they are not alone and who want fairness and justice in burden-sharing. The economic and hidden emotional costs of caregiving, which remain embedded in perceptions that people's problems are of 'domestic' 'interests' or 'needs', allow politically established, formal helping systems to justify their continuing limited responsibility for care and support. It is important that formal helping systems take account of the hidden costs of caregiving—the economic burdens, the social stigma, the expenditure and loss of energy, the conflictual relationships. We as professionals may make a difference when we define situations as having multiple dimensions, including political and economic interests and rights, rather than justify our non-intervention by defining situations solely as domestic matters.

Caregivers may benefit from an understanding of their situations if these are explained beyond the narrow confines of domestic interests and needs. Caregivers need information, lots of it, and they need to have information available and repeated frequently as the care situation changes, as it often does rapidly and unexpectedly. The type of information needed goes well beyond that provided by public health or physician-based systems. The stigma, societal ignorance, and secondary traumatization that caregivers find themselves dealing with does not belong with them alone, although it may be comforting at times to believe one has control even of this:

> It was partly because of the isolation I put myself in, which needn't have happened really. It could have been dealt with. . . . My parents had no idea what I was going through. My father said when he found out that [my husband] had AIDS, he never slept for wondering when the kids and I would die. And he never said anything. It's almost as if people have to be taught different ways.

In contrast to Folkman et al. (1994), who believe people need to be taught nursing skills, the caregiver whose words are cited here believed it would have been helpful to learn how to deal with family conflicts, how to reassure and take support from family members, how to ask for help, how to preserve precious energy resources in the face of personal tragedy and social ostracism.

Social work directed to the tasks of facilitating the caregiving role will address the inevitable outcomes of broad social interpretations as well as clients' own interpretations of their tasks. The contextual framework emerging from the 'switch point' might indicate that social work tasks should address caregiving experiences on three dimensions: (1) the multitude and range of necessary adaptations and actions on the part of caregivers dealing with *complexity* in the role; (2) the *constraints* of the role because of the social context in which it is being implemented; and (3) the *resilience* necessary to balance the multiple dimensions of the caregiving role. Some of these dimensions are represented in Figure 2. Several of these tasks may not be the exclusive domain of caregivers dealing with HIV/AIDS patients in a home setting. However, the particular ways in which these factors play out in each unique human situation can and should be the concern of professional social workers.

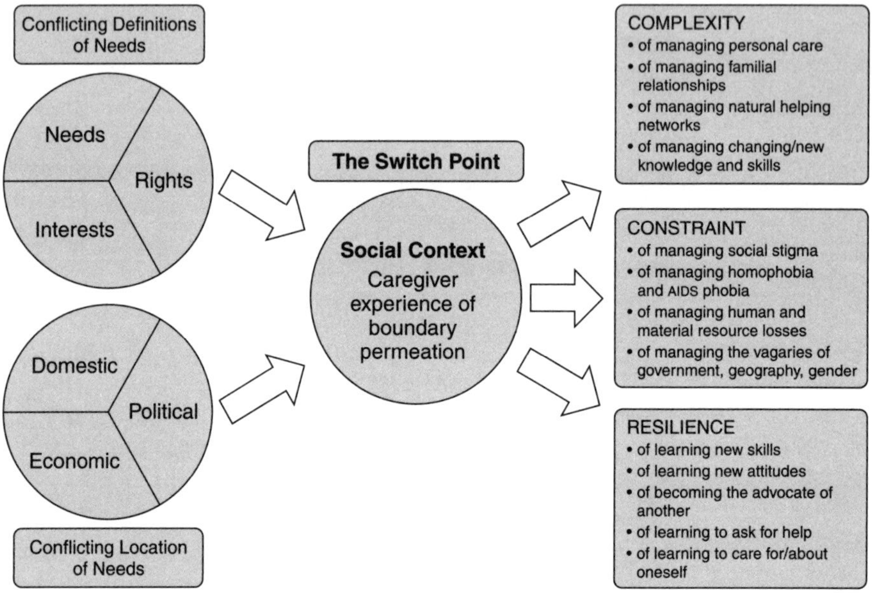

Figure 2 Individual Factors Influencing Social-Structural Shifts

Here, our perception of and experience with the notion of community, and the fair and just distribution of resources, can and should provide guidance. It is useful to explore the availability of *real* support systems rather than those we may assume, hope, or interpret to exist. For example, it is inadequate (for a variety of reasons) to assume that all gay men are part of a gay community or that this 'community' can and should take care of its own. Similarly, it is important to understand that a support group within the gay community that allows for partner grieving may not be appropriate for parents or for wives, ex-wives, children, or siblings. While all of these grievers may suffer a common stigma, their experience of loss is unique, and the likelihood of finding others in exactly the same situation is limited.

Finally, most caregivers put their own lives on hold as they demonstrated their commitment to the care receiver. Little evidence is available in the literature on the process caregivers experience as they re-enter the larger society from the cloister of caregiving. Many in the study believed that the caregiving experience taught them difficult though meaningful lessons. Some believed they were changed in significant and positive ways:

> Regardless of how that time was, I survived it, and I didn't think I could. . . . and now I can perceive it as a learning experience whereas before it was just too clouded to be able to perceive that in any other way than just hell.

> There was a great caregiver in me!
>
> I think caring for a person that way cannot help but to make you stronger both emotionally and spiritually . . . you come out a better person.

Caregivers' comments underline the need for the profession to work towards balancing the creative resolution of personal and social issues. What we are capable of hearing from caregivers, if we choose to listen, will demonstrate their capacity to balance the complexities and constraints of the caregiving tasks with their enormous resilience. Our task is to honour and support this spirit.

Note: This chapter is adapted from a poster presentation entitled: 'Complexity, Constraint, Resilience: Issues Beyond Caregiver Coping', developed for the Eleventh International Conference on AIDS, Vancouver, July 1996.

REFERENCES

Britton, P., J. Zarski, and S. Hobfoll. 1993. 'Psychological Distress and the Role of Significant Others in a Population of Gay/Bisexual Men in the Era of HIV', *AIDS Care* 5, 1: 43–54.

Delgado, J., and M. Rose. 1994. 'Caregiver Constellations: Caring for Persons with AIDS', *Journal of Gay and Lesbian Social Services* 1, 1: 1–14.

Folkman, S., M. Chesney, M. Cooke, A. Boccellari, et al. 1994. 'Caregiver Burden in HIV-Positive and HIV-Negative Partners of Men with AIDS', *Journal of Consulting and Clinical Psychology* 62, 4: 746–56.

Fraser, N. 1989. 'Struggle over Needs', in Fraser, *Unruly Practices: Power, Discourse, and Gender in Contemporary Social Theory*. Cambridge: Polity Press, 161–87.

Green, G. 1993. 'Editorial Review: Social Support and HIV', *AIDS Care* 5, 1: 87–104.

Grosser, S. 1996. 'Seeking Entitlement: Service Provision and the Act of Asking', *The Social Worker* 64, 4: 85–100.

Kadushin, G. 1996. 'Gay Men with AIDS and Their Families of Origin: An Analysis of Social Support', *Health and Social Work* 21, 2: 141–9.

Packenham, K., M. Dadds, and D. Terry. 1994. 'Relationship between Adjustment to HIV and Both Social Support and Coping', *Journal of Consulting and Clinical Psychology* 62, 6: 1194–1203.

Powell-Cope, G. 1995. 'The Experiences of Gay Couples Affected by HIV Infection', *Qualitative Health Research* 5, 1: 36–62.

Wardlaw, L. 1994. 'Sustaining Informal Caregivers for Persons with AIDS', *Families in Society: The Journal of Contemporary Human Services* 75, 6: 373–83.

Chapter 6

Diversity in a Context of Adversity

Issues in Working with HIV-Positive Women

LOIS JACKSON

INTRODUCTION

We know relatively little about HIV infection in women or of the social, behavioural, and psychological impacts of HIV for women. The unique features of HIV infection in women have been subject to neglect in both the Canadian research agenda and policy decisions related to funding and access to resources. This has had implications for program development and for the delivery of services for HIV-positive women. As we move into the twenty-first century we can expect that greater attention will be given to the needs and experiences of HIV-positive women as an understanding of the gender differences in HIV infection and the impact of HIV develops. We can also hope that social workers will play an important role in the HIV epidemic and will be attuned to the diversity of issues affecting women, how these issues differ from those of men, as well as the wide variations in experiences for women from diverse social and economic backgrounds.

I will discuss here the relative lack of attention to women and HIV, particularly in terms of research, and point to some of the implications of this relative void in terms of care and treatment issues for HIV-positive women. I will also explore some of the more salient issues facing HIV-positive women that constantly draw attention to the unique place of women in the HIV epidemic and the diversity of their experiences. HIV-positive women are not a homogeneous group. They come from varied socio-economic backgrounds, are at different stages of the life cycle, have different health/illness experiences related to HIV, and have varied access to therapies and information related to HIV (Levy et al., 1994). We must be sensitive to this diversity while recognizing that we live in a divided society and inequities related to class, race, and sexual orientation, as well as gender, play a major role in health-related beliefs and practices.

WOMEN AND HIV RESEARCH IN THE FIRST DECADE

During the first decade of the HIV epidemic, the research focused almost exclusively on men as HIV was viewed through a male prism (Campbell, 1990; Crystal and Sambamoorthi, 1996). The focus on men occurred despite the fact that women have been infected with HIV, and at risk of HIV, from early in the epidemic (Hankins, 1990; Sherr, 1996; Richardson, 1994; Doyal, 1994). Indeed, women are at greater risk than men as they have a higher risk of contracting HIV both from an individual act of intercourse and from each sexual partnership (Doyal, 1994: 13). Women have also been very much a part of the HIV epidemic insofar as they have been primary caregivers to HIV-infected individuals (Bennett et al., 1996), but much of this work has remained invisible and has not been the focus of research. As late as the 1991–5 period, publications on women and HIV/AIDS, as found in a Medline search, comprised only 7 per cent of all publications on HIV/AIDS, pointing to the relative lack of attention to issues specifically related to women (Sherr, 1996).

In the early years of the HIV epidemic, women tended to be viewed as at risk of HIV only if they were located within a defined high-risk group such as injection drug users or female prostitutes (Jackson and Highcrest, 1996; Kitts and Roberts, 1996; Padian, 1988). Examining issues related to women as a social group was, according to some, a waste of resources since epidemiologic data and the official HIV/AIDS statistics pointed to the fact that the greatest number of infected individuals were gay men and injection drug users. Even when women did want to participate in research studies, particularly clinical drug trials, exclusion criteria ensured that they were not considered. Gender exclusion criteria were frequently defended on the grounds that women might become pregnant while in the drug trial and the drug might do damage to the foetus (Doyal, 1994) or, alternatively, that a pregnant woman might contaminate the results of the trial because of the interaction between the drug and the woman's hormonal levels.

The lack of attention to women's health needs is not unique to HIV but has historically been evident in the context of other diseases and disorders. For example, heart disease is the leading cause of death of women in the United States, yet 'most of the research on the natural history of the disease, risk factors, pharmacological and behavioural interventions and rehabilitation has been conducted on men' (Shumaker and Smith, 1994: 198). As Kitts and Roberts (1996: 3) note, 'Health research has tended to overlook the specific consequences of disease and illness on women and men, and neglected to examine fully the different social, cultural, and economic contexts within which women and men work and live.'

In a context of relatively little research on women, there has been a tendency to generalize findings based on studies with men (Walmsley, 1996). This has assumed a 'universal' person, which is clearly antithetical to what we know about the differences between men and women in terms of their social location within our society and how their roles influence health and well-being, including emotional and psychological health, variations in the experiences of diseases, and the needs associated with illnesses (Doyal, 1994; Jackson et al., 1997; Love et al., 1997; Walters, 1993). Men and women inhabit different structural positions, and the 'meanings of their bodies, their health expectations and relevancies, their typical sickness profiles, and their illness reports differ' (Clarke, 1992: S55). The androcentric view that White males represent the norm upon which medical facts are established, and all other groups represent a deviation from this norm (Achilles, 1987; Shumaker and Smith, 1994), has until quite recently been firmly entrenched in medical research. However, as Shumaker and Smith (1994: 191) note, the possibility that a clinical trial would ever be conducted on an all-female or African-American population and the findings extrapolated to White men was unimaginable. Only now is the norm, and the structures through which this norm has been sustained, under attack by diverse groups demanding to have their health concerns addressed.

WOMEN AND HIV RESEARCH IN THE SECOND DECADE

In the early 1990s epidemiologic studies began to suggest that an increasing number of women were becoming HIV-infected and that many of these women were not situated within the traditionally defined high-risk groups of injection drug users and prostitutes. The need for research that included women began to be raised within policy circles. HIV-positive women and (primarily) female researchers became more vocal about the importance of research specifically examining issues of relevance to HIV-positive women, and there was a move to include women in research—to include them in treatment trials and to track the natural history of HIV in women. As Lorraine Sherr (1996: 17–18) notes, the first era of the HIV epidemic was characterized by 'oversight' and, despite the fact that women were becoming infected and dying from HIV, their situation was overlooked, but in the second phase there was an 'awakening' and women were acknowledged, and the response was noticeable. Within Canada, the addition of female-specific manifestations of HIV disease as part of an AIDS-defining condition occurred in July 1993 during this awakening phase.

Much of the research, particularly clinical research, initiated and implemented during this phase was limited, however, as it understood women almost exclusively in terms of their role as mothers. Many studies were designed based on the conceptualization of women as reproductive agents rather than as individuals with multiple roles and interests. HIV seroprevalence studies of vertical transmission and studies of the effects of AZT on reducing the chances of vertical transmission, for example, dominated much of the clinical research on women. In health research in general, reproductive health and women's health have been treated as conterminous and interest in women has tended to be in terms of their relation to their children—unborn or living—thus reinforcing the dominant cultural construct of women as unworthy of attention in and for themselves. The tendency to reduce women to their reproductive capabilities has also marked much of the HIV research agenda.

When women have been conceptualized as more than reproductive agents, they have all too often been viewed as the same as men. The social construction of gender and the multiple ways in which gender differences are created and reinforced have been noticeably absent. This has meant, for example, that often the same measurements are used to test the psychological well-being of HIV-infected men and women even though human lives are not homogeneous in a gender-divided society. As Sandra Harding notes, women and men are assigned different kinds of activities so that they lead different kinds of lives with significantly different contours and patterns (Harding, 1991: 121). Creating a questionnaire that is supposed to be universally applicable fails to capture the unique situations of men and women and the diversity among individuals given their socio-economic and ethno-racial backgrounds. It assumes that there is a 'norm' from which certain individuals or groups of individuals differ, and the norm has historically been created using the White adult male as the yardstick. Rather than beginning from the position of gender differences and inequities, and the unique socio-economic situations of men and women that can influence their psychological well-being and emotional issues, these universal psychological tools often assume sameness.

Much of the research within the field of HIV, as well as in other areas of health, has also failed to recognize gender differences in barriers to participating in research because the assumption is that gender differences are simply physiological. For women, however, there are many barriers that underscore their position of inequality within our society and that serve to further marginalize them in terms of their place in health research. Some women, for example, have partners or husbands who object to their participation in research studies, and because of their economic and/or emotional dependence on a man, these women feel unable to protest and, consequently, acquiesce to their partners' demands. Other women face obstacles related to child-care responsibilities and language and educational barriers. Such barriers may be particularly pronounced for women from poorer backgrounds and different ethno-racial groups (Walmsley, 1996).

MEDICAL CARE AND HIV-POSITIVE WOMEN

Adam and Sears report that in their study of HIV-positive individuals living in Canada and the United States it was primarily gay men who sought voluntary testing in the absence of symptoms. They suggest that this is because gay men are more likely to see themselves as at risk of HIV, have the resources for testing, and perceive AIDS as having immediacy in their lives. The immediacy derives both from the overall level of AIDS education in the gay community and from the proximity of friends' experiences with testing and HIV infection (Adam and Sears, 1996: 5).

In contrast to gay men, studies of HIV-positive women have found that women are much less likely to seek voluntary testing in the absence of symptoms. In a recent study involving interviews with 40 HIV-positive women living in the Metropolitan Toronto area, Jackson et al. (1997: 21) found that the most common reported reason for testing was because the woman had some direct knowledge that someone with whom she had been intimate (sexually or through the sharing of injection drug equipment) was symptomatic or had died of AIDS, or because the woman was symptomatic or her child was symptomatic. Most of the women (36, or 90 per cent) in this study either had no perception of any great health risk prior to HIV testing or perceived themselves to be at risk of diseases and disorders other than HIV. Women's knowledge of serostatus therefore often precedes their realization that they might be at risk. Heterosexual women may not perceive themselves to be at risk because they view themselves as engaging in 'ordinary' or 'normal' and therefore 'safe' heterosexual intercourse (Adam and Sears, 1996; Jackson et al., 1997). For lesbian women there may also be a perception of being safe because HIV has been characterized predominantly as a gay male disease, and lesbian women have been noticeably absent from the HIV/AIDS discourse on risk.

Testing for HIV relatively late in the progression of the disease can potentially influence access to life-prolonging therapies. The preponderance of available evidence suggests that the survival time for women following an AIDS diagnosis is generally shorter than for men (Blum et al., 1994; Siegel and Gorey, 1997), and there may be a number of reasons for this, including gender differences both in the time of testing and in obtaining a correct diagnosis. As Lesley Doyal (1994: 23) points out, existing guidelines often pay 'little attention to symptoms such as thrush, herpes, menstrual problems and cervical cell abnormalities that seem to characterize the early states of the disease process in many women'. This may mean that physicians' ability to be attuned to HIV in women is muted because of the lack of attention to gender differences in many guidelines. There is also some evidence that women may be underrepresented among patients offered antiviral agents and prophylactic treatments, even after controlling for a variety of factors such as time since diagnosis, race, and exposure category (Siegel and Gorey, 1997: 15). This suggests that gender differences in survival time may be a product of an array of gender disparities in research, treatment and care, and access to appropriate therapies. Crystal and Sambamoorthi (1996) also argue that HIV-positive women may have greater difficulties negotiating the health-care system than men because of competing claims on their time, especially their caregiving responsibilities to children and others. This may be a further factor in differences in survival time.

Given the relative lack of research attention to the needs and experiences of HIV-positive women, women will also tend to face even greater uncertainty than infected men about their medical situation, the most optimal medical treatment, and the best options available to them. Relatively little is known about how the disease is manifested in women and the efficacy of different therapeutic agents for women. Decisions about therapeutic interventions are thus made more difficult for women. Gendered differences in pay and the fact that women on average only earn approximately 67 per cent of what men earn may also mean that women are not readily able to access many of the complementary treatments and therapies that might contribute to their physical and emotional well-being (Levy, 1995: 1).

STIGMA AND HIV-POSITIVE WOMEN

HIV-positive women, especially women who have contracted HIV through sexual transmission, are often blamed for contracting HIV and for not practising safer sex. Even if their partners are not responsible enough to use a condom, the women are somehow supposed to know better than to have unsafe sex. Within our society, women are culturally represented as more responsible than men, and this translates into their being the ones who are to be knowledgeable about birth control and responsible for protection against sexually transmitted diseases (Campbell, 1995). If there is a birth-control/condom failure women are to 'blame', and not infrequently this blame is internalized by women who become burdened by feelings of regret.

The self-blame is often further reinforced by the stigma attached to the vertical transmission of HIV from mother to child in the womb. Even well into the second decade of the epidemic, HIV remains a stigmatizing sexually transmitted disease, and intersecting with this stigma are the strong negative attitudes associated with vertical transmission. In our society, women are targeted by health education campaigns because they are assumed to be responsible for the health of others, especially children (Daykin and Naidoo, 1995), and in the area of HIV this means that women are held responsible for having HIV-infected children. As mothers, the women are characterized as personal failures because they have failed to protect their child(ren). Moreover, to even consider pregnancy when one knows that one is HIV-positive is considered, in some circles, heresy. Indeed, Lawless et al. found that in the area of reproduction some of the most blatant forms of discrimination occurred. HIV-positive women report being denied the right to have children and forced to have abortions even against their will (Lawless et al., 1996; Bennett et al., 1996). The strong cultural taboos against women causing harm to their children frequently turn into practices denying them their reproductive rights. Pregnant women affected by HIV or AIDS need positive help with housing, employment, and income support as well as health care, but all too often they become the objects of negative medical surveillance, receiving fragmented and inappropriate treatment (Doyal, 1994: 23).

For many HIV-positive women there is often a tension between the need to access medical and social services, on the one hand, and the fear of discrimination and stigma, on the other. There are numerous accounts of women diagnosed with HIV being confronted by a judgemental health-care worker who questions them about their 'sexual promiscuity' or their drug use. Even in the face of evidence to the contrary, health professionals often question the woman's truthfulness (Lawless et al., 1996). HIV-positive women, like many HIV-positive men, often change their physician or dentist after their diagnosis because of unkind remarks and discriminatory behaviour. Women who do not feel comfortable with their physician or other health-care professionals may visit irregularly or miss potentially beneficial treatments (Levy, 1995). Or, they may 'shop around' to find a health-care worker who is sensitive to their situation and with whom they can feel comfortable discussing their health concerns and problems.

In some instances, HIV-positive individuals fail to disclose their health status to health-care professionals and social service agencies because of fears of stigma or discrimination. This fear may be heightened for women who are considered to be in marginalized groups, such as injection drug users or prostitutes, because of the negative attitudes most professionals, as well as others, hold concerning the 'underclass'. Even among HIV-positive women, there have been reports of discrimination between women from different backgrounds reflecting societal discriminatory patterns based on sexual orientation, class, or ethno-racial background. As Lawless et al. (1996: 1375) note, 'Although all HIV-positive women are affected either directly or indirectly [by stigma], the increased social isolation and poorer health of positive women who are also injecting drug users makes them particularly vulnerable to the effects of discrimination.'

HIV-POSITIVE WOMEN AND SOCIAL SUPPORTS

Women have often been characterized as having more social supports than men in terms of family relations and informal ties with friends and community organizations. For many HIV-positive women, however, these supports may not be operative because the women are afraid to disclose their HIV-positive status for fear of reprisals, particularly discrimination directed at their children or other family members. In many large urban centres gay men have available to them well-established community groups that offer support and services in the absence of strong traditional nuclear or extended family ties. Some HIV-positive women may feel estranged from such organizations, and the social isolation of living with HIV may make them especially dependent on medical practitioners or other health-care professionals. Having children may decrease the woman's sense of isolation, but the extra burden of concern about eventual placement of children, disclosure of HIV status or AIDS diagnosis to children, and possible rejection by older children remain (Green, 1996).

Many HIV-positive women may also have strong feelings of anger if infected by a partner, and working through this anger may require an extensive network of support that may be difficult to access if they have fears related to stigmatization and ostracism. Other women may have internalized guilt over having an infected child and this may result in either 'inappropriate rigid boundaries, "caring too much", resulting in over-protection of the child, or loose boundaries, whereby child or siblings are in control and exhibit behavioural disturbance' (Bennett et al., 1996: 179). Regardless of the woman's specific response pattern, however, many women will require support systems to assist them in coping with the complexities of the feelings associated with being infected and having an HIV-positive child.

Crystal and Sambamoorthi found in their study of HIV-positive women that even when women did participate in support groups, they were much more likely than men to discontinue. They suggest that this is perhaps because of domestic conflicts or child-care responsibilities, or because the groups were unable to meet the women's needs (Crystal and Sambamoorthi, 1996). In this study, the women's 'personal care needs were great but their own needs for care were complicated by their responsibility for others, especially children with whom most resided' (1996: 195). HIV-infected women may also have greater difficulty than men in travelling to group locations for a variety of reasons—inability to secure child care, domestic responsibilities, or concerns about travelling on public transportation at night (Adam and Sears, 1996). Adam and Sears (1996: 45–6) found that some women in Detroit overcame such obstacles by supplementing structured support groups with an informal telephone group, which suggests that different forms of support are needed if one is to be sensitive to the particular situation of varied groups.

Even in cases where a woman has disclosed her HIV-positive status and has a supportive network of family and friends, this may not be reflected in her psychological and emotional well-being. Vivian Walters (1993: 401), in a study of 356 Canadian women, reports that such issues as 'gendered caring roles, family structure, women's position in the labour market and financial resources are all intertwined and threaten women's mental health.' For HIV-positive women these issues may include, as well, the burden of coping with a disease that remains highly stigmatized in spite of clear and definite improvements in the public's understanding of the disease.

In countries such as Canada, where there is an extensive health-care system, there still remains an emphasis on women as caregivers, as the ones primarily responsible for helping friends and family in hospitals or individuals ill at home or in a hospice. This role may take a heavy toll on HIV-positive women, who may neglect their own health to care for others. The gendered division of labour between the private and public spheres has meant that women tend to carry the primary responsibility for domestic work even if they are working in the paid labour force, and this may have further serious implications for the health of some HIV-positive women. The cultural expectations concerning women as the caregivers may also, at times, make it difficult for some women to abdicate caregiving responsibilities to others, especially professionals. As Bennett et al. (1996) note, often a woman's personal identity is defined by her role as caregiver, and passing this responsibility to another is traumatic. Some women may feel in conflict over the need to obtain help to cope with their many responsibilities and duties and the sense of failure associated with passing responsibilities to others.

HIV-POSITIVE WOMEN AND SEX PRACTICES

Women living with HIV have to face complex choices concerning being sexually active, practising safer sex, and communicating their status to partners. For many HIV-positive women it is unclear if it is acceptable to have sexual relations after an HIV diagnosis because of risks of transmission, and many face a disruption in their sexual desire, arousal, and orgasmic functioning after diagnosis (see Hankins, 1996). Although for some women the disruptions in their sexual desires and sexual activity may be long term, for others it is a temporary state following diagnosis and for yet others the disruption is episodic.

There is a clear and substantiated link between a woman's economic dependence on a husband or partner and her belief that she owes him sexually (Luxton, 1980). This sense of dependency may influence a woman's decision concerning disclosure of her HIV-positive status. Women with children who are economically dependent may be especially prone to fear about revealing their status. Even for women who are relatively independent economically, however, there may be fears related to disclosure of HIV status because of the potential for abuse if a partner becomes angry when hearing of his partner's HIV-positive status. Zierler et al. suggest that violence against women, including sexual violence, occurs in a context that overlaps with the HIV epidemic among women. The conditions that serve to engender violence against women appear to be similar to the conditions that increase women's susceptibility to HIV infection, and include poverty as well as social inequality due to class position, gender, and race/ethnicity. As these authors note, these conditions create 'extreme vulnerability to violence victimization as well as to sexual activities that may not be expressions of shared desire, particularly among women who are homeless or dependent on men for economic support whether through sex work or domestic partnerships' (Zierler et al., 1996: 304).

For HIV-positive women, as for other women, the ability to practise safer sex is not simply a matter of having condoms available and having information about condom use. Condom use involves a relationship between (usually) two individuals. The forces influencing condom use are mediated through community and societal relations that many researchers, public health officials, and policy-makers often fail to acknowledge (Jackson and Highcrest, 1996). For women, their sexuality and their sense of agency around condom use are connected to cultural notions of femininity. Dominant constructions of femininity may actually contradict the need to play an active role in sexual relations with one's partner, particularly if one's partner is male. In our society, primacy is accorded to male desire and 'women are cast as the passive recipients of male passion' (Doyal, 1994: 14). Many heterosexual women feel that they do not have a right to assert their own needs and desires in a situation where their partner's wants are seen to be paramount. As Lesley Doyal notes, 'They feel unable to assert their wish for safe sex, for fidelity, or for no sex at all' (1994: 14). At the same time, since female sexuality is strongly associated with reproduction, for which many women feel they are personally responsible, it is often difficult for women to develop a 'positive image of female sexuality or their own ideas of what might constitute pleasurable sex' (Holland et al., 1994: 67).

WOMEN, HIV, AND PREGNANCY

There are multiple losses associated with HIV that all HIV-positive individuals have to cope with—loss of life expectancy; loss of health; and loss of friends, some of whom may have died from the complications arising from HIV and others who are not able to deal with HIV. These losses require supportive relations and an understanding of the meaning of the losses for the individual. Although not exclusively issues affecting women, additional losses that many women may face, which can greatly influence how they respond to an HIV diagnosis and their ability to cope with the diagnosis as well as the types of services that they need, include the loss of childbearing, the loss of a child, or the loss of one's future that was to include having a family. Women who have never had a child and who decide not to conceive or are not in a situation that is conducive to having a family may be particularly prone to strong feelings of loss and sadness.

A number of factors influence the decision not to become pregnant or to terminate a pregnancy. These include the 'fear of inability to care for the child and a lack of options for adoption of the child within the family or circle of friends should illness in the mother intervene' (Hankins, 1996: 5). If the woman has a previous experience with an HIV-positive child this may greatly affect the decision to have another child, although the cultural importance the woman attaches to childbirth and child-rearing may override other considerations about pregnancy (Richardson, 1990). Whether or not a partner is HIV-positive may impinge on the decision, as can concerns about the mother's own health and the possibility that pregnancy may exacerbate HIV-related illnesses. As Hankins (1996: 5) suggests, 'Among the reasons for conceiving a child are the desire to experience motherhood for women who have yet to have a child, a gender self-image that requires childbearing in order to be complete, an evaluation of the risk as acceptable, personal optimism, and previous experience with a child that sero-reverted and that lost maternal antibodies to HIV and was found to have not become infected.' In the realm of mother-to-child transmission a 'complex web' of scientific advances and ethical/legal debates can serve to make reproductive choices overwhelming and difficult. Counselling requires sensitivity to the factors that can influence women's decisions as well as a commitment to keep abreast of this rapidly advancing field.

CONCLUSION: THE ROLE OF THE SOCIAL WORKER IN RESPONDING TO THE NEEDS OF HIV-POSITIVE WOMEN

The medical and social needs of HIV-positive women living in Canada have frequently been improperly addressed by health-care professionals, service agencies, and policy makers (Allen, 1994; Hankins, 1990, 1995; Jackson et al., 1997). This situation has developed at least in part because of the failure to recognize that the HIV epidemic in Canada includes women from diverse groups and that women are often different from men in terms of their experiences and needs related to HIV. When women have been identified as different from men, however, they have often been conceptualized only in relation to others—especially in relation to children—rather than as unique human beings attempting to juggle diverse and often conflicting roles. Some women have internalized the dominant cultural representation of women as carers of others, and as a consequence often deny their own needs. As Travers and Bennett (1996: 72) note, 'Women are typically concerned about the effect that diagnosis will have on others and how they can help reduce the negative impact of their diagnosis.'

Social workers can assist HIV-positive women by helping them explore their own needs related to HIV and the options and choices available to them in responding to the challenges created by HIV. Women need to be seen by social workers as individuals who are not necessarily living in a nuclear family (Gavigan, 1996) and whose relations with lovers/partners/spouses may change over time and are often based on economic need because of women's subordinate role in the paid labour force and pay inequities based on gender. In our society and in our work, gender differences and inequities of class, race, and sexual orientation also need to be acknowledged rather than glossed over if we are to provide appropriate supports and services to HIV-positive women. By recognizing the similarities and differences among women and the health needs and experiences of different women, we can begin to work towards developing the required supports and services that can assist women living with HIV.

Social workers can play an important role in counselling HIV-positive women and in guiding them to form a positive sense of self. To do so, social workers need to have positive attitudes and learn the skills required to explore different, often highly charged and difficult issues. Social workers also need to be sensitive to the potential power differential between themselves and their female clients and to how this can affect the degree of comfort the woman feels with the social worker and, hence, her ability to disclose her problems and concerns. Listening to what the women are saying about issues that are important to them and placing the women's needs at the centre of attention (Ruzek, 1993; Ulin, 1992), rather than imposing on them ideas and strategies developed through professional bodies, will help to ensure relevance to the women's lives. To deny women a collective voice and role in the construction of appropriate responses only serves to further disempower them.

By providing HIV-positive women with information in a supportive environment and by advocating for access to needed supports and services, social workers can help HIV-positive women address the many and varied issues they must confront over the course of the illness. Specific supports are required by women, such as the provision of child care, transportation, interpreters, and so forth, as the unavailability of such supports often keeps women from attending to their own medical and social needs. Locating appropriate services and supports that can provide for the psychosocial needs of HIV-positive women requires an understanding of the multiple and often conflicting roles of women in our society. Individually helping women to develop needed communication skills and conducting workshops to assist with self-esteem and conflict resolution are crucial, for these will help women with some of their feelings of anger and frustration and will be important in their coping with HIV as an illness.

It is equally important, however, to challenge the social structures that sustain inequities (Heis and Elias, 1995; Lucke and Raphael, 1995). Health, illness, and wellness are located within individuals in social relations, and the inequities of these relations must be addressed if we are to move towards more positive, healthy lives for all women (Arber, 1997), including HIV-positive women. Economic and political inequities serve to create the conditions that place enormous obstacles in front of individuals seeking to live with HIV. Women, including HIV-positive women, bear a heavy burden in terms of caregiving, and are often unable to access the needed supports and services because of their socio-economic position. Challenges to these and other inequities need to be mounted to create more humane organizational structures (England et al., 1997). Only by addressing the many intersecting inequities related to women's position in our society can we hope to develop optimal conditions of existence for HIV-positive women.

REFERENCES

Achilles, R. 1987. 'Beyond His and Her: Detecting Sexist Research in Health', *Health Promotion*: 9–10.

Adam, B., and A. Sears. 1996. *Experiencing HIV: Personal, Family and Work Relationships*. New York: Columbia University Press.

Allen, J. 1994. *Women and HIV/AIDS in Nova Scotia Needs Assessment Report*. Halifax: Nova Scotia Women and AIDS Project.

Arber, S. 1997. 'Comparing Inequalities in Women's and Men's Health: Britain in the 1990s', *Social Science in Medicine* 44, 6: 773–87.

Bennett, L., K. Casey, and P. Austin. 1996. 'Issues for Women as Carers in HIV/AIDS', in L. Sherr, C. Hankins, and L. Bennett, eds, *AIDS as a Gender Issue: Psychosocial Perspectives*. London: Taylor & Francis, 177–90.

Blum, S., et al. 1994. 'Trends in Survival among Persons with Acquired Immunodeficiency Syndrome in New York City', *American Journal of Epidemiology* 139, 4: 351–61.

Campbell, C. 1990. 'Women and AIDS', *Social Science in Medicine* 30, 4: 407–15.

———. 1995. 'Male Gender Roles and Sexuality: Implications for Women's AIDS Risk and Prevention', *Social Science in Medicine* 41, 2: 197–210.

Clarke, J. 1992. 'Feminist Methods in Health Promotion Research', *Canadian Journal of Public Health* Supp. 1: S54–7.

Crystal, S., and U. Sambamoorthi. 1996. 'Care Needs and Access to Care among Women Living with HIV', in L. Sherr, C. Hankins, and L. Bennett, eds, *AIDS as a Gender Issue: Psychosocial Perspectives*. London: Taylor & Francis, 191–6.

Daykin, N., and J. Naidoo. 1995. 'Feminist Critiques of Health Promotion', in R. Bunton, S. Nettleton, and R. Burrows, eds, *The Sociology of Health Promotion: Critical Analyses of Consumption, Lifestyle and Risk*. London: Routledge, 59–69.

Doyal, L. 1994. 'HIV and AIDS: Putting Women on the Global Agenda', in L. Doyal, J. Naidoo, and T. Wilton, eds, *AIDS: Setting a Feminist Agenda*. London: Taylor & Francis, 11–29.

England, S., S. Kreigher, B. Miller, and N. Linsk. 1997. 'Community Care Policies and Gender Justice', *International Journal of Health Services* 17, 2: 217–32.

Gavigan, S. 1996. 'Familial Ideology and the Limits of Difference', in J. Brodie, ed., *Women and Canadian Public Policy*. Toronto: Harcourt and Company, 255–78.

Green, G. 1996. 'Stigma and Social Relationships of People with HIV: Does Gender Make a Difference?', in L. Sherr, C. Hankins, and L. Bennett, eds, *AIDS as a Gender Issue: Psychosocial Perspectives*. London: Taylor & Francis, 46–63.

Hankins, C. 1990. 'Issues Involving Women, Children and AIDS Primarily in the Developed World', *Journal of Acquired Immune Deficiency Syndromes* 3, 4: 443–8.

———. 1995. 'HIV Counselling and Testing Issues for Women—Testing Experiences', presentation to Women and HIV National Workshop, Montreal.

———. 1996. 'Sexuality Issues, Reproductive Choices and Gynaecological Concerns Affecting Women Living with HIV', in L. Sherr, C. Hankins, and L. Bennett, eds, *AIDS as a Gender Issue: Psychosocial Perspectives*. London: Taylor & Francis, 1–15.

Harding, S. 1991. *Whose Science? Whose Knowledge? Thinking From Women's Lives*. Ithaca, NY: Cornell University Press.

Heis, L., and C. Elias. 1995. 'Transforming AIDS Prevention to Meet Women's Needs: A Focus on Developing Countries', *Social Science in Medicine* 40, 7: 931–43.

Holland, J., C. Ramazanoglu, S. Scott, and R. Thomson. 1994. 'Desire, Risk and Control: The Body as a Site of Contestation', in L. Doyal, J. Naidoo, and T. Wilton, eds, *AIDS: Setting a Feminist Agenda*. London: Taylor & Francis, 61–79.

Jackson, L., and A. Highcrest. 1996. 'Female Prostitutes: What Are Their Risks of HIV Infection?', in L. Sherr, C. Hankins, and L. Bennett, eds, *AIDS as a Gender Issue: Psychosocial Perspectives*. London: Taylor & Francis, 149–62.

———, P. Millson, L. Calzavara, A. Rachlis, C. Rowe, S. Strathdee, C. Wagner, S. Walmsley, and the HIV Women's Study Group. 1997. 'HIV-positive Women Living in the Metropolitan Toronto Area: Their Experiences and Perceptions Related to HIV Testing', *Canadian Journal of Public Health* 88, 1: 18–22.

Kitts, J., and J. Roberts. 1996. *The Health Gap: Beyond Pregnancy and Reproduction*. Ottawa: International Development Research Centre.

Lawless, S., S. Kippax, and J. Crawford. 1996. 'Dirty, Diseased and Undeserving: The Positioning of HIV-positive Women', *Social Science in Medicine* 43, 9: 1371–7.

Levy, L. 1995. 'Clinical Care and Treatment for HIV-positive Women: Treatment Barriers', presentation to Women and HIV National Workshop, Montreal.

———, R. Foley, and S. Forer. 1994. *Taking Care of Our Health: A Study of Women Living with HIV/AIDS and the Treatments They Use*. Toronto: Voices of Positive Women.

Love, R., L. Jackson, R. Edwards, and A. Pederson, with the Critical Social Science and Health Group. 1997. 'Gender and Its Inter-relationship with Other Determinants of Health', Fifth National Health Promotion Research Conference, synthesis paper. Halifax, Dalhousie University.

Lucke, J., and B. Raphael. 1995. 'HIV and AIDS: Issues for Women in Australia', *Health Care for Women International* 16: 221–8.

Luxton, M. 1980. *More Than a Labour of Love: Three Generations of Women's Work in the Home*. Toronto: Women's Press.

Padian, N. 1988. 'Prostitute Women and AIDS: Epidemiology', *AIDS* 2: 413–19.

Richardson, D. 1990. 'AIDS Education and Women: Sexual and Reproductive Issues', in P. Aggleton, P. Davies, and G. Hart, eds, *AIDS: Individual, Cultural and Policy Dimensions*. New York: Falmer Press, 169–79.

———. 1994. 'AIDS: Issues for Feminism in the UK', in L. Doyal, J. Naidoo, and T. Wilton, eds, *AIDS: Setting a Feminist Agenda*. London: Taylor & Francis, 42–57.

Ruzek, S. 1993. 'Towards a More Inclusive Model of Women's Health', *American Journal of Public Health* 83, 1: 6–7.

Sherr, L. 1996. 'Tomorrow's Era: Gender, Psychology and HIV Infection', in L. Sherr, C. Hankins, and L. Bennett, eds, *AIDS as a Gender Issue: Psychosocial Perspectives*. London: Taylor & Francis, 16–45.

Shumaker, S., and T. Smith. 1994. 'The Politics of Women's Health', *Journal of Social Issues* 50, 4: 189–202.

Siegel, K., and E. Gorey. 1997. 'HIV-Infected Women: Barriers to AZT Use', *Social Science in Medicine* 45, 1: 15–22.

Travers, M., and L. Bennett. 1996. 'AIDS, Women and Power', in L. Sherr, C. Hankins, and L. Bennett, eds, *AIDS as a Gender Issue: Psychosocial Perspectives*. London: Taylor & Francis, 64–77.

Ulin, P. 1992. 'African Women and AIDS: Negotiating Behavioural Change', *Social Science in Medicine* 34, 1: 63–73.

Walmsley, S. 1996. 'Medical Care of Women Living with HIV', in L. Sherr, C. Hankins, and L. Bennett, eds, *AIDS as a Gender Issue: Psychosocial Perspectives*. London: Taylor & Francis, 119–48.

Walters, V. 1993. 'Stress, Anxiety and Depression: Women's Accounts of their Health Problems', *Social Science in Medicine* 36, 4: 393–402.

Zierler, S., B. Witbeck, and K. Mayer. 1996. 'Sexual Violence Against Women Living with or At Risk of HIV', *American Journal of Preventive Medicine* 12, 5: 304–10.

Chapter 7

Families with Children

Issues Arising from HIV

Lillian Wells, Robyn Salter-Goldie, Dale D'Amatteo, and Susan King

As HIV/AIDS spreads in the heterosexual population, women of childbearing age and their children are at particular high risk. We do not know how many women in Canada have HIV or how many of these women have had children exposed to HIV perinatally. This is partly due to the reporting system (in terms of AIDS rather than HIV), but also reflects the fact that some parents may not know they or their children are infected.

A recent study of 110 families across Canada in which the mother with HIV had subsequently had a child illustrated the complexity of the health status within these families (Salter-Goldie et al., 1996, 1997). There were 23 different configurations of HIV-positive or -negative status among mother, father, and children, with some families having more than one child in HIV-positive or -negative categories. A total of 172 living children were being cared for in these families and eight had died of AIDS-related illnesses. The 68 per cent of children in this sample who are HIV-negative and some of the HIV-positive children will outlive one or both parents. While new treatments are extending the lives of people with HIV, at this time all of these children could eventually lose their mothers through AIDS-related death and many, their fathers and one or more siblings as well.

It should be remembered that, with improved treatments during pregnancy, the proportion of HIV-negative children born to HIV-positive mothers is increasing. Also, newer tests facilitate earlier diagnosis of a baby's HIV status. While people with HIV now may live longer, the complexity and range of social and emotional needs continue over time.

Studies of family HIV in the United States have focused on inner-city mothers and children, mostly infected through IV drug use. The Canadian study (Salter-Goldie et al., 1997) found that our population crossed socio-economic class and reflected the multicultural make-up of the country. Parents had the same pattern of educational background as the Canadian population but had lower incomes. Poverty, added to the extra costs associated with HIV, was a major stress for many families.

Many parents were in long-standing marital relationships. There were some single-parent fathers due to spousal death or, less frequently, separation. About one-third of the families consisted of a lone-parent mother and her children. Several mothers had developed new partnerships after the death of or separation from the previous partner.

In our study, while children's ages ranged from infants to older teenagers, most were between one and five years old. Over the next few years the impact on the school system and the need for planning future care are only two aspects that will increase. Studies elsewhere have documented the special difficulties that infected and affected teenagers face (Rotheram Borus et al., 1996): services will be required for this population.

Our study was based on children exposed perinatally to HIV who were living with their biological parents. It was not fully reflective of families where the children were in the care of child welfare because the parents were not able to care for them due to drug use, ill health, or other reasons. Orphans living with grandparents or other relatives and children adopted or living in foster care are growing populations who will need social and health services and social work intervention.

The vignettes used here to illustrate the range and depth of social work service that families require are from the perspective of social work in health care since this is the arena where most practice has been developed. The link to social work practice in other fields such as child welfare, the school system, family counselling, and children's mental health is clear. There is a growing need for workers in a variety of specific HIV/AIDS and mainstream agencies to have expertise for work with these families.

Our general knowledge of the needs of families affected by illness has developed from situations where one member has health problems. With HIV, the degree of stigma, the uncertain course of HIV/AIDS, the possibility of premature death, the number of family members infected, and the gap between need and availability of services add to the complexity of the help required from the social work profession.

Social work practice in situations where HIV affects parents and children is characterized by the following features:

- A family-centred approach based on knowledge of family dynamics and how family functioning and child development are affected by chronic disease and by death of close family members.
- A holistic perspective that takes into account biological, psychological, social, economic, and spiritual dimensions of life.
- An ecological approach to practice requiring skills in dealing with intrapsychic and interpersonal issues, combined with skills for active involvement in addressing social and physical environmental and structural issues.
- A philosophy of outreach with special skill in developing relationships and 'working at the client's pace' and in responding to the diverse needs of individual members of both nuclear and extended family.
- Social work roles that encompass enabling, mobilizing, teaching, coaching, mediating, negotiating, advocating, collaborating, co-ordinating, consulting. Functions include: psychotherapeutic assessment and treatment (with individuals, families, and groups); case management; community development and social action; community planning and imple-

mentation; administration and organizational change; policy development; quality assurance and establishment of standards of practice.

- A program of long-term service. Families identified the importance of the help and personal support of social work and other health professionals (Salter-Goldie et al., 1997). A consistent relationship and availability of service from the same individual, possibly over a number of years, are critical features identified in this and other research (Reidy, Taggart, and Asselin, 1994).
- The need to work differentially with the family as a whole and individual members over time as situations and issues change. This is founded on respect for their unique world-views, values, and strengths, and requires cultural competence and understanding of racism and other oppressions.

The following two case studies illustrate features of social work practice in dealing with families affected by HIV/AIDS.

VIGNETTE #1

B is a mother and D a father, both living with AIDS. They have three children, the two eldest, M, aged 15, and R, 10, are not infected. G, aged 5, is HIV-positive with some symptoms. The family came to Canada five years ago from an African country. One year ago B became ill, was admitted to hospital, and tested positive for HIV. She had an AIDS-defining illness. Her positive test led to all other family members being tested: within a month of the mother's initial illness the parents discovered that three of their family (mother, father, and youngest child) were all infected.

After 5-year-old G's positive test, she was referred to a children's hospital HIV/AIDS program. The social worker met with the mother to assess the current needs and begin a long-term working relationship. The immediate need was for adequate housing and a telephone. The family was living in severe poverty so the first social work contacts with the mother addressed resource needs and also provided information about HIV in children and adults. The mother was able to tell the social worker that her husband would not come to the hospital, did not want anyone to visit the home, and had a drinking problem, and that his style of coping was to try to avoid thinking about HIV and its effects on the family. The mother's style of coping was to seek information and resources. She wanted to know how one child could be infected and not the other two, how the medications would affect the child, what other services were available to help the family cope with the uncertain health and poverty, and who could care for all three children if the parents became ill and if they died. B was aware that her husband was feeling guilty about how the HIV came into the family and that she herself had feelings of anger about this.

The social worker's first approach was to develop a trustful, helping relationship with the mother, starting with her immediate needs for better housing and a telephone and viewing the needs of the whole family as the mother felt ready. The social worker referred her to two HIV/AIDS volunteer agencies, working collaboratively with them to meet these practical needs.

B had many strong coping skills, among them an optimistic outlook, a strong faith, and an ability to accept and appreciate help in such a way that she rewarded her supporters with her thanks. However, she was also coping with serious isolation, having no family or friends in Canada and having told no one about the family HIV except the health-care staff and the staff of the volunteer agencies. The social worker asked if she would like to attend a support group for mothers with HIV, but she felt this would be difficult because she was afraid of meeting anyone from her country who would find out about her HIV. Also, she thought her husband would strongly oppose her going out in the evening. She did accept the idea of talking anonymously on the phone with another HIV-positive mother who was involved with HIV activities in the community. Eventually, she was able to attend a mother's group, which she found very helpful.

Another issue for B was disclosure to her children. She had made a firm decision not to tell any of them, but her 10-year-old overheard a phone conversation about HIV and asked her about it in front of the 15-year-old. She told them the truth and asked them not to tell anyone; however, the younger of the two told a friend who told their teacher.

Soon the school principal called the social worker, asking what to do about the presence of the 5-year-old infected child in the school. He wanted to know what policies the school should have in place, who needed to know about the family's HIV, and whether there was any risk of HIV transmission if the infected child was bleeding at school. With the mother's permission, the social worker visited the school and provided information about HIV to the principal and teacher. She advised them that no one needs to know about the infected child's HIV and that there have been no reported cases of HIV transmission in schools or day-care centres. She gave verbal and written information about how HIV is transmitted, answers to questions people often ask, universal precautions and teaching resources for these, and where to get information on developing HIV policies for schools.

She also met with the two affected children and their mother to give immediate and ongoing support and information about HIV, their parents' and sister's health, and living with the secret.

When B was ready, she and the social worker discussed the issues of planning for the future care of all three children if the parents became ill and if they died. B was able to discuss this difficult subject because she felt she would be relieved of the stress of worry if she had some idea what could happen. Her first desire was to sponsor her sister, who lived in her home country, to come to Canada and live with the family, with the role of looking after the parents if and when they were ill and if and when they might die. The sister, who was 19 years old, did not know about the family HIV, and the mother's dilemma was whether or not to tell her. She believed that if she told her sister the whole family in Africa would know, and this was very difficult to consider. On the other hand, not telling her and expecting her to come as a major caregiver seemed unrealistic, too. The worker suggested that the International Social Service could be a resource by having a social worker in the home country talk to the sister about this difficult issue.

To date, the father has not come himself to see the social worker, but the mother and worker have discussed aspects of parental and marital relationships, such as the anger and emotional reactions in the family, including the father's violence, sexual issues such as condom use, fear of pregnancy, reinfection between infected partners, and whether B is safe from abuse if she refuses sexual relations without condoms.

VIGNETTE #2

H and R are the parents of a 4-year-old girl, M, who is HIV-negative and a 2-year-old boy, T, who is HIV-positive. H, the mother, has AIDS and has had several serious illnesses. She is now unable to work even though she would like to continue. R, the father, has some minor symptoms and a T4 count in the 200s, but he does not take any anti-retroviral medications. He works full-time, earning about $16,000 per year. T requires anti-retroviral medications and monthly intravenous gamma globulin to boost his immune system. This treatment is successful, and he is developing normally and has few symptoms.

Both children attend day care full-time. The cost is subsidized because their mother is not able to care for them alone while the father is at work. Their father is now the primary caregiver, taking them to day care and picking them up after work, bringing T to the hospital every month, and providing most of the care at home. The children have had some emotional difficulties associated with their mother's illness, showing symptoms common to young children in distress. M is bedwetting, wetting her pants during the day, and has oppositional behaviour and distractibility. T is crying more often and having difficulty leaving his mother. H and R are very loving parents who do all they can to support their children to cope with their problems and they work very well together to support each other and to maintain a hopeful attitude and cheerful family life. They were diagnosed four years ago, when H was pregnant with M. H became ill during the pregnancy and both parents were diagnosed with HIV. When M was born they brought her to the children's hospital to have her tested. They met regularly with the social worker when they came to the hospital and later, when T was born and diagnosed with HIV, they continued working with the social worker.

During the four years of knowing about their HIV, this young couple has coped with many difficult issues while trying to live as normally as possible. They have had to deal with severe stress in many areas of their lives, which has sometimes led to serious tension in their relationship. At a particularly difficult time they used crisis couple counselling and subsequently saw the social worker regularly for marital counselling. They have coped with sexual issues such as practising safer sex, unplanned pregnancy, and learning about the issues of reinfection when both partners have HIV. They have also coped with the painful emotional issues of having an infected child, their own and each other's health problems, uncertainty for the future of all three infected family members, and special needs of the uninfected child. They have had to learn to work with health-care staff, understand medical treatments, and co-ordinate all their health-care appointments. Living on a low income while having medically related expenses has been an added burden.

For the first two years that they knew of their HIV this couple was very isolated with this information, having told no one except the health-care staff. They have no family living near them and no family or friends who can care for their children if they are unable to raise them. They have found that talking to other people with HIV, beginning with the support group for mothers with HIV, and telling some of their non-infected friends give them a sense of much more support now, but it was a risk to disclose their HIV status and they had to make each decision with care in regard to telling each of their friends.

In working with this family, social work service has featured (1) ongoing supportive counselling individually and with both parents to validate their feelings, to listen, and, in some ways, to serve as an older extended family member, which was what the parents desired since they had no family living near them. The parents and worker discussed HIV-related decisions such as disclosure to friends and to agencies in order to obtain services. Parenting was another major topic—raising children under these circumstances, ways of supporting the children's emotional needs, and planning their current and future care. Another feature has been (2) a period of intensive marital counselling, dealing with ways to cope with stress and tension that are non-destructive and mutually supportive and improving communication and sexual relations. Finally, intervention has included (3) referral, communication, and interagency co-ordination in working with the parents and agencies to provide information and to act as broker and advocate in arranging a variety of services. These include:

1. mothers' support group, child care, financial help, food, infant formula, clothing through HIV/AIDS organizations;
2. health-care services, homemaking through the Home Care program;
3. medical information through the family doctor and HIV specialists for parents and child—working from an interdisciplinary perspective to integrate medical and psychosocial care;
4. income supplements, drug coverage through social assistance;
5. day-care services, with a subsidy, through the municipal program;
6. subsidized housing;
7. legal services for arranging power of attorney and wills;
8. future care planning with child welfare services.

While the sources of these services vary in different jurisdictions, this list illustrates the range and complexity of arrangements needed and achieved, which also included linking H with other parents with HIV (she is one of the parents who provides telephone support to other parents who are not yet ready to disclose their HIV except through phone calls) and future care planning and legacy planning for the children.

H accepts that she may not live long and wants to leave a legacy of information and love for her children. She has written a diary for them and kept photos and mementoes. She made them a videotape with help from the social worker, carefully planning what she wanted to say, courageously overcoming her own grief well enough to leave them a message of love and support for the future. H and R also worked with the social worker to plan a referral to the child welfare agency requesting an unusual type of foster care. They asked for foster parents who would be like an extended family in helping the parents care for the children, especially during times of illness, and eventually these foster parents would become full-time caregivers if both parents die. They wanted this support for their children to ease the potential loss of both parents and so they could help select the foster parents and work with them as much as possible. They and the social workers from the children's hospital and child welfare collaborated on the plans to find such a family and on other immediate needs, such as respite care so the parents could have some time alone.

Social work with families who are affected and infected by HIV calls for a broad range of activities and well-developed skills (Beauger, Dupuy-Godin, and Jumelle, 1990; Bor and Elford, 1994; Bor, Miller, and Goldman, 1992; Boyd-Franklin, Steiner, and Boland, 1995; Children and Family AIDS Task-force, 1993; Hackel et al., 1997; Kaplan, Marks, and Mertens, 1997; Littrell, 1996). These are outlined in the following sections.

CRISIS INTERVENTION

People who are newly diagnosed often experience overwhelming stress and crisis characterized by overpowering emotions and a range of problems that overtax normal coping skills and personal and social resources. Crisis intervention can be important at this stage and through other difficult periods. Many parents describe how, over time, they experience a roller-coaster of stress, emotional upset, and insurmountable problems. The worker must also be alert to the potential for violence or suicide as two responses in such periods of high stress. Parents do report that the needs of their children and the pleasure children bring provide help for them in overcoming negative thoughts, including those of suicide.

Germain (1984) cautions that many crisis states actually present long-term demands. She notes, however, that the elements of crisis intervention emphasizing the rapid response to need, active helping, help in cognitive restructuring of the situation and in problem-solving, and help mobilizing social, emotional, and material supports are all important factors for practice related to chronic health problems.

EDUCATION AND CONSULTATION FOR THE NUCLEAR AND EXTENDED FAMILY: VARIOUS DOMAINS

Social workers have traditionally played key roles in helping families integrate medical and health-care information into their lifestyles. The families described in the two vignettes do not have extended families available. For those that do, mothers and sisters often play special roles as confidantes and in providing a range of social and practical support (Salter-Goldie et al., 1997). Typically, social workers act as teachers, coaches, and mediators in assisting the empowerment of families and their individual members. It is often critical, also, to reach out to members of the extended family to help them incorporate information on transmission and treatment and how this impacts on their family relationships.

WITH COMMUNITY SERVICES, EMPLOYERS

Vignette #2 illustrates social work activities when the school principal requested information and guidance regarding a specific client situation and relating to policies that the school should follow. A school social worker seeing children where there is illness or death in the family may need information and consultation to work with the children and to support teachers.

WITH COMMUNITY SERVICES AND THE PUBLIC: GENERAL ASPECTS OF HIV/AIDS IN FAMILIES

Social workers with expertise in this area have a responsibility to contribute to public education and the knowledge of the wide variety of service providers who may be serving families affected by HIV. This education may serve to dispel stigma, discrimination, and misinformation that cause problems for affected and infected family members.

IN-DEPTH CLINICAL TREATMENT

Vignette #2 illustrates the use of supportive counselling over a broad range of issues as well as a period of more intense work that focused on the relationship of the couple (Goldstein, 1996). In this case the hospital social worker provided the service. In other cases it may be more appropriate for family therapy and in-depth treatment to be provided through adult or children's mental health settings, family service organizations, etc.

At the interpersonal level there are often concerns about family relationships and child-rearing, couple relationships, parent-child relationships, and child behaviour issues. At both intrapsychic and interpersonal levels frequent concerns may relate to coping with stress, addressing existential issues and finding meaning in life, building on strengths and solving problems, building mutual support systems, and dealing with intense emotions such as guilt, anger, and depression (Brookins, 1993; Littrell, 1996; Septimus, 1989).

Members of the extended family may also want counselling. They may have emotional and practical concerns, need an opportunity to discuss what the family HIV infection means to them, and want to address issues of family relationships. Counselling around the implications of the HIV education they have received may be indicated.

GROUP WORK AND PEER SUPPORT

Social work with groups can be a very powerful means of reducing isolation and developing mutual support, with group members working together to address emotional issues and find solutions or ways of coping with problems. Groups for parents, especially mothers, are most common. However, as in many illnesses, children's emotional issues may tend to be neglected (Dowdy et al., 1997). Groups for infected children and for affected children have been shown to have a positive impact (Goldstein, 1996). Periodic reunions for former group members can be key features of the program and illustrate the need for a continuity of service and relationships.

While groups can provide a safe place to discuss sensitive issues, they can also be a threat for those concerned about keeping the HIV status of their family confidential. Parent-to-parent support by telephone was an acceptable alternative for the mother in Vignette #1. Another risk factor in group work with this population is that developing close attachments to someone who becomes ill or dies can exacerbate loss.

Parents in our study who had participated in a special summer camp spoke of the long-lasting and even transformative impact this had for them (Salter-Goldie et al., 1997). This relaxed, recreational setting provided an opportunity for discussions and sharing of experiences. It enabled people (some who had never met others with HIV) to reduce their profound sense of isolation. This was especially highlighted by mothers. Further, for some, camp facilitated a meaningful re-evaluation of their lives and relationships.

SEXUAL RELATIONSHIPS

As noted in the vignettes, sexual relations involve issues of safer sex and decisions about pregnancy and perhaps abortion. Feelings of guilt, anger, and blame may be aroused, depending on how HIV came into the family. How, when, and whether to disclose to potential new sexual partners is another area for thoughtful decision.

STIGMA, DISCRIMINATION, AND DISCLOSURE

Parents worry about the possible negative impact of disclosure on themselves and their children when people in the community and certain members of their family know about the HIV. They are concerned about potential hurtful reactions and loss of friendships for their children. They may be concerned that their own children will think badly of them. They are often concerned about bringing shame and dishonour to the wider family and, especially those who are visible minorities, about bringing disgrace to their community and an increase in societal racism.

Some parents are concerned that knowing about the HIV status may be a difficult burden for children or that a child, as in Vignette #1, may tell others. While most parents tell older children, one study found that teenagers who knew about the diagnosis but did not know who could care for them and be substitute parents if their own parents became ill or died had more serious emotional and behavioural problems than those who did not know about the HIV (Rotheram Borus et al., 1996). This highlights the need for children to feel secure about plans for future care from the time of disclosure.

Disclosure is a serious decision that, once acted on, cannot be withdrawn. Some parents are open publicly and gain strength from their contributions to social change; others are convinced that secrecy is the best for them and their children. This is clearly a decision that must be taken by the parents in the light of their personal circumstances and values.

THE POSSIBILITY OF PREMATURE DEATH

A major theme identified by parents (Salter-Goldie et al., 1996, 1997) was the deep sense of loss for their anticipated future as a family and concern that centred on the needs of their children. One father said, 'There's two [of four] that might survive in this family. I have a responsibility to keep myself sane and economically viable. How will I measure up to that responsibility?' A mother said that she worries about her daughter: 'How will she react when I die, whether the supports [at that time] will be the right ones . . . her ability to move on?'

Parents work to find new meaning in life and to reconstitute their identity, to grieve with their families for those who have died, to prepare children through 'focused parenting', and to make the most of the 'precious time' they have with their children.

FUTURE CARE PLANNING AND PREPARING A FAMILY LEGACY

Parents work to provide a legacy for their children—happy memories, souvenirs, and internal resources and social skills to enable them to cope with future difficulties. They worry about financial security and a stable home and alternate family life. Some feel secure that when the time comes the extended family will decide who is best able to care for the children. Others worry about the burden that caring for the children could place on relatives or friends and whether siblings (especially if they have different fathers) can remain together. Issues of custody and guardianship can be dynamic and complex from emotional, practical, and legal perspectives.

Such issues are usually very difficult for parents to consider, especially if no suitable family is available. Mason (1996) studied the permanency planning of 19 mothers and identified six activities mothers said they needed to complete before permanency plans for children could be put in place. These are: (1) identify potential caregiver and screen, select, and reach agreement with that person; (2) talk to the potential caregiver about the mother's HIV status; (3) talk to the children about HIV, including mother's status, child's status, safer sex, and death and dying; (4) develop a relationship with potential caregiver around children; (5) make legal arrangements, including a will, stand-by guardianship, guardianship, and adoption; (6) permanently transfer children to the caregiver's home while the mother is alive or at her death, depending on preference. These activities are not completed in order—they overlap and can vary in time from a month to years. The process is dynamic and subject to disruption by the mother or potential caregiver at any point. These mothers gave the following advice to social workers:

> Be there for us. Keep in contact and develop a relationship. Be genuine, honest and sincere. Get in touch with your feelings. Help us understand our feelings. Keep talking to us. Know where we are in the process of planning

> but do not push too hard. Raise the issue, back off if we resist and bring it up later. Stay on us about planning but realize that you cannot make people do something if they are not ready. (Mason, 1996)

Planning for future care with families living with HIV/AIDS can require the involvement of child welfare services. Creativity in finding resources for respite care for infected and affected children, foster parenting, and potential adoptive parents was illustrated in Vignette #2. In other instances, support may be needed to help extended family members to provide for the best interests of the children. New programs to address these very specific issues are required.

SOCIAL WORK AND THE HIV FAMILY

CREATIVITY AND INNOVATION IN RESOURCE ACCESS

The new and unmet needs of this population require active outreach by the social worker to initiate and forge links with a variety of services. The desire of the mother in Vignette #1 to have her sister come to Canada sparked the need for the worker to contact senior-level people in Citizenship and Immigration to see what special arrangements were possible on humanitarian grounds. She could then help the parents reach a decision, advocate on their behalf, and help them develop their own ability for advocacy.

Babies of HIV-positive mothers should not be breast-fed but the costs of formula may be too much for low-income (employed or unemployed) families and these costs may not be part of government funding for families on social assistance. The worker will need connections and skills, and possibly an advocacy network of AIDS organizations. Child welfare and public health may be required to obtain government funding, and perhaps baby formula companies could be approached to provide support in the interim.

REFERRAL

This area is complicated by issues of disclosure and trust, which can predominate, especially for newly diagnosed people. The need to have services and at the same time protect privacy raises dilemmas. The social worker can help parents work out the implications and make an informed decision. For example, does the mother decide to disclose her HIV status to get a subsidy or does she use a secondary diagnosis? How does she decide to deal with information about her positive child's diagnosis? Some services can be arranged without disclosure or with limited health information that still preserves privacy but presents the situation honestly through partial truth-telling.

COLLABORATIVE PRACTICE

The importance of collaboration within and among service sectors is indicated by the complexity of issues related to family HIV/AIDS, its impact on so many realms of life, the fact that most current services were not designed to address the particular needs of these families, and the changing nature of HIV/AIDS treatment. Issues of stigma and discrimination and of privacy and confidentiality can complicate this process, as they do with referral. Salter-Goldie et al. (1997) found that many parents identified professionals as key members of their social support network. Skills of conferring, co-operating, and consulting are needed in a variety of multidisciplinary and interdisciplinary contexts (Germain, 1984). The need for comprehensive services challenges service providers to work with families and with each other in new ways.

NEGOTIATION, MEDIATION, ADVOCACY

Social work as a profession has a responsibility to influence service providers and organizations to be more responsive to the biopsychosocial needs of people. Empowerment practice recognizes the importance of: both the personal and the political dimensions of the situation; collaborative partnerships with clients, client groups, and others; recognizing that clients are active subjects and claimants and that the practice emphasis is on the expansion of client capacities, strengths, and resources (Simon, 1994).

POLICY AND PROGRAM DEVELOPMENT

The service infrastructure must adapt to the challenge of HIV/AIDS (Rowe, 1993). Needs of families cut across traditional health and social service sectors and extend into domains such as work, school, housing, religious practice, and the legal system. Needs can be quite different when two generations have a health problem as opposed to when only one family member does. Family HIV raises issues that illustrate limitations of our service system and the advantages of a proactive family policy as advocated by Baker (1995), rather than a series of residual programs. Social workers (individually and in coalitions with clients, service providers, and others) can influence policy and raise awareness of the complex intergenerational issues and the need for comprehensive, flexible, family-centred care.

CONCLUSION

With HIV/AIDS as a growing problem for mothers, fathers, and children, the issues challenge current social policies and institutions. Social workers need to take a strong role, in partnership with families and other groups, to develop new arrangements in community care. Over the long term this may lead to the development of family policy at the senior government level (Salter-Goldie et al., 1997; Baker, 1995). Wharf and Clague (1997: 319) describe how work towards a 'caring community' requires 'four crucial components: (1) strong national/ provincial socio-economic policies, (2) establishing caring neighbourhood institutions, (3) municipal governments dedicated to community caring, (4) an ethic of solidarity among residents'. A variety of strategies of community organizing may be needed sequentially and simultaneously: consensus strategies, when there is agreement; campaign strategies, when priorities are not recognized by the powerful; conflict strategies, when the parties disagree and values clash (Wharf and Clague, 1997).

Social work with family HIV/AIDS demands strong assessment and treatment skills and ability to address practical, socio-emotional, and spiritual dimensions of life within a family context. It requires self-awareness, application of ethical principles, and cultural competence (Dunkel and Hatfield, 1986; Gillman, 1991; Taylor-Brown and Garcia, 1995).

REFERENCES

Baker, M. 1995. *Canadian Family Policies: Cross-National Comparisons.* Toronto: University of Toronto Press.

Beauger, M., M. Dupuy-Godin, and Y. Jumelle. 1990. 'AIDS: A Clinical Approach', *The Social Worker* 57.

Bor, R., and J. Elford. 1994. *The Family and HIV.* London: Cassell.

———, R. Miller, and E. Goldman. 1992. *Theory and Practice of HIV Counselling.* London: Cassell.

Boyd-Franklin, N., G.L. Steiner, and M.G. Boland. 1995. *Children, Families, and HIV/AIDS: Psychosocial and Therapeutic Issues.* New York: Guilford.

Brookins, G. 1993. 'Culture, Ethnicity and Bicultural Competence: Implications for Children with Chronic Illness and Disability', *Pediatrics* 91: 1056–62.

Children and Family AIDS Task-force. 1993. *HIV/AIDS in Children and Families in Massachusetts: Recommendations for Policy and Programs.* Boston: Massachusetts Department of Public Health.

Dunkel, J., and S. Hatfield. 1986. 'Countertransference Issues in Working with Persons with AIDS', *Social Work* 31: 114–17.

Faithful, J. 1997. 'HIV-positive and AIDS-infected Women: Challenges and Difficulties of Mothering', *American Journal of Orthopsychiatry* 67: 144–51.

Germain, C.B. 1984. *Social Work Practice in the Health Field.* New York: Free Press.

Gillman, R. 1991. 'From Resistance to Rewards: Social Workers' Experiences and Attitudes towards AIDS', *Families in Society: The Journal of Contemporary Human Services* 72: 593–601.

Goldstein, E. 1996. *Ego Psychology and Social Work Practice.* New York: Free Press.

Hackel, K.L., A.M. Somiai, J.A. Kelly, and S.C. Kalichman. 1997. 'Women Living with HIV/AIDS: The Dual Challenge of Being a Patient and Caregiver', *Health and Social Work* 22: 53–62.

Human-Dowdy, J., C. Kiev, D. Lantz-Lathrop, and M. Winkle. 1997. 'Facilitating Adjustment to Catastrophic Illness through Involving Children in Age-appropriate Education', *Journal of Rehabilitation* 63, 2: 22–5.

Kaplan, M.S., G. Marks, and S.B. Mertens. 1997. 'Distress and Coping among Women with HIV Infection: Preliminary Findings from a Multiethnic Sample', *American Journal of Orthopsychiatry* 67: 80–91.

Littrell, J. 1996. 'How Psychological States Affect the Immune System: Implications for Intervention in the Context of HIV', *Health and Social Work* 21: 287–95.

Mason, S. 1996. 'Mothers with AIDS Planning for the Future of their Children', paper presented to the XIth International Conference on AIDS, Vancouver.

Parry, J.K. 1994. 'Death Review: An Important Component of Grief Resolution', *Social Work in Health Care* 20: 97–107.

Reidy, M., M. Taggart, and L. Asselin. 1994. 'Psychosocial Needs Expressed by the Natural Care-givers of HIV-infected Children', in R. Bor and J. Elford, eds, *The Family and HIV*. London: Cassell.

Rotheram Borus, M.J., B. Draimin, H.M. Reid, and D.A. Murphy. 1996. 'The Impact of Illness Disclosure and Custody Plans on Adolescents Whose Parents Live with AIDS', unpublished manuscript.

Rowe, W. 1993. 'HIV/AIDS Implications for the Social Service Sector', *Canadian Journal of Public Health* 84: supp. 1: 48–51.

Salter-Goldie, R., et al. 1996. 'Children Born to Mothers with HIV/AIDS: Psychosocial Issues of Families in Canada Living with HIV/AIDS—A Preliminary Report', *The Social Worker* 64: 55–66.

———, D. DeMatteo, S.M. King, L.M. Wells, et al. 1997. *Children Born to Mothers with HIV/AIDS: Psychosocial Issues of Families in Canada Living with HIV/AIDS: Final Report*. Toronto: Hospital for Sick Children.

Septimus, A. 1989. 'Psycho-social Aspects of Caring for Families of Infants Infected with HIV', *Seminars in Perinatology* 13: 49–54.

Simon, B.L. 1994. *The Empowerment Tradition in American Social Work*. New York: Columbia University Press.

Taylor-Brown, S., and A. Garcia. 1995. 'Social Workers and HIV-affected Families: Is the Profession Prepared?', *Health and Social Work* 20: 14–15.

Wharf, B., and M. Clague. 1997. *Community Organizing: Canadian Experiences*. Toronto: Oxford University Press.

Chapter 8

AIDS-Specific Social Work Practice in Rural Areas

CLAUDE OLIVIER

INTRODUCTION

This chapter presents an overview of AIDS-related social work practice with rural people. For the most part, the content comes from what has been written about AIDS work in rural Canada. While a review of the literature did enable the description of the critical issues and range of approaches and interventions being used, it also pointed to the need to document more fully this area of social work. Gaps in knowledge exist. Literature from the United States was used for purposes of comparison and to supplement certain topic areas. In addition to the literature, throughout the chapter the author shares knowledge that he has gained through eight years of social work practice with an AIDS organization that provides services in rural communities.

The chapter commences with discussion of the definition of 'rural' and the difficulties encountered in describing HIV/AIDS-related social work practice in rural areas. This is followed by a look at rates of infection and trends within rural populations. Challenges and opportunities that emerge in relation to HIV/AIDS work in rural communities are then presented. Next, the approach to social work practice is discussed in general terms and as it relates to community development and outreach. This leads to a review of services and interventions that have unique application to rural communities as well as those that have been modified in design to meet rural needs. The chapter concludes with recommendations and comments on the future of AIDS work in rural areas.

The subjective nature of the definition of 'rural' was illustrated at a recent New Brunswick conference on rural development and AIDS (AIDS New Brunswick, 1996a). Opening panel members spoke of their experiences related to HIV/AIDS. It was surprising to hear some talk about rural issues in the context of living in small to medium-sized cities. These panel members explained that they felt as though they lived in rural areas as compared to living in large Canadian cities like Montreal, Toronto, and Vancouver. Conference participants from smaller centres said that they did not have the advantages of urban life (e.g., experienced doctors, peer support, and AIDS organizations) that exist in the New Brunswick cities mentioned by the panel. It would be interesting to hear a third perspective, that of someone who resides in one of Canada's remote regions. For the most part, this chapter focuses on AIDS work in small towns and rural communities. Perhaps some of the discussion of issues and methods will also be applicable and useful to those working in more remote regions.

It is difficult to quantify or describe the HIV/AIDS-related work being carried out by social workers from within existing health, education, and social service agencies, organizations, and institutions in rural communities. There is simply not that much written about it. A Canadian study on social work and AIDS was able to identify social workers involved in AIDS work in many regions of the country (Clarke, 1995). The social workers who participated in the study were found in a variety of workplace settings, including volunteer community-based organizations (e.g., AIDS service organizations), hospitals, community social service agencies, and government departments.

Several reports produced in the past few years document the work of AIDS service organizations (ASOs) in rural communities and provide the basis for this chapter (AIDS Saskatoon, 1994; Barnsley and Bonny, 1995; Canadian Public Health Association, 1996; Truesdale and Vacon, 1996). These reports describe the range of approaches and interventions used in responding to HIV/AIDS issues. Although the activities described are not necessarily being carried out by social workers, they certainly could be interventions used by this profession. Similarly, the work being carried out by ASOs likely has application in other workplace settings.

The number of AIDS cases diagnosed in Canada up until 31 December 1997 was 15,528 (Health Canada, 1998). The number rises to an estimated 20,000 if delays in reporting are considered (Health Canada, 1998). The number of HIV positive tests diagnosed in Canada between 1985 and 1997 is 41,049 (Health Canada, 1998). It is also estimated that 42,500–45,000 Canadians were infected with HIV up to the end of 1994 (Health Canada, 1996b). Gay men, blood and blood product recipients, and persons from countries with high infection rates among heterosexuals were the groups initially most affected. Since the mid-1980s, other groups such as injection drug users, a wider segment of the heterosexual population, and women are increasingly being affected (Health Canada, 1996a); this is accompanied by a drop in the median age of new infections (Health Canada, 1996b).

Health Canada does not compile statistics on the number of reported HIV cases. This is left up to each province. Data on geographic distribution of HIV/AIDS cases, beyond province or provincial grouping, are reported by Health Canada. However, statistics for New Brunswick, a province with a high proportion of rural residents, indicate that 17 per cent of that province's HIV and AIDS cases are found outside of the larger urban regions (New Brunswick Health and Community Services, 1995).

A review of recent Canadian epidemiological reports provides some data on infection rates and trends associated with rural populations (Health Canada, 1996a, 1996c, 1996d). However, the research is limited and many of the conclusions drawn are tentative. HIV prevalence studies of pregnant women in Canada indicate an average rate of infection of about 3–4/10,000 (Health Canada, 1996a). Large cities have higher rates of infection for women, but even provinces without large urban centres have significant rates (e.g., 3.9/10,000 in New Brunswick for 1994–6). Data from Manitoba identify an increasing trend of infection among women of childbearing age (from 0.7/10,000 in 1991 to 3.2/10,000 in 1994–5).

While the epidemic among Aboriginal peoples is not well researched, evidence suggests that: they are being infected at a younger age, injection drug use is an important factor, and the rate of infection is rising (Health Canada, 1996d). Women represent a greater proportion of total adult Aboriginal AIDS cases than is found among adult non-Aboriginal AIDS cases. The movement between inner cities and rural areas means that all Aboriginal communities are vulnerable. Research indicates that transmission among injection drug users is an increasing concern and one not limited to large urban centres (Health Canada, 1996c). A survey of gay and bisexual men found that 11.8 per cent of the overall study population knew that they were HIV-positive (Myers et al., 1993). The proportions of gay men who were HIV-positive outside of Montreal, Toronto, and Vancouver were 6.2 per cent for Ontario, 7.6 per cent for Atlantic Canada, 7.7 per cent for British Columbia/Prairies, and 9.8 per cent for Quebec. Further research is needed to determine more precisely rates of infection and trends in rural communities and the population groups found therein (Health Canada, 1996a, 1996c, 1996d).

THEMES: THE CHALLENGES AND OPPORTUNITIES

The challenges that emerge in relation to HIV/AIDS in rural Canada include denial that HIV/AIDS affects rural communities; stigma and less acceptance of diversity; isolation from social supports; lack of anonymity and issues around confidentiality; lack of services; and sustainability of HIV/AIDS work (AIDS New Brunswick, 1996a; AIDS Saskatoon, 1994; Barnsley and Bonny, 1995; Beechinor, 1996; Donovan, 1996; Infolink, 1994; Manzon and Langille, 1996; Truesdale and Vacon, 1996). A migration study demonstrated a strong pattern of persons diagnosed with AIDS leaving communities of less than 100,000 population for larger population centres (Ng et al., 1996). This likely relates to the challenges associated with smaller communities. There are also positive aspects identified that impact on the lives of persons affected by HIV/AIDS and on related services and initiatives (AIDS Saskatoon, 1994; Barnsley and Bonny, 1995; Beechinor, 1996; Infolink, 1994; Truesdale and Vacon, 1996). Literature on HIV/AIDS from the United States reveals similar challenges and opportunities (Heckman et al., 1996; Hincks Reynolds and Lynch, 1994; Mancoske et al., 1995; Rounds, 1988; Shernoff, 1996; Smith, Landau, and Bahr, 1990).

DENIAL

A report on AIDS work in rural areas (Barnsley and Bonny, 1995) cites three major studies that show an overwhelming perception that HIV/AIDS is strictly an urban phenomenon specific to certain population subgroups. The report documents that ASOs from across Canada have identified the rampant denial, shared by health professionals and the general public, of HIV/AIDS in rural communities. The denial can also be about related issues such as teen sexuality, injection drug use, and the existence of community members who are gay (Beechinor, 1996). It can be difficult to get support for HIV/AIDS initiatives when people do not see their community affected by the issue.

DIVERSITY

The description of rural communities as generally possessing conservative and moralistic values and as being less tolerant of diversity comes across strongly in US literature on AIDS (Hincks Reynolds and Lynch, 1994; Rounds, 1988; Smith, Landau, and Bahr, 1990; Shernoff, 1996). Canadian reports also allude to rural communities being more conservative than their urban counterparts (Barnsley and Bonny, 1995; Beechinor, 1996). Most often this is in reference to issues of intolerance (e.g., homophobia and negative views of persons who use injection drugs) and how this can be a barrier to education and support. For Aboriginal communities, rejecting a member with HIV/AIDS may be related to protecting the community from a perceived threat (Crown et al., 1993). ASOs report struggling to develop ways to address homophobia and other manifestations of intolerance, and face challenges in trying to design and deliver programs that are inclusive of diverse groups, as well as programming specific to Aboriginal peoples, women, youth, gay men, and others (Barnsley and Bonny, 1995; Infolink, 1994).

ISOLATION

The isolation from social supports experienced by persons affected by HIV/AIDS in rural communities is well documented (AIDS Saskatoon, 1994; Barnsley and Bonny, 1995; Beechinor, 1996; Infolink, 1994; Truesdale and Vacon, 1996). A New Brunswick needs assessment of persons affected by HIV/AIDS revealed that 17 per cent of persons living with HIV/AIDS (PHAs), and 64 per cent of family members and friends of PHAs reported feeling isolated and alone (Ploem and Olivier, 1992). Geography and population distribution alone can contribute to social isolation (Collier, 1993). People may live distant from sources of support such as a PHA group, and there may be no or few other local persons affected in a similar way or at least identified. Issues around disclosure and confidentiality also contribute to the isolation experienced by persons affected by HIV/AIDS.

CONFIDENTIALITY

Confidentiality is likely to be of greater concern in rural areas than in larger centres, which by virtue of their size provide increased anonymity (Barnsley and Bonny, 1995; Crown et al., 1993; Truesdale and Vacon, 1996). PHAs and their family members fear the loss of confidentiality and the discrimination that may occur if their situations are known (Federal Centre for AIDS, 1992). A needs assessment from New Brunswick showed that 87 per cent of PHAs had fears related to discrimination (Ploem and Olivier, 1992).

The need for organizations to have policies and procedures in place to ensure confidentiality is critical. Worries about disclosure and breaches of confidentiality impede access to supports and services. For example, people may opt to go without local supports (e.g., home care) rather than disclose their HIV status to local service providers. A US report noted that confidentiality issues prevent individuals from obtaining information and services needed to avoid transmission (e.g., a youth may be inhibited to buy condoms) (Hincks Reynolds and Lynch, 1994). Issues around confidentiality also affect those trying to deliver services, for example, by making it more difficult to reach persons in most need of prevention or support (Barnsley and Bonny, 1995; AIDS New Brunswick, 1996a). As another example, communities may be so tightly knit that it is impossible to share local disguised case examples for fear of jeopardizing someone's anonymity (e.g., mentioning that a youth at the local high school is HIV-positive), thereby inadvertently reinforcing denial.

ACCESS TO SERVICES

There is a noted lack of HIV/AIDS-related medical and psychosocial services in rural communities (AIDS New Brunswick, 1996a; Barnsley and Bonny, 1995; Federal Centre for AIDS, 1992; Infolink, 1994; Ploem and Olivier, 1992; Truesdale and Vacon, 1996). A British Columbia study suggests that persons living with AIDS outside of Vancouver are not receiving needed services (Goldstone et al., 1996). Medical specialists, clinical trial sites, and volunteer programs, for instance, may not be present in rural regions and local service providers may lack experience or be unwilling to accept HIV-positive clients or patients. As a result, people may have to travel great distances for treatment and care.

Local health-care providers need the opportunity to develop effective systems of care because seeking medical services elsewhere may feed into the intolerance and insecurities that have been associated with rural health-care providers (Infolink, 1994). Furthermore, travel creates a number of stressors. For one, PHAs may not have the financial resources for travel. Taking time off work (Rounds, 1988) and locating child care or transportation also act as barriers to travel. For some PHAs, travelling may be too physically demanding and tiring. As a consequence, people may end up going without necessary care and treatment, which can lead to a faster rate of disease progression.

SUSTAINABILITY

The sustainability of AIDS work in rural communities is a concern shared by ASOs involved in this field (AIDS Saskatoon, 1994; Barnsley and Bonny, 1995; Beechinor, 1996; Infolink, 1994). ASOs and others involved in AIDS work have found that a key component in maintaining rural projects is the ongoing support of larger organizations and that providing outreach services across large geographical areas is very costly (AIDS Saskatoon, 1994; Barnsley and Bonny, 1995; Crown et al., 1993; Malenfant, 1995). Already, some AIDS groups have had to cut services to rural regions due to lack of funding. For others, securing funding is an ongoing source of stress and detracts from time spent on direct services. The shortage of resource people and funding results in less comprehensive planning. Assessing needs, setting objectives, and evaluation may be neglected in order to respond to immediate requests for education and support. It is important to note that these struggles are happening at a time when other groups, agencies, and institutions are also trying to deliver services with reduced budgets.

POSITIVE ASPECTS

Reports on AIDS work in rural areas indicate advantages of rural life. These advantages can be of a personal nature, for example, natural beauty, serenity, distance from urban sprawl, and proximity to family (Beechinor, 1996; Truesdale and Vacon, 1996). Rural communities are also associated with a strong sense of community, a tradition of volunteerism, local resource people being easily accessible, a willingness of people to rally behind a cause, and shared values (AIDS Saskatoon, 1994; Infolink, 1994). These traits can lead to opportunities for partnerships with local groups, agencies, institutions, media, and businesses. The Pictou County AIDS Coalition in Nova Scotia is a good example of possible partnerships. This group originated with a local women's centre. Even though now established, the group benefits from the ongoing support of the women's centre, which provides office space, telephone/fax, and opportunity for mutual learning (Truesdale and Vacon, 1996).

SOCIAL WORK PRACTICE: APPROACH AND INTERVENTIONS

While there are some examples of AIDS service organizations whose origins arise directly from the rural communities they serve, for the most part ASOs from larger centres are carrying out or are facilitating this work. Furthermore, ASOs are unlikely to be set up in many rural and remote areas. The reasons for this include those related to the structural issues discussed earlier (e.g., denial, unacceptance of diversity, and sustainability). AIDS Saskatoon (1994: 5), an ASO that carries out work with rural peoples, concluded that 'due to a lack of resources, neither the public health system as it exists in rural areas nor the community based ASOs have the resources to put staff in place to work full time in all the small communities solely on AIDS issues.' Reports from the United States point to the relatively low seroprevalence rates in rural areas that make developing separate agencies not practical (Rounds, 1988), and to the absence of strongly organized gay and lesbian communities that have been critical to the establishment of AIDS organizations in larger centres (Smith, Landau, and Bahr, 1990).

ASOs located in larger centres will undoubtedly continue to be a significant factor in AIDS work in rural and remote areas. Most AIDS organizations have education and support as program objectives. Education is often defined to include prevention, health promotion, and public awareness. Support generally refers to direct services to PHAs and their families and friends, such as counselling, case management, financial aid, home support, and peer support. Advocacy is another program area of importance to ASOs. Before proceeding to discuss this work, we should look at more general issues related to AIDS work in rural communities—a generalist approach to social work and the outcome objectives of interventions.

Working in rural communities may require the ability to address a range of program objectives simultaneously or in tandem. This relates to fewer specialized services in rural areas compared to urban centres and to the shifting needs of communities. For example, a volunteer group whose primary interest is in providing support to PHAs may find that there is not enough demand for its services to keep members busy on a consistent basis. To keep these groups active and cohesive, members will likely need to get involved in other program areas such as education and public awareness. The readiness of a community to respond favourably to some initiatives may also necessitate the need for a range of program options. As an example, a group that wants to do prevention work with a local high school (including the distribution of condoms) may find that it first needs to obtain public support for this initiative by doing AIDS awareness activities. Similarly, workers are recognizing the connections between education and support objectives, and that the success in one domain may have a direct bearing on the other. For example, AIDS awareness events such as the 'walks' and presentations by PHAs will likely lead to more supportive environments for PHAs and their families. As one AIDS worker from Nova Scotia put it: 'The bottom line is that most organizations are called upon to do both service delivery and do the advocacy/education necessary to move community attitudes. Perhaps we should stop drawing lines between all these activities. They consistently overlap and traditional ways of working in communities are often barriers to creating new solutions' (Truesdale and Vacon, 1996: 13).

This broad-based approach to AIDS work in rural communities fits well with a generalist approach to social work. Collier (1993) makes a strong argument for social workers adopting a generalist practice with rural peoples. He describes a generalist approach as examining the problem and solution from many vantage points, drawing on a range of conceptual and practical approaches, and then pursuing a course that is most likely to succeed. He also recommends making full use of the range of resources available in rural environments, especially since resources are often limited.

The approach taken by ASOs in larger centres when providing services in rural areas can be classified as one of either 'outreach' or 'community development'. The two approaches, however, are not mutually exclusive. While outreach services that are not necessarily based in community development have been provided by ASOs for many years, ASOs from Vancouver Island to Newfoundland report the increasing use of community development in responding to HIV/AIDS in rural communities (Barnsley and Bonny, 1995).

COMMUNITY DEVELOPMENT

Community development can encompass many ideas as reflected in the definition used at a New Brunswick rural development workshop on AIDS:

> Community development is a way to address issues locally by identifying local needs and resources and using that information, and those persons to

> find the solutions. Community development begins with local issues and local people working together. Community development is what communities have been doing throughout the ages to solve problems themselves. It involves good communication and collaboration among several persons and organizations. Community development recognizes that the social, economic, organizational, cultural, and spiritual aspects of a community must be considered when identifying both the assets in the community and the needs (Marshall-Forgie and Simpson, cited in AIDS New Brunswick, 1996a: 1).

The opportunity for ASOs in larger centres to facilitate community development is well articulated in an AIDS Saskatoon report: 'Often there is a strong desire in rural communities to "do something about AIDS". This desire is inherent despite an uncertainty of exactly what approach to take. This creates an entry point for AIDS Saskatoon's Rural Response Project. This desire and energy can then be channelled into a constructive effort and the creation of HIV/AIDS programs designed by the community for the community' (1994: 5).

The impetus for ASOs initiating community development work can come from many sources. ASO staff may recognize the need for rural development work by listening to their clients. Toll-free AIDS information lines are good vehicles for such learning. Clients (e.g., PHAs, family members, and health, education, and social service professionals) call seeking information and guidance. These sessions reveal their needs and struggles, as well as service gaps. Formal needs assessments can also demonstrate the necessity for rural initiatives. In addition, ASOs may be organized in such ways that their governing structures encourage input from rural communities. As an example, AIDS New Brunswick's board of directors is made up of members from across the province.

The initial identification of communities for development work in Saskatchewan was based on geography, location of key individuals already known to AIDS Saskatoon, and the desire to involve key community groups, agencies, and institutions. Community meetings were then held in the identified regions. In addition to the approach taken above, ASOs in New Brunswick put on a provincial workshop on rural issues and AIDS with the goals of providing participants with enhanced skills and the encouragement to begin work in their various communities (AIDS New Brunswick, 1996a). Similarly, the Newfoundland and Labrador AIDS Committee held forums in St John's to train groups of community leaders, including doctors, nurses, school counsellors, mayors, church leaders, PHAs, and family members of PHAs (Barnsley and Bonny, 1995). The community leaders' expenses were paid, and in turn they agreed to organize meetings in their home regions.

Skills associated with social work such as research, outreach, and facilitation were critical to ensuring the success of these early phases of work. AIDS Saskatoon found that the initial contact for community meetings was best done by the project worker, whose association with an ASO provided credibility. The value of her contributions and skills were underscored in an evaluation by project participants:

> She gave them [volunteers] guidance in the beginning by running the meetings and was a good facilitator by giving them ideas for displays and letting them know what materials were available from AIDS Saskatoon. . . . The initial AIDS Saskatoon initiative and facilitation was crucial since community team members had different backgrounds and did not know each other personally. It was also important to have AIDS Saskatoon involvement because teams struggled the first year not knowing which direction they were expected to go in. Many communities did not have a foundation to establish their own goals, though they felt that education and raising awareness was the key objective for them. (AIDS Saskatoon, 1994: 11)

Having targeted communities retain or assume as much responsibility and ownership of the work as possible is a goal of most community development approaches. The relationship between volunteer team or community project and ASO may change depending on the needs and level of self-reliance of the rural group. However, the experience of rural Canada is that the community projects or teams will always require, or at least benefit from, some level of facilitation or support from the larger ASO (AIDS Saskatoon, 1994; Barnsley and Bonny, 1995; Malenfant, 1995). The following descriptions of activities provide examples of how ASO resources and worker skill can support rural development work:

- Facilitation around the development of a common vision, goals, objectives, and organizational structure.
- Skills development related to: organizational process (e.g., running meetings), designing and delivering services, and program evaluation.
- Assistance in identifying needs and community resources. Of note, computer programs have been identified as useful in mapping community capacities and assets (Sandrelli, 1996).
- Assistance in procuring information, as well as in locating or developing materials.
- Provision of ongoing communication and consultation.
- Assistance in volunteer management (e.g., recruitment, training, and supervision).
- Facilitation around accessing peer support and information-sharing through conferences, newsletters, and provincial/regional networks.
- Provision of financial support, and assistance with money management, grant applications, and planning around sustainability.
- Partnership in the delivery of direct services (e.g., case management and educational projects).
- Assistance in the promotion of services (e.g., AIDS Saskatoon helped groups produce a promotional pamphlet).
- Help in securing the support and/or collaboration of other community organizations, agencies, institutions, and local media.

The relationship between larger ASOs and rural groups has also been described as reciprocal (G. Yetman, personal communication, 22 February 1997). Rural groups and volunteer teams are part of the larger ASO and assist in the overall sustainability of the larger group by fund-raising, providing direction, and delivering programs.

Evaluations of community development efforts provide support for their value. Qualitative interviews with members of rural response teams in Saskatchewan, for instance, revealed: members feeling more comfortable and knowledgeable in discussing HIV/AIDS issues with a variety of people; success in securing grants, thus enabling the teams to deliver seminars and workshops and to produce promotional materials; members perceiving an increase in awareness and willingness on the part of communities to talk about AIDS (AIDS Saskatoon, 1994).

While most of the presentation on community development has focused on geographical communities, there are also initiatives aimed at communities organized around an 'identity' or 'issue'. The AIDS Yukon Alliance, for instance, has facilitated community development with Native peoples. It looked at designing a strategy that is holistic, culturally appropriate, and respectful of both community resource people and the community's understanding of HIV/AIDS (Barnsley and Bonny, 1995). This group has hired Native workers to carry out programming (e.g., awareness events) in the predominantly Aboriginal communities in which they live. The outcome of this work has yet to be evaluated (B. Ames, personal communication, 7 February 1997). Similarly, the Atlantic First Nations AIDS Task Force uses a community development approach that is holistic and follows a model that is family-centred and respectful of the collective nature of Aboriginal societies (K. Barlow, personal communication, 22 February 1997). An evaluation of this group revealed: the holistic approach has resulted in the integration of HIV/AIDS with other community issues; information is being provided in an effective manner for Native communities (e.g., use of talking circles); significant strides have been made towards meeting its goal of education and awareness (Mi'Kmawey Communications Consultant Group, 1995). Other groups that have been organized around an identity include PHAs, gay men, and women.

Social workers are often in positions to mobilize existing community groups and resources around a shared concern or issue. The resulting networks contribute to the sharing of information, provide peer support, and may lead to better co-ordination among service providers (Barnsley and Bonny, 1995). Developing such networks rather than setting up new organizations (e.g., volunteer groups) is often more sustainable than volunteer groups, which frequently depend on one or two key individuals. Volunteer groups often become inactive when these key volunteers cease their involvement (R. Tucker, personal communication, 11 February 1997). Responding to HIV/AIDS issues through collaboration and networking has also proved successful in rural areas in the United States (Chang-Yit, Lippert, and Thielges, 1992).

OUTREACH

Since their formation, many ASOs from larger centres have been delivering services to people in rural areas. The direct delivery of services often precedes community development work. Reasons for this include: AIDS groups not being aware of the advantages of a community development approach; communities not being ready or able to get involved in such work; and the larger ASO not having the resources to facilitate or support local initiatives. The advantages of direct service delivery must not be overlooked, however, in that the most efficient way to deliver some services (e.g., toll-free AIDS lines) is still from one central point. In addition, the continuation of some services from a larger centre ensures a minimal level of service for all.

The types of outreach ASOs provide generally fall into one of two categories: services delivered directly to persons affected by HIV/AIDS and initiatives aimed at influencing other service providers or the community at large.

ASOs from larger centres deliver direct services through many of the same means. For example, many AIDS organizations provide resource materials (e.g., pamphlets, books, and videos) by mail. While this is usually done upon request, some AIDS workers have thought of novel ways to do outreach with resource materials. The AIDS Committee of Sudbury, for example, sends safer sex pamphlets to people who place personal ads in newspapers (Barnsley and Bonny, 1995). Other means of outreach include face-to-face counselling provided by support staff who travel to rural communities, and peer support facilitated by sponsoring retreat weekends and gatherings for persons affected by HIV/AIDS.

The approaches used by ASOs to influence other service providers include advocacy, education (e.g., workshops and speakers), and collaboration in the delivery of services. For instance, in the rural community of Grand Forks, British Columbia, four agencies (Public Health and organizations representing hospice, home support, and AIDS) partnered to offer an AIDS training program to home support staff and hospice volunteers (Manzon and Langille, 1996). An AIDS group in Jasper, Alberta, partnered with local businesses to deliver HIV information in staff orientation programs and safer-sex packages, including condoms, with employee pay cheques (Infolink, 1994). Another example is AIDS New Brunswick's initiation of a project to develop a pamphlet with Public Health to reach out to individuals testing newly positive for HIV. Hospital personnel who carry out HIV antibody testing agreed to send the pamphlet along with any positive test result. Working with others in outreach need not be on a big scale, however. A PHA in rural Nova Scotia explained that he gave his name to his family physician to pass on to others who might be in need of peer support (Truesdale and Vacon, 1996). A woman whose son died of AIDS asked her local church if she could reach out to other families through an announcement in the parish bulletin.

In addition, AIDS organizations try to create more favourable social environments for those affected by HIV/AIDS and more acceptance of prevention work by organizing public education and awareness events, such as speaking tours and AIDS 'walks'.

SERVICES AND INTERVENTIONS

In many ways, the interventions used in rural regions, whether through community development or outreach, are similar to those used in urban centres. Some interventions and services are virtually the same but have important application in rural communities. Others are modified in design to meet rural needs.

Social workers may not always be involved in each of the services, but the skills associated with this profession (e.g., the skill sets related to program design, delivery, and evaluation) are always present.

AIDS Information Lines

Toll-free information lines are well suited to the provision of information and support to rural peoples. Advantages for the caller include convenience, accessibility, no cost, anonymity, and control over information revealed (Parsons, Bell, and Gilchrist, 1991). There are toll-free AIDS information lines (sometimes in conjunction with STD [sexually transmitted disease] lines) operating in every province and territory. As an example, AIDS New Brunswick (1996b) has been operating a toll-free line since 1987. Demographic information on callers demonstrates that the phone line is being used by a diverse segment of the population, 25 per cent of whom reside outside of the province's three main urban centres. The nature of the requests has ranged from basic AIDS information to more in-depth questions regarding risk assessment, prevention, and testing. The information line is frequently used by PHAs, their family members and friends, and persons in helping professions. For these individuals, the information line provides access to other agency services (e.g., counselling) and referral to outside resources.

Toll-free lines are also being used for more specialized services and with specific target groups. The Atlantic First Nations AIDS Task Force, for example, operates a toll-free line accessible from anywhere in Canada. The Community AIDS Treatment Information Exchange (CATIE) provides a national HIV treatment information service. While a thorough evaluation of its 1-800 line has not been completed, anecdotal reports indicate that professionals and PHAs in rural communities are finding the service valuable (G. Brown, personal communication, 7 February 1997). Peer education and support programs, such as those directed towards 'men who have sex with men' and PHAs, are another type of targeted service being delivered through toll-free lines (AIDS New Brunswick, 1996b).

Resource Materials

Resource materials need to be chosen or designed with specific audiences in mind. For instance, a rural project worker in Ontario concluded that people in his 'area are most comfortable with the plain pamphlets produced by Health and Welfare Canada. They don't want "jazzy", big city stuff from Toronto' (Barnsley and Bonny, 1995: 90). An HIV prevention project in the Northwest Territories, as another example, recommends that materials be culturally relevant, written in plain language, and translated into local languages, as well as include illustrations to deliver the message (Crown et al., 1993). Furthermore, this project found that since some languages are primarily oral (e.g., Dene languages), audio cassettes are more appropriate than written materials. The Internet is a resource being used more and more by social workers and clients alike. Vast amounts of information can be accessed via the Internet and many of the sites are thoroughly researched (e.g., CATIE's Web site). In addition, chat lines may provide a source of both information and support (Shernoff, 1996).

Awareness Events

Theatre, mall, and health-fair displays, as well as presentations at schools, workplaces, and public forums, have been used to increase audiences' general awareness of HIV/AIDS issues. AIDS 'walks' are another means used to raise public awareness. Success in sensitizing people to issues of diversity has been reported through the involvement of PHAs and others affected by HIV/AIDS in program delivery (e.g., gay HIV-positive speakers). Speaking tours may be of particular importance in areas where no local people are able to come forward to speak publicly (Barnsley and Bonny, 1995). AIDS New Brunswick has organized several tours where PHAs have spoken to junior high and high school students. Evaluations indicate positive benefits on students' knowledge, attitudes, and intended behaviours (Ploem, 1995).

Counselling

The issues that emerge in counselling persons affected by HIV/AIDS in rural Canada include confidentiality, disclosure, isolation, establishing or enhancing support networks, accessing information and services, and advocacy.

It is worth noting again the usefulness of the telephone in addressing geographical isolation and concerns around confidentiality. This author has counselled numerous PHAs and family members by telephone. While most of this work has been episodic, centring on specific issues or problems, the worker/client relationship is often ongoing. The nature of this relationship can be illustrated by a case example.

An older man with asymptomatic HIV infection contacted an ASO support worker by telephone shortly after returning to live in the small town where he had grown up. The man explained that he preferred to keep his distance from siblings and other relatives for fear that they might suspect his homosexuality or HIV status, and that he had no intention of ever telling anyone in his small community about his illness. He saw himself as likely to commit suicide if his status became known by some breach of confidentiality or if symptoms prevented him from hiding his illness. Since distance was a barrier to in-person meetings, he and the counsellor agreed to a series of phone sessions. Their work revolved around issues related to self-esteem, suicide, homosexuality, family, illness, treatment, and available supports. Over time, the man came to the decision to move away from his community if there came a point when he could no longer keep his illness secret. He continues to have contact with the support worker every month or so, when he wants to check in or is in need of emotional support or information. While he is still reluctant to disclose his status to anyone, he does participate anonymously in a telephone support group for PHAs.

Counselling in the context of a person 'coming home' frequently arises in HIV/AIDS work in rural areas (Graham, Brownlee, and Ritchie, 1996; Shernoff, 1996; Rounds, 1988). This process is best started before the person actually moves or returns to a rural community. In this way one can ensure that the necessary supports (e.g., financial, medical, emotional, home, etc.) are in place. It can be very stressful for a PHA to move somewhere and then learn that services are not available or that there is a waiting period (which is the case for some provincial government services when a person comes from out of province). There may also be issues related to disclosure and establishing peer support, and family members will likely need some assistance in preparation for their loved one's return (e.g., finding or maintaining a support system, locating resources, and facing issues related to loss and grief).

Support Groups

Support groups for persons affected by HIV/AIDS can be difficult to start and maintain in rural areas. This is due to the small number of persons who might fit the group membership (e.g., PHAs or family members) and the reluctance on the part of those affected to participate because of concerns about confidentiality.

Two case examples illustrate these issues. In one case, a PHA and a family member from the same area asked a social worker with an ASO for assistance in setting up a support group (the two individuals were unrelated and their requests were independent of each other). Because it was unlikely that there would be other interested participants for some time, the social worker proposed starting a combined group (i.e., for both PHAs and family/friends of PHAs). The possible dynamics of a combined group (primarily related to differing needs) were factored into the decision to proceed. The members chose an open-ended group format. Over time the group increased in size to five. Members reported that the group, even with its combined membership and range of individual member issues, was meeting their needs. The social worker attended some meetings and acted as a resource person for the group facilitator (one of the original members). He was also the contact for persons inquiring about joining the group.

In the second case, a woman whose husband died of AIDS attempted, with the help of a social worker, to set up a support group for family and friends. This time the efforts were not successful as there was not the membership interest to sustain a group. However, the woman offered to provide peer support on a one-to-one basis. This format proved more popular, perhaps because it provided more security around confidentiality. The social worker connected persons with the woman and also acted as a resource person.

Support groups can also be facilitated through conference calls, thus allowing people isolated by geography, unable to travel due to illness, caregiving responsibilities, or limited transportation, or fearful of jeopardizing their anonymity the opportunity to participate (Barnsley and Bonny, 1995; Rittner and Hammons, 1992; Rounds, Galinsky, and Stevens, 1991). While there are no published reports of HIV/AIDS telephone groups in Canada, there are studies of their use in the United States with PHAs (Rittner and Hammons, 1992; Rounds, Galinsky, and Stevens, 1991); caregivers (Meier, Galinsky, and Rounds, 1995); and gay and bisexual males on reducing risks of transmission (Roffman et al., 1995). Conference call groups also allow the participation of resource persons from anywhere there is a telephone.

Practical Support

The role of the social worker will often involve assisting the client in locating and accessing services. The worker might need to take the role of an educator or client advocate to ensure that the client receives appropriate services. In addition, volunteer teams can be organized to provide practical support (e.g., visits, transportation, and help with household tasks). Models for organizing such teams have been developed specifically with rural areas in mind (Kinjerski, 1996) and a community development approach is useful in areas where there is no local ASO. The social worker may also need to provide co-ordination among the various informal and formal supports.

LOOKING TO THE FUTURE

Social workers in most fields of practice in rural Canada will likely have some contact with HIV/AIDS issues. This could take the form of prevention work or support to PHAs and their family and friends. A review of epidemiological reports provides only limited data on infection rates and trends within rural populations. Further research in this area is needed to better plan targeted education and support programs. AIDS service organizations provided ample description of their approaches to work and the services that they provide in rural communities. Information on impact or outcome evaluations is harder to find. Many ASOs do not have the resources to thoroughly evaluate the programs they deliver. Further research is critical to identify the approaches and interventions that are working and to develop even more effective ones. Topics that need to be studied include organizational structures, approaches to work, interventions, and sustainability. More needs to be written about the work being carried out by social workers in settings other than ASOs.

Research findings need to be shared with social work educators and practitioners. Information-sharing and skills-building need to be ongoing. The development of networks of persons involved in rural AIDS work is one way to share information. The importance of networking was stressed at a national gathering on rural issues and HIV/AIDS (AIDS Jasper, 1995). Vehicles suggested for networking included a national rural newsletter, communications through the Internet or a 1-800 line, and future gatherings at national, regional, and local levels.

Public policy needs to support AIDS work in general, as well as that which is specific to rural communities. The National AIDS Strategy has provided much-needed funding for a wide range of research as well as for the operation of AIDS organizations. The strategy needs to be a permanent vehicle in the fight against AIDS. Public health policy and funding at provincial levels must ensure that critical services and interventions are in place (e.g., toll-free information lines, anonymous testing sites, and treatment and care for PHAs). There is much to take comfort in with respect to AIDS work in rural communities. The interventions and services being used are creative and comprehensive in scope. Funding is needed to continue this work; research is needed to improve on it.

Acknowledgements
I wish to thank Gerard Yetman of the Newfoundland and Labrador AIDS Committee, Barbara Ames of AIDS Yukon Alliance, Kevin Barlow of Atlantic First

Nations AIDS Task Force, Ruth Ann Tucker of AIDS Vancouver Island, Glen Brown of CATIE, and Jeff Dobbs of AIDS Saskatoon, all of whom provided me with valuable updates on their respective organizations.

REFERENCES

AIDS Jasper. 1995. 'Gathering on Rural Issues and HIV/AIDS: Evaluation Summary, Analysis, and Recommendations'. Jasper, Alta: AIDS Jasper, Oct.

AIDS New Brunswick. 1996a. 'Rural Development Workshop notes'. Fredericton: AIDS New Brunswick, Nov.

———. 1996b. 'Funding Application: AIDS New Brunswick Information Line'. Fredericton: AIDS New Brunswick, July.

AIDS Saskatoon. 1994. AIDS *Saskatoon—Rural Response Project: Facilitating a Rural Response*, final report. Saskatoon: AIDS Saskatoon, Mar.

Barnsley, C., and S. Bonny. 1995. *Community Education and Development in Small Towns and Rural Areas*. Ottawa: Canadian AIDS Society, Mar.

Beechinor, K. 1996. 'AIDS Education in the West Kootenay/Boundary District of British Columbia', *Canadian AIDS News* 8, 4: 16–17.

Canadian Public Health Association. 1996. *Canadian AIDS News* 8, 4.

Chang-Yit, L., M.A. Lippert, and I. Thielges. 1992. 'Model for Rural Collaboration for AIDS Education: A Case Study', *Family and Community Health* 15, 3: 62–9.

Clarke, R.G. 1995. *Social Work Practice and Practice Wisdom in the Field of HIV/AIDS: Research Report*. Ottawa: Canadian Association of Social Workers, Oct.

Collier, K. 1993. *Social Work with Rural Peoples*, 2nd edn. Vancouver: New Star.

Crown, M., K. Duncan, M. Hurrell, R. Ootoova, R. Tremblay, and S. Yazdanmehr. 1993. 'Making HIV Prevention Work in the North', *Canadian Journal of Public Health* 84, supp. 1: 55–8.

Donovan, C. 1996. 'Small, Rural Communities Pose Unique Challenge for AIDS work', *Canadian AIDS News* 8, 4: 1–2, 21.

Federal Centre for AIDS. 1992. *Ending the Isolation: HIV Disease and Mental Health in the Second Decade*. Ottawa: Health and Welfare Canada.

Goldstone, I., A. Schilder, R. Hogg, R. Hanvelt, K. Craib, G. Bradford, T. Perry, and M. O'Shaughnessy. 1996. 'A Profile of Health Care and Informal Support Services Received by Persons with HIV and AIDS in Vancouver and British Columbia', paper presented to the XIth International AIDS Conference, Vancouver, July.

Graham, J.R., K. Brownlee, and I. Ritchie. 1996. 'AIDS, Social Work, and the Coming Home Phenomenon', *The Social Worker* 64, 4: 74–84.

Health Canada. 1996a. *HIV and AIDS among Women in Canada*. Ottawa, Dec.

———. 1996b. *HIV and AIDS in Canada*. Ottawa, Dec.

———. 1996c. *HIV/AIDS among Injection Drug Users in Canada*. Ottawa, Dec.

———. 1996d. *HIV/AIDS Epidemiology among Aboriginal Peoples in Canada*. Ottawa, Dec.

———. 1998. *HIV and AIDS in Canada: Surveillance Report to December 31, 1997*. Ottawa, Apr.

Heckman, T.G., A.M. Somlai, J.A. Kelly, L.Y. Stevenson, and K. Galdabini. 1996. 'Reducing Barriers to Care and Improving Quality of Life for Rural Persons with HIV', *AIDS Patient Care* (Feb.): 37–43.

Hincks Reynolds, J., and S. Lynch. 1994. *No Immunity: Preventing HIV Infection among Rural Youth*. Washington: Advocates for Youth, June.

Infolink. 1994. 'Proceedings of HIV/AIDS and Rural Issues Gathering'. Jasper, Alta, Oct.

King, A.J.C., R.P. Beazley, and W. Warren. 1988. *Canada Youth and AIDS: National Report to Health Canada*. Ottawa.

Kinjerski, V. 1996. 'Rural Northern Alberta Supports PWAs and Their Families, Friends', *Canadian AIDS News* 8, 4: 9–10.

Malenfant, A. 1995. *A Project to Enhance the Delivery of Support/Health Promotion, Education and Advocacy Programs from a Province-wide Volunteer Base*, final report. Fredericton: AIDS New Brunswick.

Mancoske, R.J., C. Martin Wadsworth, D.S. Dugas, and J.A. Hasney. 1995. 'Suicide Risk among People Living with AIDS', *Social Work* 40, 6: 783–7.

Manzon, L., and M. Langille. 1996. 'New Community Partnerships Provide Training in Home-centred Care for PHAs', *Canadian AIDS News* 8, 4: 17.

Meier, A., M.J. Galinsky, and K.A. Rounds. 1995. 'Telephone Support Groups for Caregivers of Persons with AIDS', *Social Work with Groups* 18, 1: 99–108.

Mi'Kmawey Communications Consultant Group. 1995. *Atlantic First Nations AIDS Task Force Evaluation*. West Dover, Nova Scotia, May.

Myers, T., G. Godin, L. Calzavara, J. Lambert, and D. Locker. 1993. *The Canadian Survey of Gay and Bisexual Men and HIV Infection: Men's Survey*. Ottawa: Canadian AIDS Society.

New Brunswick Health and Community Services. 1995. *Quarterly Surveillance Report for HIV and AIDS in New Brunswick*. Fredericton, Sept.

Ng, E., J. Whitehead, R.S. Hogg, M. Ricketts, P. Lalonde, M. Fair, T. Le, and M.T. Schechter. 1996. 'Migration Patterns of Persons with AIDS in Canada from Time of Index AIDS Diagnosis to Death', poster session presented at the XIth International AIDS Conference, Vancouver, July.

Parsons, D.C., M.A. Bell, and L.D. Gilchrist. 1991. 'Evaluation of the British Columbia AIDS Information Line', *Canadian Journal of Public Health* 82: 399–403.

Ploem, C. 1995. *HIV/AIDS Education Francophone Outreach Project, Health Regions 4 and 6*, final report and evaluation. Fredericton: AIDS New Brunswick, Jan.

———, and C. Olivier. 1992. *Meeting the Challenge: A Needs Assessment of Persons Affected by HIV/AIDS in New Brunswick*. Fredericton: AIDS New Brunswick.

Rittner, B., and K. Hammons. 1992. 'Telephone Group Work with People with End Stage AIDS', *Social Work with Groups* 15, 4: 59–72.

Roffman, R.A., B. Beadnell, R. Ryan, and L. Downey. 1995. 'Telephone Group Counseling in Reducing AIDS Risk in Gay and Bisexual Males', *Journal of Gay and Lesbian Social Services* 2, 3–4: 145–57.

Rounds, K.A. 1988. 'AIDS in Rural Areas: Challenges to Providing Care', *Social Work* 33, 3: 257–61.

———, M.J. Galinsky, and L.S. Stevens. 1991. 'Linking People with AIDS in Rural Communities: The Telephone Group', *Social Work* 36, 1: 13–18.

Sandrelli, M.A. 1996. 'Demographic Mapping of Rural Communities First Step in Empowerment', *Canadian AIDS News* 8, 4: 4–5.

Shernoff, M. 1996. 'Returning with AIDS: Supporting Rural Emigrants', *Focus*, 11, 4: 1–4.

Smith, J.E., J. Landau, and G.R. Bahr. 1990. 'AIDS in Rural and Small Town America: Making the Heartland Respond', *AIDS Patient Care* 4: 17–21.

Truesdale, D., and C. Vacon. 1996. 'The Nova Scotia Rural Development and AIDS Conference Report', Aug.

Chapter 9

Taking the Medicine Wheel to the Street

Counselling Aboriginal Street Youth about HIV/AIDS and Educating Those Who Help Them

JUDY WEISER, WITH CONNIE FIFE, ALBERT MCLEOD,
KECIA LARKIN, DOLAN BADGER, AND TIA EAGLES-CLAW

It is difficult to credit that which we perceive as overwhelming with any sense of immediacy—it's easier to say 'why bother?'

—Ken Garnhum, from 'Beuys Buoys Boys', in R. Wallace, ed., *Making Out—Plays by Gay Men* (Toronto: Coach House Press, 1993), 85–7.

INTRODUCTION

Anyone who has become HIV-positive quickly learns that it is not simply a physical problem being experienced—there are always mental, emotional, and spiritual aspects influencing the quality and direction of daily life with HIV. So often it is not AIDS itself that is the problem (i.e., its medical definition), but rather what AIDS *means* inside the mind, feelings, and spirit that will affect the path of each person's journey while living with the virus.

Frequently, only the medical aspects of treatment or prevention are given attention, as if maintaining the body's physical health is the patient's sole responsibility, while far too often there is much less preparation for encountering, understanding, or coping with the numerous psychosocial issues that may also arise. The consequences of living daily with HIV and its resulting limitations not directly connected to medical problems, such as poverty or homelessness, are sometimes harder to deal with due to their more subtle and socially isolating nature. This is especially true for individuals without a strong emotional support system of family or friends.

Many youth have grown up with AIDS already being part of their reality during adolescence—it has been an unavoidable and integral part of their life rather than something new invading the emotional security of youth. For any young person, this could easily lead to feeling defeated before ever having had a chance to get started in life. Apathy and resigned acceptance are understandable responses to feeling powerless in the face of danger. Youth, who already assume a talisman of invincibility against death, seem to be facing the threat of HIV with an increasing attitude of inevitability.

For the several hundred youth in each major Canadian city who have left home environments too abusive or emotionally toxic to stay, or who have not managed to adapt to foster homes, living on the street is their only real alternative. Surviving by any means necessary within this desperate poverty and alienation becomes their total focus:

> If you're on the street, your primary needs are getting food and a safe dry place to sleep or you have to walk around all night. You need a place to live where you can rest without fear of being attacked or having your stuff stolen. Things like a bus pass and medical insurance help, too, as does money, but simply staying alive comes first.
>
> Being HIV-positive is not so concrete a thing as eating and surviving; it can wait, unless you're sick. But when you're sick, it's hard to know if it's from eating out of dumpsters, drugs, street abuse, or what. So the idea that there's this slow-growing virus is no big thing—you'll deal with it later when the problem gets bigger. In the meantime, you just lock it away in a closet in your mind and keep focusing on more urgent things like getting food or a place to sleep for that night.
>
> My life's already been screwed by HIV anyway, so why should I worry about infecting a trick? He's using me; why should I care about him? Nobody ever did anything nice for me, except my brothers on the street—why should I have to look out for somebody else? If they demand a condom, fine; if they don't and I can get more money that way, why not? (R.S., 1997)

In the case of street youth, and particularly First Nations street youth (most of whom initially thought themselves invulnerable because rumour had it that only White men got AIDS), HIV is often considered just one more of many personal crises to be dealt with alone and outside the usual social support systems available to those less marginalized and more societally integrated. 'Aboriginals account for up to 70 per cent of the street youth population in many Canadian cities. Overt racism . . . makes already harsh living conditions worse for Aboriginal youth. It also makes it harder for them to escape the vicious cycle of disconnection from family, home, history, and culture' (Gilchrist, 1995, as quoted in Ker, 1995: 1).

Street youth are often involved in prostitution or selling drugs in trade for food or shelter, and substance abuse becomes a way to numb oneself against daily horrors or loneliness. Aboriginal youth are no exception:

> I remember watching my Mom go out the door and wondering when I'd be eating again, because there'd been no food in the house for a few days already. My Dad had just beat up on her, and when she left he started punching me. Me and my sisters ran into the bush and hid out until it was dark. I woke up hungry and wet, and decided right then to just keep away, and just kept going.
>
> I came to the city with my friend and he taught me how to work the street. At least now I have a hotel room and can buy food and drugs. I don't do lots of drugs, just enough to keep me from being so afraid of the johns. (E.F., 1997)

This is a subculture with a value system quite different from those of young people securely tucked away in suburban homes with families who love them and schools that understand their needs. They are often the children of parents raised in the residential school system, whose cultural values were eroded by 'misplaced fixing'. Alienated by force from traditional ways, their only reality was marginalization and internalized racism—they were left little else of themselves and their life's purpose (Chrisjohn and Young, 1996). Self-esteem is usually close to being non-existent in most of the Aboriginal street youth I have encountered, as is even the concept of there being something called a 'self' in the first place, never mind one that has the right to be treated decently. As one such youth explained it:

> There was 'Indian', and there was 'White'—and an entire universe between them. I only knew what I'd lived, and that was, at least on my reserve, that 'Native' was real second-class, full of despair, danger, and no future.
>
> If you'd told me a few years ago that some day I'd come to a point where I'd feel some pride in my culture, I'd have laughed you off the street. No way! If I could have turned my skin white I would have, immediately. Now I'm beginning to meet guys like me who are succeeding and get respect, even though their skin is dark like mine—what a new concept! (N.S., 1997)

Who to trust and whose advice to believe are issues nearly insurmountable, and dependable role models who can bridge the gap between youth and social services, or medical personnel able to provide help, are even rarer for the Aboriginal street youth community (which in age actually ranges far wider than ages typically considered 'adolescence'—street 'youth' I have worked with have ranged from under 10 years old to sometimes past the late twenties). And it *is* a true community, family of affiliation and similarity supplanting birth family ties and replacing relatives' traditional influence. The individual's sense of obligation is to peers with whom he/she shares more in common.

> It's really frustrating because it always comes down to those things that happen: the alcoholism and sexual abuse that nobody wants to talk about. That's why we're running away. That's why we don't want to be at home. That's why we're going out and getting high so we can't feel anything, so we don't have to think about those things. That's why we're not where we're supposed to be.
>
> Because of that little piece of hell that we carry around inside that we don't want to talk about because nobody else knows how we're feeling. Yet everybody feels the same way. (Larkin, 1997)

Although Aboriginal street youth may report to non-Native medical staff for HIV-testing and treatment when there is an immediate medical crisis, large gaps still exist between current forms of delivery of treatment/prevention information and the ability of most Aboriginal street youth to understand and make use of those facts. When not in the doctor's office, most of these youth find HIV less of a priority than the basics of daily survival. When medical decline begins, they have less knowledge of how to access treatment, less successful experience doing so, and less awareness of the importance of early intervention and active partnerships with doctors.

Although, ideally, 'it is important to establish an environment of trust in which information is shared and decisions are made jointly' (Peterkin, 1996: 27), for most urban Aboriginal street youth, approaching their own health care proactively and trusting medical professionals are simply not activities they are familiar with, and so they most often deal with HIV by denial, procrastination, self-sabotaging behaviours such as substance abuse to numb or distract, and/or unabated despair:

> Teens aged fifteen to twenty-four . . . have a suicide rate three times higher than the rest of the adolescent population. . . . The role of self-esteem in the practice of safer IV drug use, alcohol abuse, and sexual behaviour is critical. . . . Abused children . . . who run away to urban centres are at a high risk for prostitution and IV drug use; such individuals have very little concern for their own safety, as they have never experienced it in the past, and have no perception that they are of any value worth protecting. (Pow, 1997: 5–6)

Peers may provide some relief but are rarely factually informed enough to provide practical help. And many simple basic facts, such as the possibility of long-term survival or that some bothersome ailments are curable along the way, are rarely available (or believed) on the street.

An HIV-positive diagnosis is an emotional rape, a violation of a person's innocence, of his/her guarantee of a future and the right to health. Once diagnosed, HIV becomes part of everything else the person does and plans and thinks about, always there, even if not always in the foreground. People with the virus become eternally vigilant for even the slightest sign of poor health, and *nothing* can replace that loss of innocence and turn their lives back to what they were like before. Feelings of helplessness and seemingly intolerable levels of anxiety become part of daily life; feelings of shame, of 'feeling dirty' or unworthy of the caring offered by friends or family, can complicate sharing the stresses even further. One youth explained it as HIV always being there, riding along on his left shoulder, whispering in his ear.

Helping these youth is difficult, but not impossible. It has become obvious to those trying to provide psychosocial or medical support that, to help most street youth change HIV-related behaviours or take more responsibility for better self-care of their health as they try to survive AIDS, methods different from those used in treating mainstream, middle-class, well-educated youth need to be found.

More precisely, an environment needs to be created that will permit these youth to initiate a desire for learning more about preventing or living with HIV, where their feelings and fears can be expressed safely and received with respect and lack of judgement by both peers and counsellors, and where need for changing behaviours or self-perceptions can be perceived as being self-initiated and done from a position of strength rather than from shame or weakness.

Very simply, they need a 'home base' where they can learn that they are not alone, where role models successful at dealing with HIV can be found *from within their own culture*, a group of people like themselves who can be trusted to help each other out and not divulge confidences shared. This need is no different from anyone else living with HIV—but it has been my experience that Aboriginal street youth do not usually initiate the founding of formal support groups. Some of them are so estranged from their communities and families that they may not even be aware of resources for counselling, visiting, or traditional healing available to them as part of their rights as band members (Peterkin, 1996: 35). Others who are non-status or Métis have no idea how to avoid being trapped in between the various support systems and need help with discovering resources they have a right to access.

Long before modern technology and scientific advancements resulted in Western medicine's current emphasis on treating specific isolated parts of the body without equal attention to its inseparable wholeness, many indigenous cultures have a long history of not making any distinction between physical healing and spiritual healing, and this is certainly true for most First Nations world-views. Many doctors and scientists are now beginning to return to focusing on these less tangible kinds of mind-body connections, as demonstrated by the growing interest in fields such as psycho-neuroimmunology. Attention is finally being paid to the evident effects of people's emotions, thoughts, and attitudes on their state of physical health and the ability of their immune systems to mobilize healing.

However, most Aboriginal people never believed otherwise, and although urban street youth may be geographically far removed from their home communities, their roots are still deeply there, even if only in rebellion to traditional ways. Because of this, some of the teachings their families have long used can still be put to effective use in the city and on the street, as long as they are presented in a non-preaching, non-judgemental, and non-coercive manner.

More specifically, two aspects of traditional Native healing practices have been used directly or indirectly for the past few years with Aboriginal street youth in Vancouver and other cities by counsellors doing group and/or one-to-one work with them (although not often in the usual kind of office or agency setting): (1) *the Medicine Wheel*, the traditional model adapted as a framework for teaching information about AIDS prevention, treatment, and self-care,[1] as well as a focus for discussion and counselling about related life issues; and (2) *the Healing Circle*, a regular (usually weekly) drop-in opportunity to share, to be listened to with respect and without judgement, to learn factual information as a serendipitous by-product of the process, to encounter healthy Aboriginal HIV-infected or affected role models, and probably most importantly, to find peers and counsellors who can be trusted and counted on for help outside the Circle event itself.

As well, both of these have been used conceptually as teaching models in various programs to train and sensitize counsellors, youth workers, and others about the different subtleties HIV/AIDS might present in the lives of their future Aboriginal clients. Of course, implications also exist for the counsellors' own self-care, especially if they are Aboriginal themselves.

Although the examples in this chapter arise from my personal experiences in counselling and teaching, this is not meant to suggest that Vancouver is the first or only place that such models have ever been used. Medicine Wheels and Healing Circles have been part of traditional teachings for centuries prior to any cities' existence in Canada, and numerous agencies across Canada (such as Healing Our Spirit BC First Nations AIDS Society in Vancouver, Manitoba Aboriginal AIDS Task Force in Winnipeg, Feather of Hope in Edmonton, Atlantic First Nations AIDS Task Force in Halifax, and others) have used these and other traditional teachings, such as the Teaching Turtle (McLeod et al., 1996), as models for successful interventions with Aboriginal street youth for many years prior to my having started my specific work with them.

I wish to be clear that the cultural information summarized below did not originate with me, but rather is my best attempt at distilling and sharing learnings from a variety of teachers, such as Leonard Johnston and Frederick Haineault, who were the first to use the Wheel for HIV/AIDS education when they began Healing Our Spirit in 1991, and Dolan Badger (a recent educator for that organization, who clarified many of its details for me), and also from the many clients and friends whose teachings through informal encounters provided me the best opportunities to learn through personal experience.

It is extremely important to note that there is a big difference between my becoming sensitized to the cultural information that helps me to better help my clients (and myself) and my assumption that this awareness now gives me an inherent right or role to present this information as if I now 'own' it. I am the student here, and I am not Aboriginal, nor do I wish to pretend that I am. However, this is the community in which I feel most at home and prefer to be. I help any time that I am asked or invited to, but this is far different from assuming that help is needed before it is asked for, or that I have a right or obligation to inflict my ideas just because I might be well intentioned.

It is with deep respect that I offer reflections on what I have learned so far, in the hope that this may help others—but I am not suggesting that people like me should take on any active sole-leadership roles in activities like the Circle described below. Sometimes the best kind of help that can be offered is supportive silence and background 'invisible' helping. Most Aboriginal people I know are tired of Euro-Canadians assuming Native People are not educated in the first place just because they have been educated differently.

> It is not suggested that non-Natives presume to teach Aboriginal youth about their world, but rather that non-Natives need to become more sensitized not only to the reasons that such awareness is so vitally necessary, but also to the reasons that it really won't work for them to be doing this activation from their inalterably outside position. (Fife, 1997)

THE MEDICINE WHEEL

Explaining the Medicine Wheel as 'a traditional conceptual model for teaching numerous understandings about life' is a *vast* understatement of the fullness and richness of its meaning to the many First Nations people whose cultures use it as a rich source of knowledge about the cycles, rhythms, and meaning of life itself. Its significance lies not only in the concepts its framework maps, but also in their interrelatedness and further connections to other levels of living and being.

The Wheel, also known as the 'Circle of Life' or 'Cycle of Life', represents time and seasons of nature and humans, demonstrating their connection to Mother Earth and to the lives of all inhabiting and being nurtured by her. It also describes the parts of a person that exist within the reciprocity of other parts, as well as their goal of harmony and relationship—and thus also shows the path towards healing by striving to better balance all the aspects to the greater good of the whole-beyond-its-parts.

The model is an unbroken circle, ever cycling in life's eternal revolutions; the goal is not to drive out disharmonious or potentially destructive parts, but rather to encompass them as natural contrasting components coexisting within the larger, flexibly adjusting balance. ' "Evil" cannot be eradicated, but turned into something that is more in balance with the universe, and indeed, the universe would not be in balance without the "Evil". . . . Evil doesn't disappear . . . it takes on more manageable form that a person can live with on a daily basis' (Tafoya, 1997: 2).

Along with the traditionally important symbol of a wheel, a circle, a full wholeness of cycles, the number 'four' assumes a powerful place in most Aboriginal cultures, playing an important role in every aspect of being. The Medicine Wheel encompasses many interrelated levels of the four aspects of things; for example, the four directions (East, South, West, North), each representing cycles of seasons and stages of life, each with its own animal symbols and spirit colours connecting to the natural aspect it relates to, or as another example, the four races (red, yellow, black, and white). Over time, occasional variations have evolved between different descriptions of the Wheel, depending on each Native nation's tradition of application, so the following examples (from Cree teachings) may not match other models exactly, but all Wheels have a similar overall structure and content. The details may vary from nation to nation; what is most important is that the concept of the Wheel and the way it is used is known to all.

At the right is East, which begins the quadrant of yellow (daybreak), turning next to South. From South to West is white (high noon when the sun is at its hottest), moving to West. From West is red (the colour of the setting sun), and the final turning is to North (black for night).[2] These are also seasonally representative from the new yellow-green young growth of spring, the dry high sun of summer, the autumnal colours of leaves, and the dark long nights of winter and nature's resting.[3]

The Wheel also describes the four stages of human life (child, youth, adult, and elder) as well as the four aspects of life itself (physical, emotional, mental, and spiritual). These four aspects are part of every individual, whether or not the person actually accesses them or is consciously aware of their internal existence.

East to South is child/physical (children being very active, touching and experiencing all things as directly as possible). From South to West is youth/

emotional (adolescence being well known as a time of turbulence with strong body/emotional changes). West to North is adult/mental (a time for more rational, cognitive experiencing through thinking), and North back again to East is elder/spiritual (like winter, a time for endings and rebirth, as Mother Earth prepares once again for separating, and then rejoining, spirit and matter).

Each stage and each aspect of human life is necessary for the formation of a fully healthy person; to neglect or diminish the worth of any of them throws health and/or life itself out of balance. To be whole, each aspect needs specialized attention for growth and healing, and each needs to be focused on every day of one's life. 'There is not just one fixed "correct" traditional Medicine Wheel—it's a learning tool where different peoples have adapted it to fit their own particular culture. . . . It's not each exact detail that's so important as the recognition of the whole, that the Wheel is universal . . . that we are all on that Wheel together, and the transitions are not fixed passages' (McLeod, 1997).

Most First Nations also have some tradition of using smoke from burning special plants as a means of cleansing, purification, grounding 'negative energy', keeping away harmful spirits and welcoming in good ones. This smoke-covering/bathing ritual, often called 'smudging' (also sometimes called 'brushing' or 'wiping', since an eagle feather is usually used to rhythmically move the smoke around), is used to clear and harmonize the physical environment (including one's body), and is also often done to prepare a room, or the people in it, for special events, ceremonies, or discussions to occur.

The substances used in smudging (the 'medicines') differ among various Native nations, particularly those geographically separated, but there are traditionally also four of these medicines, each representing one of the four directions (though, again, each nation will have evolved its own unique variations over time): sweetgrass from the East, sage from the South, cedar or tobacco from the West, and from the North, a fungus that grows on the north side of weeping willows.[4]

People of many (but not all) Aboriginal nations will be accustomed to smudging themselves and/or brushing their environments with different medicines, depending on each nation's cultural traditions. Those nations whose traditions do include smudging will usually begin ceremonies (including Healing and other kinds of Circles) with each person being offered the opportunity to take part by smudging themselves either as they enter the door or in turn around the Circle as they stand at its beginning. Even if a particular medicine is not available in a specific territory, or if people of a particular nation do not smudge at all, most are still aware of what others have traditionally used, even if not done that way in their own territory. Again, it is the process and overall concept that matters more than any particular details.

The Medicine Wheel also must be conceived of as an integrated whole that is so much more than the sum of its individual parts. All four aspects and the quadrant areas connecting them have a place on the Wheel and are deeply interconnected. Every part is needed to complete the whole, yet each is different. Each provides context for the others but all are not the same. They connect through the middle, as well as through each other, since even the centre is made up of all parts without them losing their distinct identities even while blended. The full model must be conceptualized in a minimum of four dimensions.

Thus, each aspect of life is an integral part of life itself, which cannot continue without all of them doing their parts to keep the entire wholeness alive, healthy, balanced, nurturing, and supportive of life itself. People are their own agents of healing, and the goal is to attain balance not only among all the parts but also in their relationships with others. 'A person is a mental, emotional, physical, and spiritual being who grows and changes through the existence of vision and will. All these relationships affect each other' (Young and Paul, 1995: 100). And when HIV/AIDS is perceived through the Medicine Wheel's framework, implicit in the middle where all these connect in wholeness and balance can be found the immune system, functioning as a natural fusion of mental, emotional, and spiritual with physical.[5]

Similarly, in the circle of individuals, families, and communities, everyone is a part of the Medicine Wheel of life. Each is somehow different, yet equal, and each is needed to form the whole, like individual links in a chain joined together even though no two are exactly alike. In terms of using this model in HIV/AIDS treatment and education, this message also carries the signal that even though people's HIV status might make them 'different', all persons living with the virus are nevertheless part of the circle and should not be excluded. This also subtly signals that discriminating against some people, cutting their links with others based on their differences, will break the chain and leave the Wheel no longer whole.

Although not all Aboriginal cultures use the Medicine Wheel, they certainly incorporate aspects of its underlying concepts and teachings in their daily lives. Therefore, even though Aboriginal youth may come from nations where the Wheel was not part of their upbringing, they nevertheless will understand what it is about, even if only at the deeper level of collective unconscious. And using it is a way to join together street youth from east of the mountains with those with whom they might not initially think they would share much in common. Finding these deeper connections can be a beginning towards reunification with cultural traditions and the family ties bridging them.

Aboriginal people's traditional sources (and definitions) of help usually involved relationships with nature, spirituality, tradition, and culture (which, in their world-view, were much the same anyway). 'In western culture, children are shaped with values to help that individual strive for individualism. The Aboriginal prepare and mould their children through a process of collective consciousness, within a world where they can see their relationships to all life: human, animal, and plant' (Young and Paul, 1995: 107). Healing was traditionally more collectively oriented and focused more on reconnections with others, rather than on individual ego-accomplishments, and even today people seem to be returning to nature, spirituality, and family to heal and find balance in their lives (McCormick, 1995).

Non-Natives need to realize that Aboriginal thought process, philosophy, and world-view are intrinsically opposite to most Western/European/non-Native values and ways of thinking: 'We are non-linear in our thinking, which is directly opposite to the way that most social workers are educated. Furthermore, to us, *relationship* is central, not our accomplishments or the material world' (Fife, 1997).

THE MEDICINE WHEEL AS A MODEL FOR AIDS EDUCATION

The Medicine Wheel has proven to be a useful model for teaching about HIV and its progression, as well as a method of explaining why prevention and treatment efforts must be aimed at the whole person (and at all four races!), not just at their medical symptoms. As Leonard Johnston explained it, the four stages of the medical model commonly used to explain the progression of the virus once it enters a person's body can be seen to fit quite well into the parts of the Medicine Wheel.

Window period. Starting in the East, where there are new beginnings and new experiences, the virus gets into our bodies and, like a little child, it wants to touch everything and get into everything, exploring everywhere it can find. Like a small child, the virus is very physical, but with its effects reaching not much farther into the world than its own personal sphere of influence. At this stage, a time of innocence, most people do not even realize they might have been infected and may, in fact, be unknowingly infecting others through high-risk behaviour (or, they are so angry or desperate that they don't care who they infect).

Asymptomatic stage. From the direction of the South comes involvement with the here-and-now, like a youth exploring everything in the immediate world around them, but not yet aware of larger influences of the complex world surrounding it. It is at this stage that the person finds out that they are HIV-positive, and it becomes a very emotional time as one confronts one's own mortality (often for the first time). A wide range of feelings erupt, such as anger, fear, loss, hatred, self-hatred, apathy, isolation, shame, denial, sadness, anxiety, and many others. Like a youth who is dealing with the pressures of growing up, the infected person experiences these numerous complex emotions and becomes similarly self-absorbed. It is at this stage that an HIV-positive person may appear fine and feel healthy, but nevertheless, the immune system is slowly being broken down.

Symptomatic stage. From the direction of the West comes reflection and contemplation. The virus has slowly broken down the immune system, and it is getting harder and harder to fight off common infections. Signs of sickness may have begun to appear, and the person usually wants to learn more about what is happening to their body. For some people previously unaware they had been infected, the appearance of various HIV-related illnesses may be the first time they even realize the virus is inside them.

This is the stage where mental processes start to become more active, where people often try to educate themselves and those around them about the effects of the virus, and where they try to mentally adapt to internal emotional and physical changes. They try to deal with it rationally, but this is usually not enough by itself.

This is the adult stage, often accompanied by increased responsibilities and commitment to struggle to assist and educate others as well as self. People begin to take stock of their lives, to deal with unfinished business and relationship difficulties, to mend broken ties or unmet obligations, as a means of 'preparing the way' and beginning to try to understand their particular life's journey.

AIDS stage. From the direction of the North comes understanding, wisdom, and often, acceptance of inevitable decline. The virus has broken down the immune system so much that the body develops various life-threatening opportunistic infections. Treatment drugs may help for a while, but for many people these do not succeed forever, and so death approaches closer, faster. Much like elders realizing the end is drawing near, people dying from AIDS-related causes often gain in wisdom as they begin to look inside and contemplate the larger aspects of life. It is not uncommon for earlier anger, fear, denial, or bitterness to give way to more peaceful resolution and readiness for whatever will come after physical death.

In this stage, people who are HIV-positive begin to review their life's path and reflect upon what they have accomplished, who they are, and how they have affected others, as well as what might still be necessary for completing the final steps towards resolution and closure. It can be a time of understanding what one's value has been and for discarding less meaningful things or feelings.

Death may not be 'the end', but it is a termination of this particular journey, and this can give much reason to examine its meaning. It is at this time that spirituality frequently increases in importance, along with a return to more traditional roots and ceremonies. Contemplating one's death is rarely easy, particularly for youth who may still carry the blush of invulnerability. But all elders are not necessarily aged, and some youth become quite wise as they approach the end of their current life path.

Going through the stages. Just like the maturing of a human being, this path/progression is not a smooth linear one but one of frequent backsliding, of reaching one stage while perhaps still feeling part of an earlier or later one, or even sometimes of being in two stages at the same time. Growing older is not a simple step-by-step progression, and sometimes the journey pauses a long time before getting moving again. Everyone travels the wheel at their own individual pace; so, too, life with HIV!

Viewing AIDS from a Western/European medical model, we appear to see a linear decline downward towards death—which is usually viewed primarily negatively, as if a disappointing failure or defeat. One message of viewing life alternatively as a continually turning circle is that things can be seen as not inevitably proceeding down some straight-line path to a finishing point (after which there is nothing), but rather a model whereby death can be seen as being an integral part of life still ongoing. Ending is also beginning, and the spirit continues onward even though we have no explanation for this from within the limits of our human knowledge. It is all a cycle: the body goes back to Mother Earth and new things grow from it, while the spirit and the circle continue onward.

HEALING CIRCLES

The Healing Circle is a way for a group of people to meet together for support and problem-solving in a manner in which each participant is on equal footing with the others. It is a 'Circle' because all people are seated in a big circle,[6] so that there is less power imbalance among all participants and all can learn from each other. Someone may initiate calling the Circle together, but it is a true circle with no teacher-student foreground/background prioritization.

All listen to whoever is speaking, without interrupting. Each person speaks only for themselves alone, owning their feelings and making 'I' statements rather than trying to speak for other people. The speaking travels around the Circle clockwise as many times as needed, with no time limit set, but although one has the right not to speak, no one can be interrupted once they have started talking.

> There is no set time length for sharing circles; you stay however long it takes. This is part of the discipline. So you need to be aware of the time factor about sharing circles, that they can take as long as they want, that they *are* a natural rhythm, and that silence is still participation too. Silence is a way of communicating—even if people are not talking, they are still an active part of all that is happening. (McLeod, 1997)

To symbolize visually each person's right to speak in turn, some iconic object is usually passed from speaker to speaker, such as an eagle feather, special stone, or talking stick—whoever holds this may speak uninterrupted until deciding to pass it to the next speaker. Talking, Sharing, or Healing Circles in any Aboriginal tradition may differ slightly as to specific patterns or rules (such as how many 'rounds' occur); however, similar to Medicine Wheels, their concept is still used in most First Nations communities.

> A Circle is a universal way of celebration, a way for us to look at ourselves as an entity. We call the attention of the Creator through drum and song and prayer. We are presenting ourselves to the Creator in this way, so it doesn't matter who you are. We are celebrating that we exist; it's a celebration of all on the physical plane, that all that has been created is good and there should be no shame. Reality is what is there—it is not to be judged; all is sacred. In any Circle, there is no preconceived idea of what will come from it. If the elements are there, then when they come together there *will* be answers in the Circle. So you must come without expectations. You're there to receive whatever will come. (McLeod, 1997)

HEALING CIRCLES FOR ABORIGINAL STREET YOUTH IN VANCOUVER

For many months, I was involved with a weekly Circle (support group) for Aboriginal street youth in Vancouver, which can serve as a good illustration of applying the above concepts to real-life situations.

This group began its meetings initially as a result of the AIDS-related deaths of several youth within a three-week period and the resulting effects on their friends. Their formal memorial services had been well attended; several youth had spoken caring messages at the services and expressed some of their feelings. But once these were over, there still seemed to be a need to grapple with the despair and emptiness felt on the street by both street kids and various youth counsellors—there was a general feeling that something else was needed to honour the deceased in a way that marked their passing in a meaningful and more positive way.

Since two Aboriginal street youth workers, Dolan Badger and Greg Scofield, had just begun a group for HIV-positive Aboriginal street youth, they decided to try the approach of calling an evening Healing Circle for the HIV-affected street community, including counsellors and other workers, as a way to help everyone process what had been happening. 'It was better when they opened the circle wider; there was more of a family feeling that way' (Eagles-Claw, 1997).

For most street youth, there is no family other than themselves with whom to grieve a death and share the turbulent feelings of being left behind by those who have passed on, while they must still try to survive a daily life that is often quite brutal. Yet it is often at times like this that they search their memories to grasp traditions long ago rejected, in some awkward attempt to 'do the right thing' ritually, even if unclear on its actual details or reasons. Doing something is preferable to doing nothing, and anything that feels at all right can provide some amount of comfort:

> Group ritual provides a structure for powerful open expression of emotion in a way that is not uncontrollable and overwhelming to those involved. It also provides a community-sanctioned role for the participants . . . [and it] moves us from stranded individual confrontation with unknown forces to community participation in their harnessing and adaptation. (McKusick and Tafoya, 1992: 5)

Although each youth attending was not necessarily familiar with various components of a traditional Healing Circle, such as smudging, opening prayer, singing songs, passing the eagle feather to each speaker, and so forth, every one of them had memories of having seen such things before, or at least of hearing about them from their elders, even if many years earlier.

The Circle provided a way for these youth to connect with each other on common ground, even though they might come from different backgrounds individually. And the informal environment certainly felt more like home than the fluorescent-lit funeral parlours from earlier in the month or the agency offices of counsellors trying to help each individual client in isolation from their circle of friends. Non-Native people were also welcome to attend, as long as traditional ways were followed. Some of these were other youth, while others were their counsellors—but all were equal in the group since all were attending for personal rather than professional reasons, and this had its own benefits in keeping things Aboriginal-focused.

Although the Circle was initially conceived of as a one-time event, those attending requested to meet again on a regular basis, and so a weekly Circle for HIV-infected or -affected First Nations street youth was born. The group continued for many months under the leadership of Dolan Badger and with the background involvement of myself, a non-Native psychologist and art therapist who has been counselling HIV-positive, gay and two-spirited First Nations people (most of whom are street-involved) for the past eight years.

I attended the weekly group but stayed less active than the Aboriginal leader(s), often just listening intently unless I had something personal to share (a Circle is *not* a therapy group needing any 'outside expert' guidance!). Instead, I was connected through being permitted to hear the experiences, thoughts, and feelings shared by youth, who then would frequently seek me out for more private individual counselling regarding how to handle what personally/emotionally arose during their Circle sharing. The weekly gatherings varied in group size, usually containing about a dozen 'regulars' and a random dozen or so more who dropped in for most but not all of the evenings.

For street youth, this type of attendance record can be considered a success, especially when this became obvious from seeing them together outside the group in mutually supportive situations, such as going together to funerals or AIDS information evenings, which previously they would not have considered risking attending alone. They finally had an environment where it was all right to talk about HIV—and acceptable to discuss, or even show, their feelings. The Circle became a safe place, a family whose members were now traditionally related and 'raised', not unlike traditional family training or upbringing:

> Throughout the years that Aboriginal youth become street-involved, there are wide gaps that separate each majority group. It all differs depending upon which category and first friends you knew and hung around with (such as drag queens, trannies, fems, straight or gay, butch, s & m, lesbian, alcohol and/or drug addicts, *and most importantly, street-involved or not*).
>
> Each person would recognize one another by gestures, but interaction was non-existent. Each category deeply expressed their family values, taking on family roles such as mothers, daughters, sons, aunties, and so on, and we would adopt any newcomer to the scene and take them under our wing.
>
> As violence accelerated in the streets, each family branch slowly combined together to make a more larger support system, which, with the healing circles, gave the opportunity for them to educate and experience themselves in the various needs, lifestyles, and family network that each group possessed.
>
> Healing circles were an ideal place for them to grasp and take in the knowledge that each group possessed in a non-judgemental, open-minded, and safe environment outside the street and bar establishment. (Eagles-Claw, 1997)

Without the Aboriginal 'activators' the Circle could not have happened, but neither they nor I presented (or even considered) ourselves as its 'leaders'—each week the group found its own topic evolving and its own goals being planned naturally. We found that our presence in the Circle or in more private encounters with the youth individually was not solely in the role of counsellors, but also, since we were members of the Circle ourselves, we were 'practically family'. In speaking just as human beings instead of facilitators, our own stories taught and our ears learned from lessons taught by the stories related by the youth around us—it turned out that it was not just the youth who learned more about the effects of HIV on daily life and found some much-needed healing!

In seeing their role models express feelings and demonstrate skills needed for self-care and processing personal grief, the youth learned more about how their own feelings and problems were connected and new ways to process AIDS-related losses in a context of understanding and support. These are good skills to have learned, and are especially effective because the learning happened as a natural process instead of a planned lesson. In the fullness of the Circle everyone, including facilitators, gave as well as received, helped as well as learned, and formed bonds for surviving when solitude was not able to provide answers. It was another lesson on the journey to self-esteem and self-trust that these youth needed in order to be confident enough to request information, seek treatment, and trust medical professionals if only they were willing to risk trying.

USING THE MEDICINE WHEEL FOR REACHING STREET YOUTH

We found the Medicine Wheel model useful not only as an underlying conceptual model for AIDS-related helping and teaching, but also actively helpful as a visible reference for stimulating discussion or self-reflection in both private individual counselling sessions and in the Circle/group.

I believe that the success of this group demonstrated that adapting traditional rituals and practices, such as the Medicine Wheel, Healing Circles, smudging, and so forth, to both street culture and current issues of HIV awareness and self-care, can result in clients' increased sensitivity to HIV-related medical, emotional, and spiritual needs, as well as better self-respect, self-empowerment, awareness of cultural and spiritual roots, and thus healthier lifestyles. Not insignificantly, their willingness to use existing medical services and help peers do the same increased as a result of these traditional practices and ceremonies.

Various other workers have also confirmed that the youth in the group, in addition to regularly attending the weekly Circle, began not only to improve their record of keeping medical and counselling appointments, but also to take a more active role in these sessions, demonstrating more sophisticated knowledge and greater interest in maintaining better health care for themselves and their peers. More than a few times we were pleasantly surprised to find one of 'our' youths being already aware of an upcoming AIDS information session or conference event we wanted to alert them to, or spontaneously offering to go along to speak 'from the heart' when we mentioned teaching various workshops to AIDS counsellors-in-training.

And although these youth could not be expected to become medical experts or prevention specialists overnight, we were pleased to note the increasing occurrence of the occasional medically correct statement or clean-needle lecture being spontaneously delivered by one or another of these youths to peers outside our Circle. All of these may be small measures of success, perhaps, but they are still important steps on the path to taking care of oneself and not harming others.

It is important to recognize that our group was not unique. All across Canada for many years different AIDS agencies and organizations have been using different approaches to try to reach youth, and some of these approaches will work with any young people seeking survival and family on the street. Many Aboriginal AIDS organizations have had similar groups ongoing for years, and I encourage readers to contact those listed at the end of this chapter for their stories and advice. 'It is important for social workers to educate themselves about existing Native organizations, and their various approaches, in order to refer clients appropriately. Not knowing about them is no excuse; "not knowing" is far too often a matter of simply "not caring enough to find out" ' (Fife, 1997).

USING THE MEDICINE WHEEL TO TEACH YOUTH COUNSELLORS ABOUT HIV/AIDS

As explained previously, the Medicine Wheel can be an excellent model for teaching many things about life and has been used successfully by many Aboriginal AIDS organizations as a foundation for integrating AIDS-related information into a culturally appropriate context and providing a less threatening educational framework for getting these urgently needed facts into a community usually resistant to such attempts. And I have just discussed above how well these concepts succeed when applied to working with Aboriginal street youth.

So when I received a request from the Native Youth Worker Training Program (of the Urban Native Youth Association) for Dolan Badger and myself to share our HIV-related knowledge, counselling experiences, and intervention methods in a six-day course for counsellors-in-training, I knew that much more needed to be taught than just the usual 'AIDS-101' medical facts or prevention information. To teach only the physical/medical aspects of AIDS would have provided a good start, but this by itself would not have been sufficient, in that doing this would neglect the complex psychosocial, emotional, and even spiritual issues involved in understanding how HIV affects the whole person. Counsellors hoping to help those living with HIV must be taught how these other factors directly influence the way the virus is experienced physically, especially when considering AIDS in Aboriginal communities, even urban ones.

The Medicine Wheel model was an obvious vehicle for teaching the subject matter. As well, its concepts were important at a meta-level as the foundation for planning the course layout as an integration of such applications. Balancing the components of the Wheel in scheduling the topics and experiential components each day of the course would automatically produce a comprehensive training package that would include all aspects necessary for understanding the numerous interrelated complexities involved. The students would encounter learning in all four quadrants and have personal experiences from each part, which would help them integrate cognitive learning with their own individual discoveries about feelings, beliefs, and attitudes. And they would better understand, viscerally, the interrelationships involved in people's resulting behaviours and consequences.

The course was taught to 25 students ranging in age from late teens to mid-forties, and from almost as many different Native nations, who were midway through their 10-month training to become Aboriginal youth workers. Some were deeply spiritual; others culturally urban and not practising any of the traditional ways. Their diversity reflected the complex mixture of youth they would later be encountering as clients.

The model of delivering information during this course was conversational rather than formal lecturing, and was done in a Circle format where the two of us sat among them (and usually not next to each other). Although there were six full teaching days, these were scheduled across several weeks, so that there was time to absorb the information without being overwhelmed and so that questions could emerge naturally. Each day began with a smudge and a checking-in around the Circle to see how people were and what they wanted from the day. The first day this was done more formally, with people introducing themselves and where they were from (both familially and geographically), and sharing what they chose to about any HIV-related personal experiences. They were told that all their questions would be answered by the end of the course, but that the first day was for focusing on the other-than-medical aspects because these were needed first in order to make use of the factual parts taught later, and that this schedule reflected the way things usually happen naturally—emotionally before medically.

I co-ordinated the first day, which was oriented totally to psychosocial issues (such as the feelings at testing or diagnosis, family concerns, partners and children, what happens after death, and so forth). Students learned about these cognitively in the morning and experienced many of them during the afternoon, when they not only viewed and discussed videotapes of Aboriginal people living with HIV talking about their life experiences, but also had some private time with their inner thoughts and feelings during an 'art-therapy' kind of assignment for which they were asked to draw what HIV/AIDS means to them. After drawing, they could volunteer to discuss why they drew what they did, what it meant to them, and how they felt. At the end of the day, they discussed in the Circle how there were more mental, emotional, and spiritual elements to HIV knowledge and treatment than they had realized, and how this might affect not only their work, but their own personal lives.

The second and third days were given over to basic AIDS information and were taught by Badger, based on his past work as an Aboriginal AIDS educator. The Medicine Wheel was used throughout, not only for explaining the stages of AIDS but also as a model for integrating the physical with the other components.

Throughout this course, we collaborated in presenting the information, with an easy conversational tone, and deferring to each other when not knowing an answer. On days one of us co-ordinated, the other still took active part. In this way, our major cultural differences were openly acknowledged, yet treated respectfully. Thus, our comfortable interchanges served as a clear message that cultural differences can coexist and be noted when they make a significant difference, but also that there is benefit from using the best of both worlds without this difference devaluing or threatening either one of them.

On the fourth day, we returned to more personal integration of fact with feeling. The morning consisted of guest speakers from various Aboriginal AIDS organizations and agencies: an educator and client counsellor from Healing Our Spirit; an educator from the BC Native AIDS Awareness Program; the Native social worker from St Paul's Hospital; an educator from the Transgendered/Transsexual High Risk Project; and two speakers from the YouthCO (Positive Youth Counselling and Outreach) Project. All these people were invited so that the class could meet those they were most likely to be networking with regarding their future clients, once they began actively working with street youth.

In the afternoon, Aboriginal youth and adults who are themselves living with HIV came to speak directly with the class and tell their stories. This was a very powerful session, as one young woman (with her child) and four young men spoke from their hearts, giving real-life pictures of what it is like to live with HIV as Aboriginal persons who had 'come from the streets' (or, in the case of two speakers, were actually still there). The questions the class asked afterwards clearly indicated not only that they had heard about future clients' situations, but also that they had very quickly internalized the message about how HIV might eventually affect them personally and the risks they might need to be aware of in their own personal non-work-related lives.

That day ended with the usual closing Circle, but the class was so moved that two members spontaneously asked people to wait while a drum was brought so that an Honour Song could be sung for the guests and teachers. It was a moving ending to a deeply emotional, mental, and spiritual day.

On the fifth day the class went to the building where most HIV-positive people in Vancouver eventually go for services because it houses the Persons With AIDS Society, AIDS Vancouver, Positive Women's Network, Wings Housing Society, the food bank, and library. Representatives from these groups spoke to the class and gave informal tours (often accompanied, at our request, by Aboriginal workers or volunteers associated with these organizations). Additional site visits were done at a nearby street-oriented community health centre and the office of the Street Youth Services organization. By the end of that day, the class had been to most places their clients might go and had seen first-hand the human faces inside what might have previously been perceived of as doors too overwhelming to walk through.

On the final day, the invited speaker was a mother from a village in northern British Columbia, accompanied by her daughter and granddaughter, who spoke about the death of her son from AIDS-related causes and how this affected not only his immediate family but also the entire community. They spoke about stigma, shame, healing, and breaking the silence surrounding it all—and the class learned a lot more about the personal face of HIV and its 'psychosocial ramifications'. These guests also explained their involvement in contributing a panel about him to the Canadian AIDS Memorial Quilt, and how it was used at his Stone Feast a year later as well as in a Display of Quilts for Aboriginals at the Friendship Centre in Vancouver several months later. After that introduction to the Quilt's prevention/awareness educational possibilities, in addition to its grieving and memorializing functions, the class was shown a real piece of the AIDS Quilt, along with short videos relating to it. Finally, the class participated in another art-therapy exercise for closure, showing what HIV/AIDS means to them now that they have completed the course.

Course evaluations demonstrated students' enthusiastic response to this more encompassing way of learning about HIV that integrated the psychosocial and medical aspects by addressing all four components of the Medicine Wheel. Many emphasized that they had heard the warnings and facts before, but never before understood the complexity behind them or the feelings involved. As well, they had not previously recognized their own personal risks. This kind of feedback, combined with our own experiences during the course, suggests that teaching the Aboriginal counsellors of Aboriginal street youth using a model based on the Medicine Wheel, Healing Circles, and other First Nations traditions can greatly benefit the healing work done with Aboriginal street youth.

CONCLUSION

Aboriginal street youth live in both street and First Nations cultures simultaneously and are at extreme risk of HIV infection. They need culturally sensitive and non-judgemental counselling, education, and treatment—but first must come their internal desire to seek these (and their willingness to actually experience the accompanying feelings). These youth will trust most those who are most familiar with their underlying culture and its traditional value system, regardless of how long ago *they* think they left such things behind. Aboriginal spirituality is so much more than just religion—it is an entire way of life, with involvement all day long every day, not simply once a week inside a building—and this is as true for street youth as it is for their elders.

Many traditional healing models and spiritual considerations still have an important place in HIV work with today's Aboriginal street youth. In addition, they provide a foundation for teaching others how to do this work. Medicine Wheel teachings and Healing Circles can serve as an excellent means of beginning the connecting and reconnecting necessary for these youths' survival. 'Fear attacks us physically, trying to kidnap our spirits, our souls. But two against one—you and the spirit within—have better odds to challenge fear' (Ward, 1997: 14).

Even if not actively pursued as interventions, deeper meanings flowing within the Wheel and the concepts rooted in the Circle approach can help Aboriginal youth improve their self-understanding and their connections with friends, families, and traditions, as well as with a network of counsellors and other workers who are better sensitized and therefore offering deeper understanding of the complex net their lives are caught up in. In the best of all possible worlds, these services would be offered by Aboriginal helpers; however, in the meantime, the information in this chapter may hopefully suggest ways that non-Natives can also help, and still do so in appropriate ways.

> It is important to understand that learning all these techniques in these pages is a goal for respectful awareness, not a certificate qualifying non-Native readers to now go out and start up Healing Circles for Native youth. Rather, such learnings teach sensitivity to the ways such things are done, and thus can help, and that there are certain ways to begin them, such as contacting local elders who can then decide what should or should not be started, by whom, and how. It may turn out that the more non-Native social workers truly understand, the more they will realize how much of a back seat they should take.
>
> Ceremony is so very private, and is best done by those traditionally trained and entrusted to do it. Sometimes it may be better to help assist the formation of Healing Circles from a background position, and actually not participate in them at all. *This is a difficult understanding for people who truly care, and truly want to help: that sometimes the best 'helping' they can do is to not be seen to be helping.* By doing this, historical paternalistic attitudes can be confronted and Native people can be in control of our own empowerment. (Fife, 1997; emphasis added)

Acknowledgements

I want to acknowledge with grateful appreciation and deep respect the consultative advice from the following colleagues, who helped review this chapter for publication: Alan Mousseau (Ojibway), Speaker, Healing Our Spirit BC First Nations AIDS Society; Connie Fife (Cree), Counsellor, Urban Native Youth Association; Nikki A. Williams (Shushwap), Speaker, Healing Our Spirit BC First Nations AIDS Society; Tia Eagles-Claw (Okanagan), Street Youth Peer Counsellor; Albert McLeod (Cree and Scottish), Director, Manitoba Aboriginal AIDS Task Force; Bert Isaac (Kwakiutl and Coast Salish), Counsellor, Urban Native Youth Association; Kecia Larkin (Kwakwaka'wakw), Educator; Curtis Yellow Fly (Blackfoot Siksika), Research Worker, Aboriginal Community Health Project; Vince Smith (Cree), Street Youth Peer Counsellor; Robert Abraham (Tatla Lake), Speaker and Peer Counsellor; Nadine Caplette (Métis), Program Manager, BC Native AIDS Awareness Program; Ken Ward (Enoch Cree), Educator and Peer Counsellor; and especially Dolan Badger (Cree), Counsellor, Urban Native Youth Association Safe House, with whom an earlier version of this chapter was originally presented as a poster session at the International AIDS Conference in Vancouver, July 1996.

I also want to thank my friends Robert Cross (Oglala Lakota and Northern Cheyenne), William Belgarde (Cree), Connie Fife (Cree), and Evan Adams (Coast Salish), whose supportive understanding of my intentions in writing this helped me greatly in clarifying my personal responsibilities in creating it.

I would also like to acknowledge the pioneering work of my friend and mentor, Frederick Haineault, co-founder of Healing Our Spirit BC First Nations AIDS Society, from whom I first learned about the AIDS Medicine Wheel (and many other things as well). Though he has passed on from illness related to AIDS, his gifts of teaching and friendship are still greatly appreciated.

NOTES

1. As first conceptualized by Leonard Johnston, after going to the elders for healing and then relating their teachings about the Wheel to his personal journey with AIDS (McLeod, 1997).
2. Different Aboriginal nations may conceptualize parts or all of this differently; for example, North can represent elder and/or winter, as in resting-to-begin-again, and so its colour may be white instead of black.
3. Another version might have the four major elements rather than seasons, for example; so blue (for water) might replace black. What is most important is the overall concept and its application, even though specific details might vary.
4. Or, as another version of the model arranges it: East—tobacco (yellow), South—sage (red), West—cedar (black/blue), and North—sweetgrass (white) (Young and Paul, 1995: 40).
5. As noted in a lecture by Dr Brian Woodfall, the first doctor I am aware of who has acknowledged this understanding in public lecture.
6. There are a few exceptions, such as 'people experiencing uncontrollable outbursts, . . . like bursts of anger which might lead to physical danger or physically sick from illness or alcohol or drugs, or women in their high moon [menstruation]. They can participate and speak but not sit with others in the first circle. Such people are not considered to be dangerous or unwanted, but who possess high power and energy that could interrupt or deflect the healing process of the Circle. Both kinds go through a body cleansing period that releases high energy. They are welcome to speak from the outer circle, which surrounds the original circle. It's always preferred to have 48 hours of cleanliness [drug-free] before attending a circle; we ask people to be honest—if they're not 48-hours clean, please sit in the back' (Eagles-Claw, 1997).

AGENCIES AND ORGANIZATIONS INVOLVED IN HIV/AIDS EDUCATION AND COUNSELLING IN ABORIGINAL COMMUNITIES

AIDS Yellowknife
Box 864, Yellowknife, NWT, X1A 2N6.
Phone: (403) 873–2626; *Fax*: (403) 873–2626

AIDS Yukon Alliance
7221 7th Avenue, Whitehorse, Yukon, Y1A 1R8
Phone: (403) 633–2437; *Fax*: (403) 633–2447

All Aboriginals Against AIDS
P.O. Box 145, Lennox Island, PEI, C0B 1P0
Phone: (902) 831–2779; *Fax*: (902) 831–3153

All Nations Hope AIDS Network
1852 Angus Street, Regina, Sask., S4P 3A2
Phone: (306) 924–8424; *Fax*: (306) 525–0904

Atlantic First Nations AIDS Task Force
P.O. Box 47049, Halifax, NS, B3K 2B0
Phone: (902) 492–4255; *Fax*: (902) 492–0500

Feather of Hope Aboriginal AIDS Prevention Society
#201-11456 Jasper Avenue, Edmonton, Alta, T5K 0M1
Phone: (403) 488–5773; *Fax*: (403) 488–3735

Healing Our Spirit BC First Nations AIDS Society
415–B West Esplanade, North Vancouver, BC, V7M 1A6
Phone: (604) 983–8774; *Fax*: (604) 983–2667

Manitoba Aboriginal AIDS Task Force
555 Broadway Avenue, 3rd Floor, Winnipeg, Man., R3C 0W4
Phone: (204) 772–6800; *Fax*: (204) 772–2784

Two-Spirited People of First Nations
Suite 201–A, 45 Charles Street East, Toronto, Ont., M4Y 1S2
Phone: (416) 944–9300; *Fax*: (416) 944–8381

Urban Aboriginal AIDS Awareness
2001 St-Laurent Boulevard, Montreal, Que., H2X 2T3
Phone: (514) 499–1854; *Fax*: (514) 499–9436

Note:
Although not a formal agency, the **Canadian Aboriginal AIDS Network** should be noted here as another very important organization to contact: 1-800-597-3809.

REFERENCES

Chrisjohn, Roland D., and Sherri L. Young. 1996. *The Circle Game: Shadows and Substance in the Indian Residential School Experience in Canada*. Report to the Royal Commission on Aboriginal Peoples, Oct. 1994.

E.F. (anonymous). 1997. Private communication, 24 Mar.

Eagles-Claw, Tia. 1997. Private communication, 28 Feb.

Fife, Connie. 1997. Private communication, 21 Feb.

Gilchrist, Lauri. 1995. 'Kapitipis e-pimohteyahk (Translation: We walk all night)', doctoral dissertation, University of British Columbia, Department of Education.

Ker, Charles. 1995. 'First Nations Grad Probes Street Life', *UBC Reports* 41, 19 (Nov.): 1–2.

Larkin, Kecia. 1997. Private communication, 9 May.

McCormick, Rod. 1995. 'The Facilitation of Healing for the First Nations People of British Columbia', doctoral thesis, University of British Columbia.

McKusick, Leonard, and Terry Tafoya. 1992. 'Steps to Survival: Cross-cultural Healing Elements in the Treatment of AIDS', *HIV Frontline* 5 (July–Aug.): 1–7.

McLeod, Albert W. 1997. Private communication, 22 Mar.

———, L. Johnson, L. Gardiner, and G. Kakeway. 1996. 'Culturally-appropriate Visual Teaching Tools Developed for Aboriginal People in Canada', *Conference Proceedings*, XIth International Conference on AIDS, Vancouver, 10 July: 52.

N.S. (anonymous). 1997. Private communication. 24 Mar.

Peterkin, Alan. 1996. 'Counselling (Adapted from: Psychosocial Issues in HIV Primary Care)', in M.A. Tobin, F.J. Chow, M.I. Bowmer, and G.A. Bailey, eds, *A Comprehensive Guide to the Care of Persons Living with HIV Disease—Module 1: Adults (Men, Women, and Adolescents)*. Mississauga, Ont.: College of Family Physicians of Canada, 27–35.

Pow, Deborah. 1997. 'HIV/AIDS Education and Prevention in Aboriginal Communities', unpublished paper, McGill School of Social Work.

R.S. (anonymous). 1997. Private communication, 20 May.

Ross, R. 1992. *Dancing with a Ghost—Exploring Indian Reality*. Toronto: Octopus Publishing Group.

Tafoya, Terry. 1989. 'Pulling Coyote's Tale: Native American Sexuality and AIDS', in V.M. Mays, G. Albee, and S. Schneider, eds, *Primary Prevention of AIDS*. Newbury Park, Calif.: Sage, 280–9.

———. 1994. 'Epistemology of Native Healing and Family Psychology', *The Family Psychologist* 10, 2: 28–31.

———. 1997. 'Native Gay and Lesbian Issues—The Two-Spirited', in B. Greene, ed., *Psychological Perspectives on Lesbian and Gay Issues, vol. 3 Ethnic and Cultural Diversity*. Thousand Oaks, Calif.: Sage, 1–10.

Young, Tuma, and Elizabeth Paul. 1994. *Healing Our Nation—A Resource Kit for Elders, Care Workers, and Educators*. Halifax: Atlantic First Nations AIDS Task Force.

———, and ———. 1995. *Healing Our Nation—Resource Manual*. Halifax: Atlantic First Nations AIDS Task Force.

Ward, Ken. 1997. 'Fear Is a Constant Companion When You Have AIDS', *Windspeaker* (Apr.): 14.

Weiser, Judy. 1996a. 'HIV/AIDS Psychotherapy—What Psychologists Need To Understand', *Canadian Health Psychologist* 4, 1: 18–23.

———. 1996b. 'Psychosocial Consequences of Living with HIV/AIDS—Or, What I Learned from My Clients and Friends', *The Social Worker* 64, 4 (Winter): 18–33.

Chapter 10

Care and the Context of Injection Drug Use

ANNE BOWLBY

Injection drug use is the second most likely means of HIV transmission in Canada and is growing rapidly in major cities. Models of care developed for previous populations seldom meet the needs or respond adequately to people who inject drugs. This chapter considers care in the context of clients who are injection drug users, the social work skills needed to respond, the challenges of providing care, and the kinds of programs that have been most effective.

BACKGROUND—SCOPE OF THE PROBLEM

As of the end of 1996 between 19,000 and 20,000 people in Canada had been diagnosed with AIDS; 8.2 per cent of these were as a result of injection drug use (approximately 1,560 to 1,640 people) (Health Canada, 1996). This is only the tip of the iceberg. As a result of the long incubation period from HIV infection to AIDS and with evidence coming from a number of Canadian cities of the massive increases in the number of people who inject drugs and are testing positive for HIV, it is likely that there are thousands more injection drug users with HIV in Canada, some of whom are unaware they are infected. In Ontario, the number of people diagnosed with HIV is approximately three times that of those who have been reported with AIDS. In addition, from Ontario data, it is known that only 50–60 per cent of people who inject drugs acknowledge injection drug use as a risk factor when being tested for HIV. Due to stigma and fear of the law, injection drug users (IDUs) may be reluctant to use health-care services, let alone be tested for HIV.

According to researchers, when the rate of HIV infection among IDUs goes over 10 per cent, there is a greatly increased risk of transmission of HIV (Magner, 1997: 1) in this group because of the ease with which the virus is transmitted through needle-sharing. The experience in a number of international cities is that it is extremely difficult to control the spread of HIV among IDUs once this critical percentage is reached.

THE PREVALENCE OF INJECTION DRUG USE IN CANADA

In Vancouver, there has been an ongoing progression to the outbreak of HIV among injection drug users (Patrick et al., 1997: 27A). In Montreal, HIV prevalence among IDUs is 19.7 per cent and incidence is 8.2 per cent per person year (Hankins et al., 1997: 28A). In Toronto, the incidence of HIV among this group seems to have remained stable at approximately 8 per cent. In Ottawa, the preliminary analysis of HIV rates among IDUs is extremely high (estimated at 18 per cent). Smaller communities are also reporting higher rates of HIV infection among injection drug users. One of the most difficult challenges for addressing the problem of HIV among IDUs is that there are not accurate estimates of how many people inject drugs. While injection drug use is not necessarily a lifelong activity, the time during which a person spends injecting drugs can be critical. Equally critical is whether unsterilized needles and drug equipment are shared and with whom.

WHO IS BECOMING INFECTED?

When voluntary HIV testing began in 1985, men having sex with men comprised the majority of people who tested positive. As of 1995, the trend had changed as more and more women tested positive, as well as injection drug users and men having sex with men and using injection drugs (Wright et al., 1997: 29A). While heroin is often thought to be the main drug of choice among IDUs and, therefore, responsible for the spread of HIV, it appears that cocaine use is far more serious (Magner, 1997). With the frequency of injections required by people who inject cocaine and the problems of obtaining enough new or sterilized needles, transmission of HIV is very efficient for this type of activity. Further, addiction treatment for people who use cocaine presents unique challenges.

Injection drug users are not a connected community of people like the gay community. While it is unlikely that any group can be considered homogeneous, IDUs tend to be more isolated than others due to the stigma associated with injecting drugs, fear of arrest, and criminality. Unlike members of the gay community, IDUs are likely to have been arrested and incarcerated. In addition, while in correctional facilities, prisoners are unlikely to have access to clean needles or bleach for cleaning needles and needle-sharing happens. In addition, many people report that the only time they have shared needles is while incarcerated (Myers et al., 1995).

Women are particularly vulnerable to HIV infection. Sexual and/or physical abuse as children and as adults is common among women who use substances. It has been estimated that as many as two-thirds of women who present for addiction treatment have experienced abuse (Harrison, 1997). Women testing HIV-positive report injection drug use as a risk factor as well as sex with men. In addition, men tend to be the gatekeepers to illicit injection drugs, which adds to women's vulnerability.

While injection drug use is a very efficient method of transmitting HIV, most drug users report use of multiple drugs (and methods) as well as use of alcohol. Many community-based AIDS organizations are reporting that the majority of their clients have or have had a history of drug and alcohol use. While the challenge for stemming HIV among IDUs consists of innovative methods of outreach to teach safe injection methods and to ensure an adequate supply of clean needles and access to appropriate treatment, the issue is firmly based in drug use itself, not just injecting behaviour.

It is well known that at the time of seroconversion (the change in status from seronegative to seropositive), HIV is extremely active and the possibility for transmission is high. Given the efficacy of transmission through needle-sharing, it is extremely important to reach IDUs at the point of seroconversion. This also means a concerted effort to increase access to HIV testing, particularly when seroconversion is suspected. From a traditional HIV prevention education standpoint, this information is somewhat contrary to the messages about always being infectious, regardless of stage of disease, and always practising safer sex and needle use. However, this is one of the challenges that must be met if we are to stem HIV infection in injection drug users.

People who inject drugs need education about the signs and symptoms associated with seroconversion. Staff working with people who inject drugs need to be trained to assess and advise clients who may have recently seroconverted.

BASIC ASSUMPTIONS

1. People who use injection drugs are worthy of our attention and intervention. Although this may seem very basic, there is a wave of conservatism across Canada that tends to blame addicts in general for their problem, and, in particular, those who inject drugs. Criminality, stigma, and the attitude of professionals towards people who inject drugs continue to marginalize this population.
2. Drugs and alcohol impair judgement and, thus, the commitment to safer injecting and safer sex practices. To address injection drug use only addresses a part of the problem, which must be put in the broader context of substance use, addictions, and other high-risk activities.
3. People who use injection drugs are likely to use more than one substance. While each person may have his/her own substance of choice (drugs or alcohol), the choice is often what is most immediately available at the least cost. In addition, substance users may use a variety of methods (e.g., injection, pills, smoking) to consume their drugs.
4. Substance use interventions must include a range of harm-reduction techniques, including abstinence from all substances, safe injection, methadone for opiate users, and safer sex practices. Most clients report that they are not successful the first time they enter addiction treatment. Relapse management is a critical part of addiction treatment and harm reduction must be part of relapse management.
5. Interventions must be client-centred. A client may choose to reduce the amount of injecting he/she engages in and social workers or other human service professionals must be able to support the changes. For example, a client may choose to abstain from only one substance while continuing to use other substances.
6. A variety of methods and approaches are likely to be successful. As with other areas of social work, it is extremely important to be flexible in order to be successful. Clients are likely to be the best resources of what will work for them.

7. Injection drug users, as with other people who use substances, have a variety of dreams, hopes, achievements, and problems. It is important to listen to clients and to address their lives as they see them. A client may, for example, only wish to deal with a housing problem and not be interested initially in methadone as an option to heroin.
8. Attitudes of social workers dealing with people who are dependent on drugs or alcohol are extremely important. The ability to be non-judgemental is critical in dealing with people who are dependent. It is vital for the worker to develop an understanding of his/her own values, attitudes, and beliefs about people who use drugs, have been to jail, have HIV, are gay or lesbian, and/or have worked in the sex trade. How a social worker projects her or his own comfort with these issues will be evident to the client and will affect the outcome of the counselling.

DEFINITIONS

The use of language in HIV and substance use is extremely important. The language often perpetuates stigma and reinforces the feeling of unworthiness of clients. Distinctions are made that to the lay person are only fine lines, but in discussions about HIV they become extremely important. In the discussion of HIV and injection drug use, it is important to define the words. There are differences between the person who uses drugs, the person who overuses drugs, and the person who abuses drugs. Many times, these distinctions are blurred and anyone who uses drugs is labelled an abuser or an addict; conversely, when a person's life is being controlled by substances, they are labelled a user. The definition of a drug abuser could be someone whose life is dependent on use of the substance. The definition of an overuser could be someone who, due to circumstances, overuses a particular substance but has the control to reduce or abstain when the crisis is over. The definition of a user could be someone who uses occasionally but can walk away at any time without suffering any loss of identity or meaning. For those who are dependent on substances, the substances have taken on a meaning in their lives that is not easily replaced, nor is it easy to change the pattern of use. The use has the control. However, irrespective of the terms, in a client-centred practice, the client is the person in charge of the definitions. For some clients, use of substances can be a positive coping strategy when dealing with traumatic situations.

Addiction services, by and large, provide treatment to people who self-identify as dependent on substances. While early intervention and secondary prevention programs have shown a great deal of success in diverting people who are overusing before they become dependent, the number of these programs is minimal. Often for those who overuse, the resolution of the underlying issues becomes the resolution of the overuse. Overuse in the case of a person with HIV may be as a result of coping with the diagnosis and can be transitory. For those who are dependent on substances, the substance may take on a life of its own and, while there are likely to be many other issues that should be dealt with, overcoming substance dependency is likely to be only one of many issues to be resolved.

CURRENT INTERVENTIONS

Addiction treatment services have traditionally been based on the premise that when a client is ready, he or she will voluntarily make the contact. This assumption presumes that people know how to access systems. In addition, in most instances, clients are asked to be clean or sober to attend assessment in the addiction service office. In recent years, more social and health-care service outreach programs have been developed to provide a variety of services to people on the street and in other isolated situations. When appropriate and possible, referrals to office-based services may be facilitated and made. Referral may involve actually meeting the client and accompanying him/her. By and large, however, the majority of social and health-care services do not 'go where the clients are', but wait for the clients to find and come into the service. Addiction treatment services are not atypical in this respect, with the exception of needle exchange programs.

The addiction treatment system offers a broad range of services, including assessment, case co-ordination, detoxification, long- and short-term residential programs, and non-residential individual and group counselling. In addition, after-care programs may be offered in the community or in recovery homes or other supportive housing arrangements. The goals of the programs are to reduce or eliminate the use of alcohol or drugs as a contributing factor to physical, psychological, and social dysfunction and to stop, slow down, or reverse the progress of associated problems (Corbett, 1997). Many of the programs, in fact, strive to eliminate the use of alcohol and drugs for life. While this goal is what many people who are dependent on substances strive for in the long term, most people are not successful on their first attempt to remain sober or clean and may experience a sense of failure with each 'failed' attempt. Some programs are very harsh on those who are not successful and do not acknowledge the difficulties for people trying to change their lives or recognize the progress the person may have made in spite of a relapse.

Relapse prevention and management are an integral part of addiction treatment. However, few programs offer harm reduction within the context of relapse management. When the goal is total abstinence, talking about harm-reduction strategies if a person decides to use substances seems to be contrary. It is a difficult balance to maintain, but it is similar to the discussion of teaching condom use in schools, irrespective of whether the students are sexually active or not. If programs are in fact client-centred, then the decision must be left to the client and the client has a right to as much information as possible on which to base a decision. Harm reduction in the context of relapse prevention may help the person to seek assistance earlier if relapse occurs and may prevent HIV infection.

Most addiction programs have been based on an abstinence model, which includes abstinence while in the program. Incorporating people who only wish to reduce their use into these programs has proved to be a challenge. It is extremely difficult to run a group session where some participants are abstaining and others are reducing. The issues and goals for the two types of participants are not the same and there may not be common ground. Some programs are offering alternative programming for people who wish to reduce rather than abstain, and these programs appear to meet better the needs of these clients.

Two types of programs have emerged in the broad spectrum of addiction treatment programs as also providing an HIV prevention benefit. The first is the needle exchange program, which grew out of HIV prevention efforts. The program offers a multifaceted service to people who use injection drugs. The impetus for the programs grew out of the emergence of HIV among people who inject drugs and the fear, in some communities, the reality, of the rapid spread of HIV in this community. While needle exchange programs are not considered addiction treatment, they do fill the needed function of going where the clients are, offering service in a non-judgemental fashion, and assisting those clients who wish to attend more traditional addiction treatment programs. Ontario needle exchanges are offered by public health units but are often also located in existing community-based organizations (e.g., services for street youth). People who use the services of these agencies can exchange their needles in locations where they already receive services. Stand-alone needle exchanges also offer a variety of services, including assessment and referral to a variety of other resources such as addiction treatment, health care, and prevention and risk-reduction counselling.

The second program that has emerged as an addiction intervention for reducing HIV infection is methadone treatment. Methadone has been used since the 1960s as a method for reducing crime related to drug use and to allow drug users to maintain employment (Canadian Centre on Substance Abuse, 1994). Methadone is used as a substitute for opiates and assists people who inject heroin to reduce their risk of complications arising from injection and of HIV infection. Methadone does not seem to be particularly effective for people who inject cocaine. With the onset of HIV infection within the injection drug-using population, methadone has taken on a new significance.

From a traditional addiction treatment standpoint, both of these programs are quite radical. The first, needle exchange programs, do not have a goal of abstinence, but rather have the goal of harm reduction. Needle exchanges provide an opportunity to connect with people who are using injection drugs. This opportunity may lead to connections to the health and social services system and reduce the isolation of users. The second, methadone programs, also have the goal of harm reduction. As methadone replaces heroin, it allows the user to organize other parts of his/her life so that this life is no longer chaotic, marginalized, or criminalized. Again, it may lead to greater stability for clients.

HIV programs have been characterized by innovation. When the first cases of AIDS were diagnosed among gay men, the gay community rallied to provide information for treatment and prevention. Community-based AIDS organizations were formed and offered both HIV prevention and support services. Because of the prevention focus, there were clear connections with the broader client group and prevention provided a type of outreach to those who could be at risk. As HIV spread to other populations, attempts have been made to incorporate HIV prevention and support into existing community-based AIDS programs. Outside of larger urban centres, these attempts have been fairly successful. In larger urban areas, programs addressing the specific needs of population groups have been developed. In many of the provinces, public health services have also been very involved in prevention work and hospital HIV out-patient clinics in providing treatment and counselling. However, none of these organizations has been particularly effective in dealing with injection drug users. This is not overly surprising, as addiction programs that have been providing treatment to IDUs for years also report that IDUs are the hardest to reach and programs have the most difficulty engaging clients in treatment.

CASE HISTORIES AND INTERVENTIONS

For people who are chronically dependent on substances, it is not unusual for their lives to be chaotic and for them to be facing complex and numerous issues. It is extremely important to address financial, legal, housing, employment, relationship, and other psychosocial issues with the client. The following case histories are intended to inform and challenge social workers about the multiplicity of competing issues for clients who use substances including injection drugs.

George is 45 years old, White, and gay. He describes himself as middle-class, as a respected member of the community with tremendous social support. When he reached puberty, he had to deal with his sexual attraction to men. He felt profoundly that he did not belong anywhere. He entered an emotionally stressful period and his grades dropped. He went to university in the 1960s, discovered drugs, and eventually started using injection drugs with his friends. Initially, his injection drug use was recreational, but soon it became the method of choice due to the availability and the need for a quick high.

In an attempt to organize his life, he eventually stopped using, completed school, married, and got a good job. At that point, he had never dealt with his feelings about his sexual orientation. The confusion and the stress of not having dealt with this led to a real identity crisis. He was unsure about where he was going. His wife could not understand what he was going through. He separated from his wife and family, went for counselling, and moved into the gay community.

He did not allow himself to have any problems in his new life. With the losses of his family, his home, and his job for the sake of his new life, he set out to make this new life perfect. When it was not, he returned to drugs, looking for ways outside himself to make the life better. When he tested HIV-positive he went into crisis, shock, and denial, and when he finally found himself in another city with no idea of how he got there, he knew he had to turn his life around.

He entered drug treatment again. This time, George's goals were quite different from the first time he had been through treatment. He focused on his current life as he was living it. Because he was no longer confused about his sexuality, he was able to discuss it openly and could look at his current life realistically. He found people who listened. He found a sense of belonging, a connection with other people and himself that he had not found previously. He discovered ways to express himself and to talk about himself that he had not known in the past.

There are probably many reasons why George was successful. Not the least important was his desire to succeed, to stop looking outside himself for happiness and perfection. He learned to accept himself. George made a critical decision about his life, who he was, and how he wanted to live, and he made a commitment to change. The diagnosis of HIV may have been the catalyst for change, but George's own determination to continue was essential to maintaining the change.

Warren is a 25-year-old Aboriginal. He is heterosexual, but is not involved in a relationship. He describes his family as dysfunctional. Alcohol abuse and physical and sexual abuse were the norm. His family moved to a large urban centre when he was quite young and although the physical and sexual abuse stopped, the alcohol abuse did not. He left home in his teens and never finished high school. As the middle child, he was viewed as the pet. When he was 20, his father asked him to move home again and go back to school. He tried, but he was still using alcohol and going to school never really worked out.

Warren drifted to a northern town for college. Unable to find a summer job, he returned to the city and lived with his brother, who was using cocaine and other drugs. Warren tried drugs and really liked the experience. Three months later, he was selling to fund his own use. In addition to paying for his habit through selling drugs, Warren worked as a prostitute. He was arrested for prostitution.

Warren has tried in the past to get help for his drinking and drug use, but has problems talking to counsellors. He relies on his friends and his younger siblings to discuss his problems. He has also found it very difficult to access services. As an Aboriginal man, he was raised to keep silent about his problems and often uses metaphors to describe himself, his feelings, and his life. As he is still using drugs and alcohol, many services do not know how to engage him. His goal is to reduce his use of drugs but, at this point, he is not interested in dealing with his drinking. He is uncomfortable with 'talk therapy' with a total stranger who does not appreciate his background or culture.

Warren is in the final stages of HIV. He does not know how much longer he will have to live. He cannot afford the drugs that are recommended by the doctor. His relationship with the HIV medical clinic is rocky. He shows up when there is a problem and often does not follow through on the recommendations. The clinic staff do not know how to cope with the fact that Warren continues to use drugs and alcohol.

Why haven't services been able to reach Warren? The issues are very complicated. It is important to recognize his history and culture as an Aboriginal. Talking about problems with a White person is not Warren's cultural norm. The burden of abuse and dysfunction of the family means that the issues are not simply ones of substance dependency. Counsellors must be able to incorporate cultural sensitivity, especially listening to what the client is saying. Counsellors must also be able to recognize the myriad issues—both historical within himself and his family and current for himself and his family—that he is trying to deal with. Social workers also need to examine their own attitudes and biases towards Aboriginal people, as well as their attitudes towards heterosexual males who sell sex to other men. Finally, the impact of poverty on Warren's ability to follow through must be recognized and addressed.

Sandra is 21 years old. She has a three-year-old daughter. Sandra considers herself multidiagnosed—she is HIV-positive, is a substance user, and has mental health problems. She grew up in a number of foster homes, experienced physical and sexual abuse as a child, and got involved in drugs and prostitution. When she finally decided to change her life, she started with addiction treatment. Becoming clean and sober was extremely difficult—she had to create new meaning in her life. Although prostitution provided her with money to pay for her apartment and food, she found it hard to engage in prostitution unless she was high or drunk.

Sandra accessed the local community-based AIDS support program and saw a counsellor for her mental health problems at the local mental health agency. However, she could not talk about all of her problems at any one of the helping services. At each one, she would only address the issues that were relevant to the service. She felt very strongly that if she raised the others, the counsellors would not know what to do with her and she would be referred elsewhere.

What can counsellors do in this situation? As social workers, we have a responsibility to create safe places for our clients. Part of the safety for clients includes the ability to raise issues that may not be part of our explicit mandate, but are impacting on our clients' abilities to work out their issues in a holistic way.

CHALLENGES AND IMPLICATIONS FOR SOCIAL WORK PRACTICE

People with HIV pose a number of challenges for social workers, as do people who are dependent on substances, particularly those who inject drugs. The combination of HIV and injection drug use is one of the more difficult challenges for social workers. From the addictions field, there is no simple answer to reaching out to this population and ensuring that they will not harm themselves or others. Our societal attitudes towards people who inject drugs are negative. People who inject drugs often share these attitudes, which makes them feel undeserving of help.

Injection drug users, for a number of reasons, are not an organized community and do not generally seek out social or health-care services. This means that we must be creative in making connections with people who are dependent on injection drugs. One of the basic tenets of social work practice is that we 'start where the client is at'. With IDUs, we have to find ways to reach that emotional and mental place. This means that we have to be able to go out into the streets or shooting galleries or make good connections with people who are providing street-based services. To make the connections with other service providers may mean that we have to go to their agencies to meet their clients or join them on their street tours.

As one of the basic tenets of social work practice is to 'start where the client is at', we must be prepared to listen to our clients. Most people who are dependent on substances go through a number of stages before making actual changes. The stages of change include precontemplation, contemplation, preparation, action, maintenance. These stages are important. Even when a client's goal is harm reduction, if a client is looking to change, the stages still apply. The meaning a client has given to his/her dependence on substances must be articulated and addressed, and as social workers we must be able to facilitate the client in expressing this meaning. The precontemplation stage is the point at which we can provide information about the risks involved and possible risk-reduction strategies that are realistic for the client. At the contemplation stage we can continue risk reduction and outline possible options for change. The preparation stage is the stage during which we can facilitate access to options of the client's choice. During the action stage the client begins to make changes. Here, our role is to support the changes, listen for the barriers, and assist the client in finding solutions to the barriers. The maintenance stage is as important as the other stages. Although clients may have completed their addictions treatment, it is extremely important that we continue to listen. As few people succeed the first time, it is essential that clients feel comfortable talking about the challenges they face in maintaining their goals and their fears about relapse. Whether their goal is total abstinence or reduced harm, it is important that they feel safe and not judged in discussing what is happening. As with George, they may be expecting that their lives will be perfect after having made a change. The reality may not live up to their expectations. For many people, it may be easier to return to what is known rather than continue what appears to be an uphill battle.

Many people who are involved in drugs have criminal records. Knowledge of the criminal system and culture is important for social workers working in the field of HIV and injection drug use. Again, making partners with people who work in the criminal justice system is essential. Some social workers work within the criminal justice system and they have to be able to address the issues in a safe way. Although drug use is illegal and it is also illegal within correctional facilities, it is important that the issues be addressed in such a way that the social worker is not seen to be gathering specific information that will identify any person or activity but rather is perceived as imparting information that will allow the clients to make their own decisions.

RECOMMENDATIONS

Many papers on injection drug use and HIV call for wide-ranging changes to the Criminal Code to legalize drugs and drug use, to the corrections system to allow for bleach and clean needles, and to society so that people who use injection drugs will feel more accepted. While these are useful recommendations and would ameliorate some of the problems faced by people who are dependent on injection drugs, they are not particularly helpful when the worker is faced with reaching and engaging clients and assisting them in practical, day-to-day terms.

Social workers have a number of skills and responsibilities to bring to the issue. First, social workers have a history of dealing with marginalized populations. This includes counselling skills but also advocacy for better conditions for their clients. It is extremely important to deal with the client's instrumental needs, such as stable housing, employment, and food on the table.

Social workers also have a history of innovation. They must be able to go where their clients are. While many of us will not feel comfortable going to the streets, alleys, or shooting galleries, we do have the skills to partner with the service providers who are there in order to make the connections with the clients who could benefit from our expertise. Social workers, as well, have a history of negotiation. We have been able to negotiate formal systems with our clients so that they will have more stable lives.

It is also important that we work through formal social institutions to allow our clients a voice in the decision-making. HIV policy and program development and implementation have a history of involving people with HIV. Those with HIV who use injection drugs must also be involved at this level. While people who have worked in HIV do not consider it unusual to have people with HIV around the table, it is rare in other fields. We have a responsibility to ensure not only that we negotiate on behalf of our clients, but that our clients can participate in the processes themselves.

Social workers have a history of facilitation. We have been able to facilitate families to come together and take charge of their problems. We have been able to facilitate groups that empower the participants to gain strength from others and deal with their own problems. We can also facilitate the visibility of the problems facing our clients by enabling them to speak for themselves in public forums.

Finally, social workers have a responsibility through our *Code of Ethics* to be involved in social justice and change. We have a responsibility to advocate for change in the best interests of our clients and for the overall benefit of society. We have a responsibility to advocate for equal access to resources, services, and opportunities for our clients. And we have a responsibility to advocate for changes to policies and legislation at the local, provincial, federal, and international levels.

How does this translate into recommendations about HIV and injection drug use? Social workers have the skills, history, and responsibility to be involved in the challenges. We have a role to play in ensuring a humane, compassionate, and understanding response to people who use injection drugs and who have HIV.

REFERENCES

Canadian Association of Social Workers. 1997. *Comprehensive Guide for the Care of Persons with HIV Disease, Module #6: HIV Psychosocial Care and Social Work Practice: Ethical, Professional and Practical Issues*. Ottawa: CASW.

Canadian Centre on Substance Abuse. 1994. *Pragmatic Approaches To Drug Use from the Area Between Intolerance and Neglect*. Ottawa: Canadian Centre on Substance Abuse.

Canadian Journal of Infectious Diseases. 1997. *Proceedings, 6th Annual Canadian Conference on HIV/AIDS Research*. Vol. 8, supp. A (Mar.–Apr.).

Corbett, G. 1997. *Doing More for Less in Hamilton-Wentworth: The Need for Brief and Population-based Interventions in Substance Abuse Treatment*. Hamilton, Ont.: Hamilton-Wentworth Regional Public Health Department.

Hankins, C., et al. 1997. 'Moving from Surveillance to the Measurement of Programme Impact', *Canadian Journal of Infectious Diseases* 8, supp. A (Mar.–Apr.): 28A.

Harrison, S. 1997. 'Working with Women', in S. Harrison and V. Carver, *Alcohol and Drug Problems: A Practical Guide for Counsellors*, 2nd edn. Toronto: Addiction Research Foundation.

———, and V. Carver. 1997. *Alcohol and Drug Problems: A Practical Guide for Counsellors*, 2nd edn. Toronto: Addiction Research Foundation.

Health Canada. 1996. *EPI Updates*. Ottawa: Laboratory Centre for Disease Control, Health Canada, Dec.

———. 1997. *HIV/AIDS and Injection Drug Use, A National Action Plan*. Ottawa: Health Canada.

Magner, M. 1997. 'HIV Rate Critical in IDUs', *The Journal*, Addiction Research Foundation (May–June): 1.

Myers, T., M. Millson, J. Rigby, M. Ennis, J. Rankin, W. Mindell, and S. Strathdee. 1995. 'A Comparison of the Determinants of Safe Injecting and Condom Use among Injection Drug Users', paper presented to the Society for the Study of Addiction to Alcohol and Other Drugs.

Patrick, D.M., et al. 1997. 'Incidence of HIV in the Vancouver IDU Study Cohort', *Canadian Journal of Infectious Diseases* 8, supp. A (Mar.–Apr.): 27A.

Remis, R., M. Millson, and C. Major. 1997. *The HIV Epidemic among Injection Drug Users in Ontario: The Situation in 1997*. Toronto: AIDS Bureau, Ontario Ministry of Health.

Riley, D. 1994. 'The Harm Reduction Model', in Canadian Centre on Substance Abuse, *Pragmatic Approaches to Drug Use from the Area between Intolerance and Neglect*. Ottawa.

Wright, N.P., et al. 1997. 'Trends of HIV Positive Test Report Data in Canada', *Canadian Journal of Infectious Diseases* 8, supp. A (Mar.–Apr.): 29A.

Chapter 11

Home Care

Caring Together

DAVID FITZGERALD

INTRODUCTION

This chapter describes the firsthand experience of the development, implementation, and evaluation of a demonstration project of integrated community care for people with HIV. The author was hired as the co-ordinator and was responsible for developing the model in concert with a broad spectrum of community stakeholders. Perhaps the most significant aspect of the integrated community care model is that it does not revolve around additional injections of funding into the health-care system to provide new facilities or programs for people living with HIV. Nor does it advocate wholesale changes in how people living with HIV are treated medically. Rather, integrated community care is about people living with HIV having control over decisions that affect their lives.

The project used a facilitated process through which participants spelled out their visions for the project, gradually getting more specific about the outcomes. This process resulted in a detailed set of indicators for each key outcome. From this conscious and intensive process over a six-month period a clear model of integrated community care emerged to describe the vision that project participants held of a different way of doing business in the community.

The model developed is not just about agencies working together better to streamline services, fill in gaps and shortfalls, and offer clients more choices. It is about something fundamentally different—people living with HIV saying what community resources there should be, people living with HIV and people in agencies and organizations working together to decide how community resources should be used to create a supportive environment. In short, it is about finding creative solutions to difficult challenges in the community.

BACKGROUND

The response to marked increase in HIV cases throughout Canada during the late 1980s was highlighted by a rapid growth in programming and services across the country. The challenge at the time was to find frameworks, or models, to guide the responses to HIV. The experience of many organizations and communities was that the existing models and approaches were limited in their ability to respond to the unique challenges posed by this new and emerging disease. In this context the federal government established expert working groups and gave them the task of reviewing the available experience with HIV. Further, they were charged with finding solutions to problems and proposing new approaches and models. 'These models were to be based on an application of the Palliative Care model represented in the Caring Together report' (Caring Together, 1995). The expert group working on integrated palliative care for persons with HIV disease produced the report *Caring Together*. They proposed that resources be allocated for a pilot project that would seek to develop a model, then apply that model to the delivery of care in the context of HIV. The Caring Together project represented one effort to address the need for such models.

Based on the previous experience of a well-developed interagency organization and a substantial community networking process, Edmonton was chosen to be the host city for a demonstration project. Current thought at the time suggested that the existing infrastructure would support the developmental process of the project and would enhance the building of a model.

Two key factors were present at the time and influenced the direction of the project. First, the project received endorsement and key support from the interagency network. Government, particularly the Alberta government, was included as a partner, but the focus of control was held by the community—those organizations, agencies, and individuals who had experience in shared decision-making and goal-setting in the issue-area of HIV/AIDS. This community sought representation from individuals with HIV to share in the ongoing process of building a solid response to HIV. Based on this experience, the second factor came into play. The concept of developing a model of integrated palliative care then shifted to that of piloting a model of integrated community care. This decision came as a result of the experiences of community members and service providers, who believed that the quality of care and life of people with HIV would be best served with a focus on the whole life spectrum. The expert working group proposed a framework for palliative care that would begin at the time of diagnosis and develop in intensity as the treatment mode decreased over the course of the disease. This framework will likely require rethinking as the treatment of HIV dramatically changes expectations for quality of life.

The outlook became holistic. As is often the case, a service orientation was the main priority during the developmental stage of the project. The primary players and participants tended to come from the professional community. Their expectations at that time were that the project would develop a model that identified new services, along with a reorganization of the existing constellation of services. However, based on broad community consultation and the resulting information, the consumer population (those living with HIV and their personal supports) clearly indicated that their greatest concern was a loss of control and the wish to have a strong voice in the decisions affecting their lives. As well, there were the issues of the reliability of co-ordination of resources and access to services. Needs such as home care, information, and training were at risk of being lost in the maze of rules, regulations, and barriers created by key agencies.

It became clear that a model that would guide the development of the community's response was critical. New services would require continuing access to resources that might not be sustainable. Reshaping the existing network of resources, services, and relationships could be a sustainable and efficient alternative. A key development at this time was the increased attention to health promotion and its application to HIV. The clear challenge from the HIV population gave support to the adoption of a health promotion framework for the project. As Waldrop (1993) explains, 'Strategies such as: self care, mutual aid, the creation of healthy environments, fostering public participation, strengthening community services, co-ordinating health public policy, creating supportive physical and social environments and community development are all ways to address the challenges.'

An exciting movement within the project broadened the focus of model development from singular attention on services requiring long-term funding and resources to developing the entire community's ability to use its strengths, share its resources, and build a base to support long-term change and action. Health promotion provides the framework for individual and collective responsibility. Within the project, this framework fostered the shift to consumer involvement, participation, and leadership in setting priorities and sharing in the process of identifying solutions. Partners at that time included government, the organized and professional service system, and members of the HIV population. This combination of direct stakeholders provided an opportunity of shared ownership of the project, as well as shared responsibility for its outcome. Also, it provided a challenge for trust, communication, mutual learning, and respect for differences and commonalities. The professional community was challenged to view the consumer in a different light. The consumers were challenged to learn leadership and participatory skills and to discover their own sense of expertise. They possessed real-life experience and had something significant to offer. 'Having residents participate actively in all decision-making and program development structures in a community project can be a daunting challenge. . . . Residents need various ways to become involved and opportunities to take on more sophisticated challenges as they become more experienced' (Cameron, Peirson, and Pancer, 1994).

The community began to discover many things about itself. It became apparent there was the potential for creative solutions to problems with the resources then present. The social services sector was viewed as a key resource with a major *support* role to play in the process of community development. As Campfens (1987) has noted, 'Community groups, when assuming greater control over the process of decision-making in the planning of services and the deployment of resources, are known to function at a more efficient level and achieve greater satisfaction than government or institutionally delivered programs.'

Social workers believe in client empowerment and the value of strong relationships that respect mutuality and collaboration. Caring Together (the title was borrowed from the original report of the expert working group, and seemed to fit the vision, heart, and soul of the project) established operating principles that supported the primary role and centrality of consumers within the management and decision-making processes of the project. Practising and demonstrating the ideals the project set out to model to the community demanded change from the participants. One service agency manager expressed his feelings in this way:

> For me, having people living with HIV at the table was a constant reminder that organizations, no matter how client-centred we try to be, don't see the world from the client's perspective. Often when we are trying to do the best we miss the mark. We do things in a way that serves the organization. It helped me reconnect with some core personal and social work values. It offered an option for doing business differently. It's been a powerful wake-up call. (Caring Together, 1995)

An individual living with HIV recounted his experience this way: 'Now I see my input as being valuable. Being involved is a job. I feel useful and I see people listening to what I am saying. That gives me self-esteem, self-confidence' (Caring Together, 1994b). Although the basic principle of the project supported the presence of HIV-positive persons at the management table, sharing the decision-making process with individuals who might also be clients was not an easy transition for many service providers. The agency manager quoted above was greatly affected by the experience. However, this did not occur quickly or easily for many of those involved. Change is, has been, and may well always be the underlying motivation for projects like Caring Together. The need to focus energy in key areas to support changes in values, practice, and policies was very much present in Caring Together. Actually demonstrating the new model of care required 'doing business differently'. Efforts were made to progress from the mould of the project into the everyday experience of the individuals and organizations. Examples of these efforts are detailed below.

Basic preparatory work is needed within community institutions whenever strategies of community development are included in demonstration projects. Three levels of organizational change were identified by the project as being necessary to set the stage for further developments in the realization of the model:

> Level 1: greatest degree of change will be evident such that organizations will be doing things differently.
> Level 2: change would be expected in the planning toward doing things differently.
> Level 3: increased awareness and sensitivity around HIV and openness to doing things differently. (Caring Together, 1995)

It is important to note that although Caring Together was a demonstration project, it could not stay enclosed within a cocoon. It operated on the principles of shared community ownership and responsibility and, therefore, had to provide an environment for the numerous initiatives that would evolve. There was a deliberate move to apply the model as it was being developed. This was an attempt to engage the community in a change process and create the environment of integrated care. Emphasis was placed on learning from the experience of participants and adjusting the model within its original framework.

Seven points were identified as key to the process of engaging the community in change:

1. Efforts to engage the community in making change need to focus on the critical involvement of agencies and organizations in developing collaborative solutions to important community issues.
2. The experience of sitting at the same table with consumers and engaging in joint decision-making fosters engagement among community participants.
3. Efforts to engage the community in a change process need to target individuals and organizations.
4. Efforts to engage the community in change need to acknowledge that people are at different starting points in the change process.
5. Being a change agent is not something people just know how to do.
6. The challenges involved in engaging the community in the change process call for strong leadership and facilitation skills and familiarity with community development strategies.
7. Development of innovative action plans that reflect new ways of doing business calls for creative thinkers with a broad range of experience and expertise. (Caring Together, 1995)

It is clear that developing a model, and then attempting to apply a new approach to an issue within a static environment, is a difficult task. This applied to Caring Together; a new model would require a receptive community and atmosphere. In a deliberate process of preparing the community, significant time was spent setting the stage, asking tough questions, and raising challenges such as: what role would people with HIV play and how would that role be integrated into the structure of the project? how would the voice of the community be reflected in the development and implementation of the project? how would the project develop and maintain a strong community base with community direction?

New approaches, fresh thinking, a new model were critical in the development of quality community care for people with HIV. Training, value clarification, and collaborative services changed the face of care in many centres and added to the development of supportive environments and communities. These services operate within a community structure that encompasses public and private, institutional and community sectors. They are a part of the whole. To ensure that these and other supports and services are delivered with the needs of people with HIV in the forefront, resources need to be engaged and change needs to occur in policy, planning, and services. Direction from the consumer and buy-in from all key resources have shown positive results in such initiatives as the care teams and peer counsellors.

In a number of agencies, significant effort was applied to test the philosophy and principles of the project. The community was mapped into primary and secondary service sectors. Those 'first contact' or primary contact agencies were recruited to be testing grounds. It was hoped that they would pave the way for the rest of the community. Managing the process and attempting initiatives that would give some degree of success were critical. Another obvious concern was the ability of the community and service providers to integrate the activity of the project within existing structures and workloads. Some 6,000 person-hours were spent in project-related meetings. This does not include the time spent by participants in implementing the various initiatives within selected agencies. A real concern was expressed by one service agency, which questioned this time commitment and the practicality of others being able to afford the expenditure of resources, including personnel time.

Caring Together did have the benefit of federal funding. It must be noted, however, that basics such as a commitment to consumer input and realignment of resources do not require major funding initiatives. They do require planning time and a freedom to change existing practice: 'It took and continues to take a lot of conscious effort and thought to change orientation' (Caring Together, 1993b).

PROJECT INITIATIVES

From its earliest stages, a fundamental feature of the project was the input from people living with HIV, who expressed concern regarding loss of control over decisions that would affect their lives. Medical, social, and emotional interventions would be taking place as their disease progressed. These concerns were based on the perception that HIV would alter basic aspects of their lives. Fear of the unknown, along with the corresponding fear of loss of their comforting everyday existence, created a desire in people with HIV to take ground-breaking steps towards controlling their destinies.

Specifically, they feared ineffective, or insufficient, medical treatment as their disease progressed. This had a factual basis in the newness of HIV, the lack of any historical methods of treatment, and the lack of knowledge among the health-care profession. This was compounded by ever-changing standards for treatment of HIV. They also held deep-rooted concerns that medical funding for the treatment of HIV would eventually reach a cut-off point. Beyond this, patients would be left in maintenance situations, where no further progressive treatment would be given.

With this, the tone was set for developing the standards through which health care would be allocated to people with HIV. Their concerns and fears led not only to a re-examination of the type of medical care to be offered, but to a new understanding of total health care. From this, the concept of integrated community care was developed.

The standard medical model of the time spelled out the type of treatment a patient would receive and clearly indicated that the decisions for the treatment would be made by the doctor. People with HIV came to question traditional medical practices. Coincidentally, they developed a substantial level of expertise in the disease affecting them. The success of their efforts may partially be attributed to the very fact that HIV was a new disease and that there was no pool of knowledge regarding its treatment. Thus, a person with HIV could have as much knowledge as his or her medical professional. It is interesting to note that a similar approach is now being taken by breast cancer patients.

Four key areas of focus emerged from the model development process that directed the activity of the project on a community level and were viewed as critical in the realization of integrated community care:

1. Co-ordination of information, training, education.
2. Increased involvement of individuals living with HIV.
3. Creation of a supportive environment and co-ordinated resource system.
4. Enhancement of the capacity to change policies to strengthen resources for individuals living with HIV. (Caring Together 1993a)

Applying the principles of the model and testing its framework in the real world involved directing initiatives in the context of these four areas and engaging community agencies and partners in a series of pilot initiatives. AIDS service organizations, home-care programs, community social service agencies, Alberta provincial social services, and public health all took on major roles as test sites or exemplars of the model application on the community level. The mental health community, the community health-care system, addictions agencies, and others played a supportive and planning role.

To support increased *involvement of individuals with* HIV, steps were taken to link interested and skilled individuals with front-line service providers in a shared learning and service delivery strategy. Monthly meetings of front-line staff and individuals with HIV were held to further support the sharing of skills, expertise, and mutual learning/problem-solving. Advocacy training workshops were begun, HIV orientation for agency staff was presented by individuals with HIV, and an agency advisory committee with a mandate for ongoing input into policy and program development was established. A comprehensive human service agency in-service workshop was developed, with the expertise and participation of people with HIV. A Train the Trainers program was developed to continue to support skill development and ensure a future pool of qualified individuals for ongoing community training and information resourcing.

Further development of trained peer counsellors was supported. These individuals were in contact with primary service sites and enhanced the community's capacity to support persons living with HIV. Community agencies then took leading roles in supporting these developments and testing their efficacy within their own organizations. If change was to occur, a more integrated community response was necessary to provide options and support for a new way of doing business. 'Practice is built bottom up. Through talking and experience. It involves a lot of dialogue' (Caring Together, 1993b).

These approaches, or strategies, led to the realization of the need for increased involvement of individuals with HIV and to the increased ability of agencies to use resources for staff training and improved options for clients. A major challenge for any community is the ability to sustain existing resources, regardless of the provision of new resources. The key to this dilemma was the ongoing commitment and capacity of the partner organizations to anchor these approaches in their support and continuing role in the response to HIV. The increased involvement of individuals with HIV provided a major resource for the community. These individuals have a major stake in the outcome and therefore a major stake in the solutions.

The three other areas of focus—*co-ordination of information/training, development of supportive environments*, and *enhancement of capacity to change policies and influence planning*—depended on successful involvement of individuals with HIV. Information is a critical element in HIV. As one person put it: 'Information + skills + resources = control' (Caring Together, 1995).

The greater the extent of information a client possesses, the greater his/her ability is to provide input towards outcomes. An increased skill level will support more effective use of and access to resources. A common dilemma regarding the value of information is the extreme overload of data. HIV, like other health or social issues, has produced volumes of data, reports, and resource binders. The challenge faced in managing information within the context of the project was gaining an understanding of how the various organizations, individuals, and service providers could receive and use information. Interviews and focus groups were used to develop this capability. More importantly, they also enabled community participants to communicate and develop the capacity to use information as an effective tool in communication. In turn, effective knowledge and communication skills could be put to use to provide effective responses to needs, issues, and challenges. The focus on information drew attention to the need to enhance the expertise of people living with HIV so that they, in turn, could be a real resource to the community. Special attention was given to ensure that barriers were removed to create a 'level playing field' that would allow HIV-positive persons access to new or emerging information.

For an agency to be truly supportive, there must be cultural change that allows it to respond to the needs of its clients. A pilot approach used at one inner-city social service agency exemplified the challenges of building an environment to meet the diverse needs and varied life experiences of its clients. A new understanding of community and personal supports emerged from the work within this pilot project. Natural helping relationships, reduced stigmatization, increased attention to the complex lives of street-involved individuals with HIV, and unique and effective partnerships among service agencies all added to an understanding of what a supportive community environment looks like and how it functions for a diverse population. Increasingly, as individuals are managed in the community and the institutional health-care system reduces its involvement, it becomes important for street agencies to ensure that individuals function to their fullest capacity and when support is needed that it is given in a culturally and emotionally appropriate manner. The natural helpers—the peer counsellors, those with vital information, those who are key service providers—all then play a role in the constellation of the social network. These dynamics came together in this agency's approach.

The development of consumer and staff advisory committees in an AIDS service organization and in a home-care agency further advanced the concept of consumer involvement. These committees were effective in promoting the value of community input into policy and service planning and can help to create and institutionalize an ethic of responsiveness to community needs within the structure of organizations. The committee structure can be a practical way of sounding out the consumer population and getting these people to share in decision-making.

CHANGE BEYOND THE PROJECT

As a pilot project, Caring Together achieved great progress within its mandate. The model of integrated community care has proven to be a valid concept. However, outside the immediate project, the challenge of engaging the broader community and anchoring changes within organizational structures was not totally realized. In fairness, it should be noted that most participants anticipated that the application of the model would be realized over years. For evaluative benefit the impact of these projects should be reviewed three or four years after the demonstration phase. The project was successful in demonstrating that change in community response can occur. Organizations already in the process of change were open to considering the challenges posed by the project. Front-line workers, who served people with HIV, saw the value of the project, and the model, to their service delivery. They were able to recognize that HIV presents unique challenges and therefore requires new approaches and responses. More broadly, however, it was difficult to convince agencies not primarily focused on AIDS to give consideration to the value of the model. 'We were successful in the context of our cocoon (the project) but clumsy in trying to engage others' (Caring Together, 1995).

There is evidence that the model is transferable, given the amount of interest expressed by other communities throughout Canada. Within Edmonton, there are glimpses of sustained change. People with HIV are still strong in their advocacy and presence as a network. They continue to play a major role in partnership with the major AIDS service organizations. Peer counselling continues to be a viable resource for individuals, providing the option of shared learning and problem-solving. The primacy of the person with HIV continues to be supported, if not system-wide, at least by individuals and within the practice of certain agencies.

Projects like Caring Together have pushed the boundaries and challenged the frameworks that did not meet the needs of those they were intended to serve. The value of Caring Together is in applying philosophy and principles to the unique needs of any community. Such work needs to be flexible and adaptable. These projects are not recipes from a cookbook. They are templates for guiding the developments and movements of other communities. People with HIV want and need to be involved in the decisions affecting their lives. The social service sector needs to be responsive to these wants and needs. The Caring Together project is one example of how changing the dynamics between caregivers and those cared for can result in a more responsive community. Even though the long-term results are difficult to evaluate, and structural change takes place over years, not months, the Caring Together project was able to test new concepts, share their value, and suggest their viability. Most importantly, it gave hope to those who are infected and those who care for them. It sent a message to the broader community that there is another way of building a community capacity for respecting diversity, promoting collaborative solutions, and creating an environment of care through all stages of the illness.

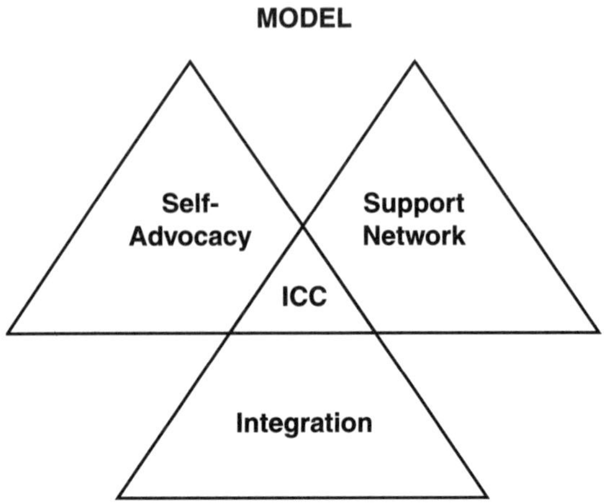

Figure 1 Integrated Community Care (ICC)

ABOUT THE MODEL

As noted above, the model developed by this demonstration project is not a cookbook recipe. It is based on a set of principles articulated by the community. The outcomes that are part of the model are in reality the outcomes established by the project. The model was to be the result of the work of participants, based on their learning and successful practical experience.

The outcomes are followed by indicators, which more clearly spell out the intent of each outcome. The model is based on three key factors which unite to form the basis for community action that will result in integrated care. If any one of these factors is missing, then the whole effort to build a strong community base is in question. These outcomes and the model itself reflect an approach to community issues regardless of their etiology. This approach is based on solid health promotion theory and community development practice. It reflects what best social work practice is about and what our *Code of Ethics* outlines. As professionals, we are challenged to walk and work with our clients. More than any other issue, HIV challenges us to follow this practice framework. We are also challenged to ensure that service organizations and the community are welcoming and supportive of clients and that they work to support individual growth. Lastly, we are called to work within community structures that seek to share resources and build partnerships, drawing on the collective skills and resources within the community. This is what the model articulates, and this is what the model challenges any community or organization or group of people to strive towards.

OUTCOMES

Following are listings of indicators for each of the three outcomes—self-advocacy, support network, and integration.

SELF-ADVOCACY

People living with HIV advocate for themselves individually and collectively to ensure that they have control over decisions about their lives and health.

- People diagnosed with HIV think it is possible to live with HIV, and they have the desire to take control over their own lives and health.
- People living with HIV believe they have the right to control their own lives and health and to make decisions about their care and treatment.
- People living with HIV are able to be in control of their lives and health; they are confident and assertive and make their own decisions.
- People living with HIV see themselves as a key resource in their own lives, trust their own experiences, and believe in their own capacities.
- People living with HIV are able to build support networks and negotiate with their personal support networks about providing support in ways that recognize that people living with HIV are in charge of their own lives and resources.
- People living with HIV challenge the community—people, agencies, and organizations—to provide a supportive environment for all people living with HIV.

SUPPORT NETWORK

The community—people, agencies, and organizations—provides a consistent supportive environment for people living with HIV and their personal and professional caregivers. Community resources have the structures and policies in place to provide a supportive environment that meets the following standards or expectations.

- They ensure access to a wide range of opportunities for involvement of people living with HIV—including serving on boards and committees, working as staff, and being peer counsellors.
- They involve people living with HIV in saying what they find supportive and in evaluating how they are doing.
- They ensure that all people working in organizations, including first-contact staff, professionals, custodians, volunteers, and managers, have basic information about HIV and are trained in universal precautions to the point that they feel confident and comfortable.
- They have identified sources of support and information for people working in organizations to contact if they need to talk about their concerns or fears.
- They recognize the stress involved in working and living with people whose health is deteriorating, and in dealing with death, and provide appropriate support to people working with those who are HIV-positive to prevent burn-out.
- They provide community-wide and agency-based opportunities for people to share their experiences of working with people living with HIV and for people living with HIV to share their experiences.

- They have explicit expectations that people working with people living with HIV make connections with those they work with, connect them with other agencies and individuals, follow up on connections, and work in ways that respect the decisions of people living with HIV.
- They ensure support for human rights generally, and specifically, for the rights of individuals who might be targets of discrimination on the basis of race, sexual orientation, socio-economic status, etc.
- Community norms and behaviours demonstrate caring support so that all people living with HIV have equal opportunities to build and have the support they choose.
- People working with people living with HIV interact with them in respectful and supportive ways built on the principle of equality.
- They believe it is the right of people living with HIV to be treated with dignity and respect and to make their own decisions about their lives.
- They respect the right of people living with HIV to be assertive about their requirements.
- They work in ways that reflect a recognition of the whole person, beyond the HIV diagnosis.
- They offer information in non-judgemental ways and present options to be explored.
- They listen to and explore information and options provided by the people living with HIV.
- They follow through with the people they work with to keep the connection alive.
- They don't see themselves as the experts, but are willing and able to seek information as required and to link people with other individuals/ resources.
- They work with clients to identify what works well for them and to find ways to maintain and build on what works.
- They support people diagnosed with HIV to see the possibility of living with HIV.
- They support people living with HIV to recognize themselves as resources in their own lives.
- They support people living with HIV to build support networks.
- They support the right of people living with HIV to choose their own personal support networks and decide how they want the support networks involved in their lives.
- They recognize and support the role and importance of personal support networks in the lives of people living with HIV.
- They feel confident in their work with people living with HIV, because they have information, skills, and support.

INTEGRATION

Community resources and people living with HIV work collaboratively to address ongoing, new, and emerging issues facing people living with HIV and their personal and professional caregivers.

- Agencies/organizations have established positive ways of working together, supported by effective communications.
- Agencies/organizations work co-operatively to decrease institutional barriers for people living with HIV and to connect them with support and services.
- Agencies/organizations know about and use a wide range of community resources, including peer counsellors, advocates, and trainers.
- All stakeholders, including people living with HIV, collaborate in making decisions about resource design and delivery.
- Funding applications and decisions reflect a co-operative and integrated way of doing business among agencies/organizations.
- Community resources work together creatively to respond to emerging populations and issues and to prepare to meet new challenges in a proactive manner.
- AIDS service organizations collaborate with other organizations in the community to work on shared concerns and issues.
- Community resources and people living with HIV work collaboratively towards changes in public policy on HIV/AIDS.

EVALUATION

The project was based on an evaluation that saw the participants engage in a learning-for-change process. The evaluators were very much partners in the process of the project and thus shared in the difference the project would make in the community. 'The evaluation was oriented to providing ongoing and intensive feedback with a view to guiding project activities' (Caring Together, 1994a). It was clear that the evaluation would not so much describe the experience of Caring Together but rather analyse and interpret the experience. For this to occur, three key areas of activity were developed. The evaluation was involved in the development and analysis of the community consultation, which provided the critical data on which the project planning based its direction and future activities. The evaluation then established the process for feedback through verbal and written format. This feedback took the form of raising questions and highlighting accomplishments and learning that would lead to a refinement of the outcomes and the strategy to reach these outcomes. Lastly, the evaluation provided discussion and issue papers and offered guidance on the development of the model of integrated community care and the project action model.

The feedback through the discussion and issue papers was particularly critical, as these formed the basis for the participants to review the impact of the project and the effect of its activities. 'The purpose of these papers was to: consolidate feedback, contribute to a climate of shared learning, reveal the differences the project was making, support the active application of the findings in the change process' (Caring Together, 1993b). This style of evaluation allowed for immediate attention to issues and encouraged the participants to analyse more critically what was being done and the impact of activity or progress. It supported the ability of all involved to be active participants and learners and thus to share in the responsibility of the evaluation. It thereby brought the project into full perspective and supported an evolving model that would be experienced in the present and reflect current experience.

A full range of topics was covered by these discussion and issue papers. They were provided at critical turning points within the project as challenges and struggles brought issues to the forefront. Key challenges included: articulating the philosophy of the project and engaging the broader community; defining involvement of consumers and the principle of 'primacy' of people living with HIV; the struggle to recruit consumers and to what end; compensation for people living with HIV involved in the project; the impact of information and its power; the implications of developing a community development approach; what had been learned about change; what had been learned from the various initiatives. Learning sessions provided a forum for these and other issues to be debated. The papers provided the information needed and raised the questions that guided these learning sessions. Based on a final submission from the evaluators, 17 conclusions were drawn from these sessions. One conclusion in particular draws attention to the struggle within many demonstration projects: 'Despite the feeling of being in a muddle, the implementation in many areas was congruent with the model that emerged. That is because the guiding principles were clear from the outset and lots of groundwork was done to understand what needed to happen' (Caring Together, 1995).

PROJECT ACTION MODEL

With the confirmation of the outcomes it became clear that a process would be needed to guide project activities to ensure that these activities were linked to the outcomes and their indicators. The evaluation guided the development of an action model as a workable framework within which to show these linkages. Program logic model theory provided the context for the development and application of the action model. 'When prepared as part of a broader program profile, a logic model helps develop a common understanding of the program between managers, staff and evaluators' (Rush and Ogborne, 1991). The project needed to state clearly what was required to achieve the indicators as a reflection of the outcomes. The task then became to identify what situation in the community would show that these indicators were present within agencies or institutions or within the skill level of individuals. Following from this, the project identified which activities were linked to support this situation—in short, what was the relationship between anything occurring in the context of the project and the movement towards the outcomes? Also, the relationship between the project demonstration activity and the daily reality of members in the community was vital in determining success. The project action model provided a concrete and visible linkage between all of these factors, and also challenged the efficacy of project activity. In other words, if a particular activity did not have a link to the outcomes, why apply resources and energy? This model/framework, in addition, allowed for a continual testing of the model of integrated community care. Does what works on paper also work in reality? Based on this approach the evaluators and the participants could ask the critical questions, raise the critical concerns, and engage in an ongoing learning process.

REFERENCES

Cameron, C., L. Peirson, and S. Pancer. 1994. 'Resident Participation in the Better Beginnings, Better Future Prevention Project: Part II—Factors that Facilitate and Hinder Involvement', *Canadian Journal of Community Mental Health* 13, 2 (Fall): 213–27.

Campfens, H. 1987. 'Nurturing Community: The Individual and Community in Development Practice', presentation to Community Development Conference, Social Planning Council, Edmonton.

Caring Together Demonstration Project. 1993a. Proposal: Application for Renewal.

———. 1993b. Evaluation Papers, Aug.

———. 1994a. 'Implications for Adapting a Community Development Approach', evaluation discussion paper, June.

———. 1994b. Participants Learning Session, Dec.

———. 1995. *Building Supportive Communities for People Living with HIV*, Final Evaluation Report, July.

Rush, B., and A. Ogborne. 1991. 'Program Logic Models: Expanding Their Role and Structure for Program Planning and Evaluation', *Canadian Journal of Program Evaluation* 6, 2: 95–106.

Waldrop, K. 1993. 'A Framework for Health Promotion . . . A Framework for AIDS', *Canadian Journal of Public Health* (Jan.-Feb.).

Working Group. 1989. *Caring Together: The Report of the Expert Working Group on Integrated Palliative Care for Persons with AIDS*. Feb.

Chapter 12

Multiple Loss and Mourning within the Gay Male Community

BILL RYAN, MARC A. HAMEL, AND CHEH CHO

I have the impression sometimes that my life is lived in a world of ghosts. As much as I seek out these ghosts in melancholy, I run from them in fear that their fate will be mine. They are my friends, all gone. Like the dinosaurs, I fear some day all gay men will be extinct.

—38-year-old man

INTRODUCTION

Few gay men of our era will forget the first time they heard of a new disease that was rearing its head in the gay villages of New York and San Francisco. In the early 1980s the illness called GRID—gay-related immune deficiency—was already taking its toll and causing widespread panic among gay men. The impact of HIV/AIDS on gay men has little parallel in the scope of loss and grief that it has signified. We invoke terms like 'war', 'holocaust', 'ravage' to try to describe the immeasurable suffering that HIV disease has unleashed on members of the gay community. As significant as the losses due to HIV disease have become, relatively little has been written on the impact that such losses have had on the gay individual and within the gay community. The aim of this chapter is to identify the various psychological and social sequelae associated with the bereaved gay individual and the gay community. Specifically, the authors wish to identify how gay men and the community have reacted to these multiple losses and how mental health professionals can lend support in circumventing these losses.

THE MAGNITUDE OF LOSS

As of December 1996, the number of reported cases of AIDS worldwide was cited as being 1,393,638 cases in 209 countries. At that time, approximately 1 per cent of these were in Canada. As of 31 March 1997, Health Canada had received reports of 14,836 cumulative cases, of which 10,837 (73 per cent) constituted cumulative deaths. To be even more specific, of the reported cases in Canada at that time, 10,815 of these (78.7 per cent) were attributed to gay men or, more broadly defined, as 'men who have sex with men' (Health Canada, 1997).

Although in North America many other populations are affected by the HIV epidemic, in Canada the overwhelming number of cases reported continues to be from the gay male community, with rising numbers of these being younger gay men (under 30 years of age) (Health Canada, 1997). In some Canadian cities up to one in four to one in five gay men may be infected with HIV (Health Canada, 1997). These statistics not only depict the continued rate of infection within the gay community but illustrate the extent of potential losses both personally and socially. Given that the rate of HIV infection has yet to decline, many other individuals (e.g., family members, lovers, and friends) may have to deal with the potential losses of their loved ones in the future.

PSYCHOLOGICAL SEQUELAE OF HIV INFECTION

Since 1981, an impressive literature on the psychosocial stressors of living with HIV has appeared (e.g., Atkinson et al., 1988; Antoni, 1991; Cassens, 1985; Catalan et al., 1992; Christ, Weiner, and Moynihan, 1986; Chuang et al., 1989; Holland and Tross, 1985; Kalichman and Sikkema, 1995; Lamping and Sewitch, 1990; Maj, 1990; Morin, Charles, and Malyon, 1984; O'Dowd, 1988; Ostrow et al., 1989; Perry and Tross, 1984; Sadovsky, 1991; Thompson, Nanni, and Levine, 1996; Tross and Hirsch, 1988). Although earlier reports had a tendency to compare the stresses of living with HIV infection with those of other diseases or chronic illness, most experts believe that the psychosocial consequences of HIV infection are more numerous and devastating than those associated with any other disease. Specifically, researchers and clinicians claim that there are numerous specific HIV stressors incomparable to those seen in cancer patients, including: the high rate of mortality among this population, the young age of those infected by the disease, the fear of contaminating others, the transmission of the disease by sexual activity, the long incubation period, and the absence of an effective cure for the illness (Christ, Weiner, and Moynihan, 1986; Wolcott et al., 1986).

Furthermore, Lamping et al. (1992) claim that persons living with HIV infection experience a double stigma: first, HIV is a potentially deadly disease and is contagious; second, the disease is associated with groups of individuals already socially stigmatized—in particular, gay men and intravenous drug users. Hence, HIV disease carries specific stressors of its own. Lamping and Sewitch (1990: 7) explain: 'AIDS-related disease is associated with a unique set of psychosocial stresses from three distinct sources, including the stresses associated with: a) a chronic illness, b) life-threatening illness, and c) AIDS-related disease.' Catalan (1995) also claims that three distinct factors explain why persons living with HIV infection may experience greater psychological distress: (1) disease-related factors following notification of a positive serostatus or presence of opportunistic infections; (2) factors related to the person's previous history of psychiatric difficulties or poor coping strategies; and (3) interpersonal and social factors, such as lack of perceived social support or adjustment. Given these HIV stressors it is not surprising that studies have suggested that seropositive individuals face a considerable amount of psychological stressors related to HIV infection, including depression,[1] hopelessness,[2] and suicidal ideations.[3]

Hence, living with HIV infection not only entails confronting one's personal losses as a result of the diagnosis; often one is asked as well to cope with those of lovers and friends. For all the above reasons, it is perhaps correct to state that individuals living with HIV infection experience specific stressors not generally seen in persons living with other chronic or terminal illnesses.

UNDERSTANDING GRIEF REACTIONS

The typical response to any loss is grief. Grief is generally defined as the 'process of psychological, social and somatic reactions to the perception of loss' (Rando, 1984).[4] Given the intensity, implications, and consequences of experiencing a loss (see Parkes, 1972; Stroebe, Stroebe, and Hansson, 1988), as well as the universality of its occurrence, much effort has been expended in identifying the leitmotif underlying the human experience of loss. Lindemann (1944) was the first researcher to investigate systematically the grieving process related to loss. After studying grief reactions among 101 recently bereaved patients, Lindemann found some common patterns of grieving, including somatic or bodily distress, preoccupation with the image of the deceased, guilt reactions related to the deceased, hostile reactions, and inability to function as before the loss. In addition to these responses, Lindemann added that many grievers seemed to develop symptoms that closely resemble those of the deceased. The belief that all bereaved individuals exhibit similar features persisted throughout the grieving literature. As an illustration, Averill's (1968: 744) description of grief responses during bereavement reflects this 'stereotypical response hypothesis' in which he states that grief responses are:

i) A complex but *stereotyped* response pattern which includes such psychological and physiological symptoms as withdrawal, fatigue, sleep disturbances, and loss of appetite;
ii) Elicited by a rather well-defined stimulus situation, namely, the real or imagined loss of a significant object (or role), and it is resolved when new object relations are established;
iii) A ubiquitous phenomenon among human beings and appears in other social species as well, especially in higher primates;
iv) An extremely stressful emotion, both psychologically and physiologically, and yet behavior during grief is often antithetical to the establishment of new relations, and hence the alleviation of the stress.

The apparent stereotypical or predictable manifestations of grief observed by Lindemann and others incited an array of researchers to propose stage theories of 'normal grief' reactions.

STAGE THEORIES OF GRIEVING

Engel (1964) proposed that the process of grieving involved three stages. The first stage is shock and disbelief. This stage is characterized by the bereaved's inability to recognize and accept the reality of the loss. Denial is suggested as the primary response during this first stage. The second stage, developing awareness, is typified as a gradual acceptance and significance of the loss. Physiological and psychological reactions are said to result. Finally, Engel asserts that resolution is achieved whereby the bereaved re-enters into daily activities, completing the three-stage model.

Bowlby and Parkes (1970) suggested a similar three-stage grieving process but divided Engel's second stage into two distinct phases. During this second phase, *pining*, which involves the bereaved's yearning for the presence of the deceased, and *disorganization and despair*, characterized by depressed affect ensuing from having failed to relocate the deceased, are said to be common experiences. Finally, Kübler-Ross's (1969) model of the grieving process is perhaps the best known of the stage models of grieving. Derived from her work with cancer patients, she views the sequence of response to loss as following five stages. The grieving process begins with denial and isolation characterized by a period of shock. Anger ensues at the second stage. Pleas made to supernatural forces or beings and to others characterize the third stage; in other words, bargaining. The ineffectual quest to regain the lost object or person results in depressive episodes, which colour the fourth stage. Kübler-Ross's final stage, acceptance, is identical to the aforementioned three-stage models of grief whereby the bereaved person re-enters one's social arena and activities.

As attractive as the stage models appear, they have received much warranted criticism. Bugen (1977: 196–7) states:

> First, the stages are not separate entities, but subsume one another or blend dynamically. Secondly, the stages are not successive; any individual may experience anger for instance, prior to denial, or perhaps disorganization before shock. Thirdly, it is not necessary to experience every stage. Depression, or for that matter any volatile emotion, may never be a recognizable response to loss. Fourthly, the intensity and duration of any stage may vary idiosyncratically among those who grieve. For one mourner, sadness may be a short-lived experience, while anger is a more protracted stage; the duration of these two emotional stages might be reversed for someone else. Finally, little empirical evidence is offered by proponents to substantiate the theory of stages.

In addition to the above criticisms of the stage models of grieving is their failure to conceptualize grief responses in context. Grief reaction is a dynamic process, not a static one. Likewise, grief responses are very much under stimulus control, which renders bereaved individuals vulnerable to their environmental and contextual stimuli. As such, certain stimuli (e.g., listening to a piece of music or residing in the same household as that shared with the deceased) may elicit grief reactions that may lead the bereaved person to 'regress' to previous stages. In turn, certain stimuli (e.g., a network of social support) may be sufficient for a bereaved person to adapt placidly to the loss without going through any of the predetermined stages.

DIMENSIONS OF 'HEALTHY' GRIEVING

In reaction to such criticisms, certain researchers have opposed the notion of stages or phases of 'normal' or 'healthy'[5] grieving, opting to speak instead of components or dimensions of grief (e.g., Ramsay, 1979; Worden, 1991).[6] Given the exhaustive list of behaviours and the variety of responses related to loss, one can conceptualize grief reactions along four dimensions: *affective* (e.g., sadness, anger, guilt, anxiety, yearning, relief, etc.), *cognitive* (e.g., disbelief, confusion, preoccupation with the deceased, hallucinations, etc.), *physical sensations* (hollowness in the stomach, tightness in the chest and throat, depersonalization, weakness in the muscles, fatigue, lack of energy, etc.), and *behavioural* (sleep and appetite disturbances, alcohol or drug use, social withdrawal, avoidance, crying, overactivity, searching or calling out for the deceased, etc.) (see Worden, 1991). The advantages of conceptualizing grief reactions along such dimensions are numerous. First, unlike the stage models, dimensions of grief allow for individual variations in loss responses. Second, these components satisfy the criteria of viewing grief reactions as varying in intensity, duration, and presence. Finally, such a behavioural or multimodal model of grieving allows for an operational definition of grief behaviours for assessment purposes, empirical investigation, and intervention.

PATHOLOGICAL GRIEVING

Conflicting reports also exist in terms of what constitutes 'pathological grieving'. If researchers fail to agree as to what 'normal' grief responses include, opinions are more divided when defining pathological grief. Numerous terms have been proposed to denote pathological grief, including: 'absent' (e.g., Deutsch, 1937), 'abnormal' (e.g., Hodgkinson, 1982), 'distorted' and 'delayed' (Brown and Stoudemire, 1983), 'melancholia' (Freud, 1917), 'unexpected', 'ambivalent', and 'chronic' (Parkes, 1965; Parkes and Weiss, 1983), and 'morbid' (Mawson et al., 1981; Sireling, Cohen, and Marks, 1988). Other terms have also been suggested, such as 'abnormal', 'complicated', 'truncated', 'atypical', 'neurotic', and 'dysfunctional' (see Middleton et al., 1994, for a review). Furthermore, the lack of consensus in obtaining an operationalized definition of pathological grief is aggravated when considering other syndromes that may coexist with grief responses. Studies on the responses of the bereaved have identified manifestations of grief that can co-occur with other mental health problems, including major depressive disorder,[7] anxiety disorder,[8] and post-traumatic stress disorder.[9] At times, the presence of comorbidity with such syndromes and others also makes the validity and assessment of pathological grief difficult. Finally, the need to define what constitutes 'pathological grief' raises another important question: One's grief reaction becomes pathological for whom—the counsellor/clinician? family members and/or friends?

In summary, grief reactions are multifaceted and complex in nature. At this point, one cannot assume that grief reactions are typical, let alone stereotypical. The empirical studies seem to indicate that one's evaluation of such reactions must take place within the context of the individual and his/her social framework.

DO MEN AND WOMEN GRIEVE DIFFERENTLY?

So far, general reactions to the experience of loss have been discussed. To identify specific reactions of multiple loss of the gay individual and the gay community, it is perhaps worthwhile to ask: Do men and women grieve differently? To date, the evidence is far from conclusive.

In citing the work of Glick et al. (1974), Dershimer (1990) reported that although there are common similarities in the behaviours of the widows and widowers during mourning, some fundamental differences exist in the response patterns between the two sexes, including:

> 1) Men tended to interpret their losses in terms of dismemberment while women used terms connoting abandonment.
> 2) Men found it more difficult to give attention and energy to their work after the death whereas women tended to find solace in work.
> 3) Men, much more than women, were unable to display their grief and, as the year of bereavement progressed, men ended emotional displays more quickly than women.
> 4) Fewer men than women blamed fate or became angry with those who had not had similar misfortunes.
> 5) Men exhibited less guilt than women as time went on.
> 6) Men remarried more quickly and, in general, moved more quickly towards social recovery than women.
> 7) Men cared more about maintaining their highest levels of functioning, and were more dismayed than women by the loss of energy and competence.
> 8) The lack of a sexual partner was more bothersome to men than women.
> 9) Despite the more rapid movement of men towards social recovery, their movement towards emotional recovery was slower than that of women. (Dershimer, 1990: 30)

These sex differences can be explained by cultural forces. Culture dictates how one is expected to respond to a loss. Staudacher (1991) describes the cultural expectations of men during such times. She suggests that male sex-role conditioning acts strongly during this period. In Western society, men are generally encouraged to deal with the loss of a loved one by: (1) taking charge; (2) supporting others as they 'bear up'; and (3) accepting death as a challenge, even a test of masculinity.

Thus, death may constitute a double crisis: the loss itself and the behavioural challenge created by coping with the loss. The problem then becomes how to stay 'manly' when human needs and drives call for exhibiting 'unmanly' emotions. Lister (1991) describes the most common or typical coping styles for men during the grieving process, including:

1) Remaining Silent: A common response by men to the loss of a loved one is to bury their thoughts and emotions. Outbursts of cries and despair would indicate weakness to the onlookers and be perceived as having lost control. Hence, silence becomes a defense against being perceived as weak or out of control.
2) Engaging In Solitary Mourning Or 'Secret' Grief: Alongside this silence, many men may find it more comfortable to mourn alone. Expressions of emotions, if they occur, will most likely occur in solitude. This solitary permission allows once again others to perceive the mourner as being in control.
3) Taking Action: Sometimes, the expression of pain and sorrow may be disguised in the form of taking action. This is often seen in men who have experienced the following types of losses: the death of a child, an accidental or unexpected death, or death as a result of murder. As a means of expressing their grief, men may take on affirmative actions to somehow compensate for the loss. Filing lawsuits against the medical staff or campaigning for educational information to prevent a similar incident that caused the loss are means for men to remain in control and feed their need for action. At times, anger can ensue. Anger can be misused and simply fuel more negative emotions when violence erupts. Anger may also be directed inwardly when dealing with a loss becomes unbearable. It is not uncommon that alcohol or drug consumption increase during this period; especially if one was prone to use such substances as a means to escape reality.
4) Masking Fear: The common grief reactions of grieving men can all be grouped under the heading of 'masking fear'. Men have been socialized to hide their emotions as a means to secure their 'masculine' image; however, in doing so, the fear of one's own mortality sadly goes unexplored.

Hence, there appear to be differences in the way men and women respond to loss. Part of the sex differences identified can be largely attributed to the way both sexes have been socialized to express their emotions and experiences. In addition, the power of cultural norms on grief cannot be underestimated. There is ample evidence in cultural and anthropological studies to indicate that how members of a given society will mourn the dead is largely determined by the values of that particular culture. One only has to examine the different nuances that exist between mourning rituals in various cultures to understand such influences.

DO GAY MEN GRIEVE DIFFERENTLY?

As there appears to be some evidence that men respond differently than women to loss, can one say that gay men grieve differently than their heterosexual counterparts? Again, the influence of the culture to which one identifies oneself is crucial. If one accepts that the gay, lesbian, and bisexual communities share a distinct culture (see Pope, 1995), then the answer is probably yes. To understand why this is so, one must examine the origins of societal prejudice against gay men and lesbians. Only then can one examine how a group that is stigmatized grieves such massive losses among its own.

THE ORIGINS OF THE STIGMATIZATION OF HOMOSEXUALITY

Few human phenomena have been stigmatized as severely as homosexuality. In formal educational processes and professional training, reflected in social taboos and cultural mythology, homosexuality is seen as undesirable, perverted, abnormal, and tragic. These attitudes and values are deeply rooted in the theological, moral, and legal traditions of our culture and are still pervasive, despite being discredited scientifically.

1. *Homosexuality and religion.* Christian theologians in the Middle Ages relegated homosexuality to the realm of the unnatural, incorrectly believing that animals exhibited no homosexual (or bisexual) behaviour, which we know to be an error today. If homosexuality did not exist in nature, which was believed to be free from the stain of sin and therefore as God intended creation to be, then homosexuality in humans was seen as a sign of humanity's fall from divine grace and hence a perversion of God's will. This belief that homosexuality did not exist in nature is widely perpetuated even today by educational systems that continue to exclude correct and appropriate information about the existence of homosexuality and bisexuality in the animal kingdom, directly contributing to a conditioning of shame among young gay, lesbian, and bisexual people, leading them to believe that they are unnatural.

2. *Homosexuality within the mental health system.* In the nineteenth century, as religious domination of the sciences began to wane, the newly emerging sciences of psychology, psychiatry, and sexology began to promote the image of homosexuality as a mental illness, and through to the 1960s horrible treatments were imposed on men and women with no success of 'curing' their attractions and desires. Only in 1973 did the American Psychiatric Association remove 'homosexuality' from the *Diagnostic and Statistical Manual*—after a great deal of controversy. The World Health Organization removed 'homosexuality' from its list of mental disorders only in 1992, after overcoming years of vehement protests from the Vatican and fundamentalist Islamic countries. Still today, a small but vociferous minority of psychotherapists claim to be able to treat and cure homosexuality, with no proof in the scientific literature to bear out their claims. Religious organizations, springing from right-wing theological ideologies, also offer 'cures' and 'healing', which are no more than teaching people to lie about who they are and to adopt 'normal' (approved) behaviours.

3. *Homosexuality within the legal system.* In 1969 Canada ended centuries of legal sanctions against homosexuality and decriminalized all sexual activity between two consenting adults undertaken in private. Practically speaking, homosexuality was decriminalized without being mentioned in the bill. Most of the social discourse (and political dissent) surrounding this bill revolved around the fact that, effectively, homosexuality would no longer be considered a crimi-

nal activity. In 1977, the province of Quebec, in its provincial Charter of Rights, became the second jurisdiction in the world (after Denmark) to forbid discrimination based on sexual orientation. Most Canadian provinces have now amended their human rights codes to forbid discrimination based on sexual orientation.

The courts have obliged reluctant federal governments to interpret the Canadian Charter of Rights and Freedoms as if sexual orientation is a forbidden ground of discrimination, even though it is not explicitly enshrined as such, and the Canadian Human Rights Commission accepts complaints based on discrimination against gay men and lesbians. Recently, the federal government amended the Canadian Human Rights Code (which governs the relations between the federal government and its employees as well the relationships between employee and employer in federally regulated industries—banks, transport, communications, etc.) to outlaw discrimination based on sexual orientation. These legal changes have taken place only in the last 30 years, the majority in the last 10, which means that most adult gay men and lesbians have lived significant periods of their lives, if not in a state of illegality, at least only recently able to seek protection from discrimination under the law.

HIDDEN GRIEVERS: THE IMPACT OF STIGMA ON GRIEF

The constant stigmatization and lack of social recognition experienced by gay men have had and continue to have profound implications on how they live out their reaction to their own mortality and those of their loved ones. To a great extent and in a majority of cases, these men and their community can be considered 'hidden' grievers.

Hidden grieving implies non-legitimacy. Formal, mainstream rituals do not address the sexual orientation of those who have died, which means for the most part that their relationships are ignored. Those who belong to the gay community, even men with whom the deceased may have shared years of intimacy, are often sidelined and their situation is not recognized or affirmed. As a consequence their grief is disenfranchised. It is deemed not to be legitimate.

How do individuals react to this disenfranchisement? Often, by leaving instructions about how a funeral is to be conducted, who is to be invited, who is to be acknowledged. If this has not been arranged, the grieving life-partner may not be acknowledged in the funeral ceremony—neither by the church or synagogue representative nor by the family. Hence, alternative forms of ritualized grieving may be developed. Memorial services organized within the gay community for lovers, friends, and accepting family members may be held so that some form of public mourning may be experienced. However, such ceremonies remain outside mainstream society and can contribute to the feelings of shame experienced by the mourners.

At times, the grief of gay men may be marginalized even within their own community. Members of the gay, lesbian, and bisexual community can become tired and terrified by death and any reminder of its impact—it has been such a constant presence during the HIV epidemic. This results in further marginalization of individuals who are grieving and who need affirmation from their community and their society.

WHERE WE GO FROM HERE: IMPLICATIONS FOR RESEARCH AND PRACTICE

Numerous community organizations have been successful in providing psychological support to the gay, lesbian, and bisexual community and others to circumvent these multiple losses. In Canada, chiefly in large urban centres, psychological services are specifically designed to aid persons affected by and infected with HIV infection. In such settings, one finds support groups and individual counselling. On a more social level, the gay community has been active in keeping alive the memories of those they have lost by holding annual commemorative marches (e.g., Ça Marche in Montreal). Such events not only help to raise AIDS awareness but also give the gay community a place to express their grief. However, one cannot expect to relieve grief reactions merely by single events. Although community support is available on a continuous basis, its impact on grief reactions has largely been untested.

When HIV infection and AIDS first appeared, health professionals busied themselves to find a cure, prevent further spread of the virus, and bring psychological aid to those touched by the disease. No one was prepared for the devastating loss that would result as a consequence of the epidemic. Further still, mental health professionals and lay persons were forced to confront an issue that remained taboo, namely, death. With HIV has come renewed interest in death studies. When death is studied it is generally within the context of a single loss (e.g., death of a parent, child, spouse, partner). Today, AIDS is forcing us to name and recognize death in its entirety, in its social and community consequences. We know that individuals face multiple deaths of those close to them, and unfortunately we remain ill-equipped to help these multiple grievers. As indicated earlier, little empirical data exist on the extent of multiple loss experienced by gay men and little still has been done systematically to test effective interventions aimed at comforting this population.

Despite the lack of empirical knowledge to circumvent multiple losses, one can rely on various works that have examined strategies to deal with single losses. Consensus among researchers and clinicians exists regarding the belief that one who is confronted with a loss must undergo a process of grief (see Ramsay, 1977). For example, Hodge (1972: 230–1) states:

> The problem must be brought into the open and confronted, no matter how unpleasant it may be for the patient. *The grief work must be done.* There is no healthy escape from this. We might even add that the grief will be done. Sooner or later, correctly or incorrectly, completely or incompletely, in a clear or distorted manner, *it will be done.* People have a natural tendency to avoid the unpleasantness of grief work, but it is necessary and the more

> actively it is done the shorter will be the period of grief. If the grief work is not actively pursued, the process may be fixated or aborted or delayed, with the patient feeling that he may have escaped it. However, almost certainly a distorted form of the grief will appear at some time in the future.

This belief is independent of one's theoretical and clinical orientation. This grief work hypothesis is generally defined as 'a cognitive process of confronting a loss, of going over the events before and at the time of death, of focusing on memoring [*sic*] and working towards detachment from the deceased. It requires an active, ongoing, effortful attempt to come to terms with loss' (Stroebe, 1992–3: 19–20). Confronting a loss as opposed to denying or avoiding it is considered an adaptive response.

Evidence supporting the notion that all bereaved persons need to go through a process of 'grief work' is not unequivocal, however. The paucity of research investigating the grief work hypothesis and its efficacy in bringing about more adaptive behaviour has indicated that for some bereaved individuals the process of grief work is not always called for. For example, Stroebe and Stroebe (1991) conducted a longitudinal study on conjugal bereavement. They followed a group of 60 widows and widowers over a two-year period. Grief work was operationalized as either confrontation or avoidance. Results indicated that bereaved women who confronted their loss did not fare any better than those who used avoidance as a strategy in dealing with the death of a spouse. For widowers, the results supported the grief work hypothesis. For bereaved men, avoidance was associated with poor adjustment over the two-year period. These researchers concluded that the grief work hypothesis of the need to confront one's loss was not supported for bereaved women, although avoidance proved to be detrimental for widowers. Hence, the notion that grief work is justified for all bereaved individuals is unsupported by this empirical evidence.

Similar conclusions were reached by a recent content analysis of bereavement programs. Schneiderman et al. (1994) evaluated empirical studies on child and/or parent bereavement programs that included randomized control trials. Their analysis did not find unequivocal evidence for the grief work hypothesis. They concluded that bereavement programs appear to work for some individuals under certain conditions (see also Olders, 1989; Parkes, 1980). This result highlights an important challenge for mental health professionals. Efforts must be directed at identifying the type of bereavement program (e.g., family or group versus individual therapies), the conditions under which the counselling should be conducted (in the client's home versus the counsellor's office), as well as those clients who will benefit most from such programs (e.g., the recently bereaved versus those who experienced a loss beyond a given time period). This perspective is currently receiving more attention. For example, a content analysis of services for bereaved spouses (mostly White, middle-class females) suggested that programs that brought about adaptive change in the bereaved were of shorter duration (two to seven weeks, meeting at least weekly), were conducted in the client's or practitioner's home as opposed to an out-patient clinic, and were provided by professional counsellors as opposed to peer counsellors. Compared to ineffective programs, services that proved effective tended to tap well-defined problems, such as crying or sleeping difficulties, and had clear goals for counselling. Similar studies are needed to further our understanding on treatment strategies that would bring optimal benefits to the bereaved, particularly as they pertain to multiple bereavement (Potocky, 1993).

REASONS FOR THE INCONSISTENT SUPPORT FOR THE GRIEF WORK HYPOTHESIS

As described earlier, there is little empirical support for suggesting that all bereaved individuals must undergo a process of grief work of some type to confront a loss. Various reasons may offer an explanation.

MYTHS ABOUT COPING WITH LOSS

Perhaps no other domain in the psychosocial literature as that dealing with grief is so coloured by personal judgement. Our Western conception of grieving (i.e., mourning rituals) dictates what is 'proper' and what is 'unhealthy' grief. Although we allow for the bereaved to grieve their loss, we require these same individuals to resolve their grieving in a confined time period. We also expect the experience of loss to be similar for everyone affected. Those who fail to demonstrate any signs of 'proper grief' are quickly labelled as 'pathological', 'in denial', or 'uncaring'. It is in such labels that we understand the tremendous influence that stage models of grieving have had in shaping our social norms regarding grief behaviour. Counsellors may also share similar value judgements when confronted with grieving clients. However, the experience of grief is an individual one. The many myths surrounding grief rob the individual person of the ability and right to live this intensely intimate experience in his/her own way.

Drawing from empirical data, Wortman and Silver (1989) addressed five common myths of coping with loss, including the myth that distress or depression is inevitable, the myth that distress is necessary and failure to experience distress is indicative of pathology, the myth of working through the loss, the myth of recovery, and the myth of reaching a state of resolution. These researchers found no empirical evidence to support any of these common assumptions related to grieving. Such myths concerning coping with loss often become doctrines imposed by outsiders (counsellors, family members, friends, co-workers) on the bereaved, who, through no fault of their own, believe they must follow these milestones if they are to grieve successfully and return to normalcy. Wortman and Silver (1989: 355) concluded:

> We maintain that a complex mixture of biased input and interpretation of the data by outsiders, their own personal needs, as well as limited opportunity for open communication between parties, has led to a perpetuation of unrealistic assumptions about the normal process of coping with loss. In

addition, unrealistic assumptions held by health care professionals and the social network may also unnecessarily exacerbate feelings of distress among those who encounter loss, and lead to a self-perception that their own responses are inappropriate and abnormal under the circumstances.

The Problems with Definition, Suppression, and Detachment

In addition to the common myths surrounding the process of grieving, several other factors may explain why the grief work hypothesis has received little support (see Stroebe, 1992–3). First, the term 'grief work' is problematic. What exactly does 'working through a loss' entail? Researchers have often struggled with defining what constitutes grief work. As presented earlier, some researchers have defined confronting a loss as 'grief work' while others have used the concept 'search for meaning' (Parkes, 1972). In the absence of an operationalized definition of 'grief work', studies are bound to arrive at conflicting findings of what constitutes adaptive grieving. Second, the function of denial as a coping strategy has often been overlooked. As Stroebe (1992–3) indicated, there is some evidence that suppression of certain traumatic events may be beneficial, if not essential, for certain individuals. Lastly, the goal of many therapies is to achieve some form of detachment from the deceased. Yet, why is this a goal? 'The ties to the dead person are profound and intricate, being in death as they were in life' (Middleton et al., 1994). Perhaps the goal of grief work should not be to achieve detachment from the deceased but rather to work through a new set of more adaptive ties (i.e., cognitive schema) with the memory of the person that is no longer physically present.

Positive Features of Bereavement

Other reasons that may help to explain why the 'grief work hypothesis' lacks empirical evidence are provided by Kavanagh (1990). He has identified some positive features associated with bereavement that may help explain the great variability in grieving responses. Kavanagh notes that stimuli or reminders of the deceased are at times difficult to avoid. For instance, one who resides in the same environment as that shared with the deceased may find it difficult, if not impossible, to avoid any reminders of the loss. Constant exposure to such reminders may help the bereaved person to be desensitized naturally to the reality of the loss. A second positive feature deals with the continuation of other social roles. There are often other daily activities (i.e., occupational or child-rearing roles) that one must continue to perform. Perhaps the presence of these roles may provide not only distractions from the loss but pleasure as well, which overrides the painful experience of the loss. Finally, at times, there may be secondary gains following a loss. For instance, a bereaved person who has provided continued support to a loved one after a lengthy illness may have more personal free time, greater financial security, a sense of personal and spiritual growth, and closer ties with remaining family members. Such benefits or positive features of bereavement may be sufficient for certain individuals to confront the loss without going through a process of grief.

IMPLICATIONS FOR COUNSELLING

Given the lack of unequivocal evidence for the grief work hypothesis as a strategy to use in accompanying the bereaved, what are the implications for the individual clinician? The answer may lie in the importance of assessment. In grief counselling, assessment becomes our most important tool. With the help of the client, the counsellor assesses which grief responses are present and their consequences on daily functioning and the perception of the future. Again, we return to the importance of identifying which dimensions or components of grief, or their absence, are deemed maladaptive or intrusive to one's quality of life. The question arises as to who gauges whether a response is considered dysfunctional or not—the client, the counsellor, family members, or others. Perhaps this role belongs to both the clinician and the client as they explore together whether the response to a loss is a barrier in fulfilling the bereaved person's daily activities or personal goals. The point to be derived from the studies on the efficacy of grief work is not that providing psychological services to this population is futile. The goal of counselling for anyone who comes to seek mental health services as a result of a loss is to accompany the client in exploring how the loss has affected and continues to affect one's daily functioning and current and future plans.

The above issue brings forth the role of supportive counselling. Many counsellors place much emphasis on being active. Techniques such as grief homework are imposed at the expense of providing a more supportive approach. Perhaps clinicians need to view supportive counselling as reflecting activity, not passivity. Providing a safe environment where one can openly express one's grief to an empathic listener, where the client is able to set the pace of the counselling session, and where judgement is absent may be key to success in working with the bereaved. Future studies should explore the efficacy of supportive counselling with the bereaved.

CONCLUSION

Multiple bereavement is a common experience within the gay community in the 1990s. Its impact on the lives of these men remains poorly understood. As more and more deaths are experienced, the lives of many gay men and others will be forever changed. Unfortunately, research is lagging behind in the study of this important social reality. The following research questions urgently need to be understood to help clients manage with multiple bereavement:

- What are the psychological and social ramifications of multiple bereavement on gay men?
- Do gay men grieve differently from their heterosexual counterparts? If so, what are these differences?
- What intervention strategies are most beneficial in alleviating these losses?
- How do cultural values within the gay community help or deter the bereavement process?
- Do gay men from culturally diverse backgrounds respond differently from their mainstream counterparts?

Until we have answers to such questions, gay men and the gay community will likely remain hidden grievers, seeking support wherever they can find it, mostly relying on themselves and developing their own supportive services in an environment of exhaustion. As at the beginning of the epidemic, gay men find themselves obliged to develop, with little social support, their own caring services.

NOTES

1. The link between depression and HIV disease has been identified as the most common psychological reaction following this diagnosis (Rabkin et al., 1990). Studies suggest that between 4 and 42 per cent of persons living with HIV infection suffer from depressive disorders (Atkinson et al., 1988; Belkin et al., 1992; Rabkin et al., 1997). Studies suggest that HIV-positive individuals demonstrate higher levels of depressive symptoms than their HIV-negative counterparts (see review by Kalichman and Sikkema, 1995). These findings are robust regardless of the methodology used to assess depression, including self-reports, such as the Profile of Mood States of the Center for Epidemiological Study of Depression (see, e.g., Cochran and Mays, 1994; Kelly et al., 1993; Lyketsos et al., 1993); the Beck Depression Inventory and the Hamilton Rating Scale for Depression (e.g., Perkins et al., 1994); and the Hopkins Symptoms Checklist Depression Scale and standardized interviews such as the structured clinical interview for DSM-III-R (e.g., Belkin et al., 1992; Rabkin et al., 1997).

   Depressive symptoms often take on behavioural manifestations, including fatigue, hypersomnia, lethargy, withdrawal, forgetfulness, somatic preoccupations, anorexia, and loss of motivation. Researchers became concerned that the rates of depression assessed in this population could be contaminated with other causes of depressive-like symptoms due to side-effects of medications or physical decline related to disease activity (e.g., Belkin et al., 1992; Siegel, Karus, and Ravis, 1997; Thompson, Nanni, and Levine, 1996). However, in a prospective design study examining the relationship between depressive symptomatology and physical deterioration, a group of researchers found that after controlling for the effects of physical symptoms, baseline depression was associated with an excess decline in CD4 count (Burack et al., 1993).

   Another contaminating factor is the lifetime prevalence of depressive disorders within this population, particularly gay men. Several studies suggest that the prevalence of psychiatric problems in gay men, with or without HIV infection, is significantly higher than among other populations (e.g., Atkinson et al., 1988; Myers et al., 1984; Regier et al., 1984; Robins et al., 1984; Williams et al., 1991). For instance, one study reported that the rate of lifetime history of major depressive disorder was not statistically different in both seropositive (29 per cent) and seronegative men (45 per cent) (Perkins et al., 1994). Depression has also been associated with neuropsychiatric impairment (e.g., Heaton et al., 1994). It is estimated that 27–50 per cent of persons with an AIDS diagnosis suffer from HIV-related dementia (encephalopathy or AIDS Dementia Complex) (Ostrow, Atkinson, and Grant, 1988). Furthermore, a meta-analysis reported an association between levels of depression and immune deficiency (Herbert and Cohen, 1993).

2. Rabkin et al. (1990) define hope as 'the expectation that something worthwhile lies ahead. It implies a confidence that is positively appraised.' The maintenance of hope and the presence of uncertainty are often intertwined. The issue of uncertainty is perhaps the most distressing psychological theme in dealing and living with HIV infection (Weitz, 1989). Much uncertainty surrounds HIV disease. There is much uncertainty about issues related to (1) *the progression of the disease*: I feel fine today but what about tomorrow? Will they find a cure in time? Will there be sufficient time for me to take advantage of new medication protocols before I become too ill for the entry criteria? How long will the medication be effective?; (2) *social support*: Will my family, friends, and partner reject me? How would people at work react if they found out?; (3) *financial security*: How long will it be until I can no longer work and support myself? Who will take care of me should I become too ill and in need of constant care? How long can I afford the medication?; and (4) *death and dying*: How much pain will I endure? Will I suffer like some of my friends? Will I die alone or surrounded by my family and friends? Dealing with such uncertainties on a daily basis can often result in a loss of hope, which subsequently may lead to depression. The link between hopelessness and depression has often been cited. In the case of HIV, Rabkin et al. (1990) reported elevated scores on the Beck Hopelessness Scale.

3. The association between HIV infection and depression has led researchers to investigate the suicidal risk of persons living with HIV. Marzuk et al. (1988) were the first to examine systematically the prevalence of suicide in persons with HIV. Through a thorough review of the New York Department of Health 1985 registry, these researchers reported that the suicide risk in men with a known AIDS diagnosis was 66.15 times greater than that of the general population. This relative risk was 36.3 times greater when the sample was matched for age with men without such diagnosis.

4. 'Bereavement', 'grief', and 'mourning' are often employed interchangeably in discussing loss, thus blurring their different meanings. These three words do share distinct qualities. 'Bereavement' is defined as the 'objective situation of an individual who has recently experienced a loss, which includes a number of psychological and somatic reactions'. More succinctly, bereavement refers to the experience of having suffered a loss. 'Mourning' refers to the act of expressing grief reactions. These acts are culturally dictated and determined by the mores, values, and expectations regarding death in a given society or culture. Mourning rituals dictate the guidelines for appropriate ways of conduct following a loss. On the other hand, 'grief' refers to one's way(s) of behaving as a result of anticipated or past loss (Stroebe and Stroebe, 1987; see also Averill, 1968; Schuchter and Zisook, 1993).

5. The term 'healthy' grieving is used here instead of 'normal' grief reactions. Normality does not always imply that a behaviour is adaptive whereas healthy behaviour would always be adaptive.
6. It is worth noting that stage models of grieving continue to receive much attention, regardless of such criticisms. Ramsay (1979: 220), an advocate for using the term 'component', acknowledges that stage models are useful in that 'it is important that the counsellor knows which phases and components *can* exist so that explorations can be made to check if one component is causing problems.'
7. The *Diagnostic and Statistical Manual of Mental Disorders* (APA, 1994) distinguishes bereavement responses with a major depressive episode. The manual states: 'The presence of certain symptoms that are not characteristic of a "normal" grief reaction may be helpful in differentiating bereavement from a Major Depressive Episode. These include 1) guilt about things other than actions taken or not taken by the survivor at the time of the death; 2) thoughts of death other than the survivor feeling that he or she would be better off dead or should have died with the deceased person; 3) morbid preoccupation with worthlessness; 4) marked psychomotor retardation; 5) prolonged and marked functional impairment; and 6) hallucinatory experiences other than thinking that he or she hears the voice of, or transiently sees the image of, the deceased person' (pp. 684–5). Furthermore, empirical studies investigating whether depression and grief reaction are similar responses have been conflictual (e.g., Clayton et al., 1974; Glick, Weiss, and Parkes, 1974; Clayton, Halikas, and Maurice, 1972). The main distinctions between depression and grief reactions are the following. In grief reaction, self-esteem is generally intact, while depressed persons often exhibit signs of poor self-worth. A second feature distinguishing grief and depression is guilt. The presence of guilt feelings of not having done everything he/she could to prevent the loss is often present in the bereaved responses. This overall sense of guilt is an uncommon criterion for a diagnosis of depression (Worden, 1991).
8. Empirical studies have indicated that the severity and distress in the bereaved have often failed to reach clinical significance to warrant an anxiety disorder diagnosis (see Middleton et al., 1994).
9. When a loss has occurred via a traumatic event or unnatural death (e.g., homicide, accident, or suicide), researchers and clinicians have often identified post-traumatic stress disorder symptoms in the survivors. People bereaved with such deaths demonstrate preoccupation with the images of the deceased, replay the traumatic scene in their minds, and experience nightmares. Such behaviours related to the traumatic loss often warrant a PTSD diagnosis (see Rynearson, 1987).

REFERENCES

American Psychiatric Association. 1994. *Diagnostic and Statistical Manual of Mental Disorders*, 4th edn (DSM-MD-IV). Washington: APA.

Antoni, M.H. 1991. 'Psychosocial Stressors and Behavioral Interventions in Gay Men with HIV Infection', *International Review of Psychiatry* 3: 383–99.

Atkinson, J.H., I. Grant, C.J. Kennedy, D.D. Richman, S.A. Spector, and A. McCutchan. 1988. 'Prevalence of Psychiatric Disorders among Men Infected with Human Immunodeficiency Virus', *Archives of General Psychiatry* 45: 859–64.

Averill, J.R. 1968. 'Grief: Its Nature and Significance', *Psychological Bulletin* 70, 6: 721–48.

Belkin, G.S., J.A. Fleishman, M.D. Stein, J. Piette, and V. Mor. 1992. 'Physical Symptoms and Depressive Symptoms among Individuals with HIV Infection', *Psychosomatics* 33, 4: 416–27.

Bowlby, J., and C.M. Parkes. 1970. 'Separation and Loss', in E.J. Anthony and C. Koupernick, eds, *The Child and His Family: Volume 1. The International Yearbook of Child Psychiatry and Allied Professions*. New York: Wiley, 197–216.

Brown, J.H., P. Henteleff, S. Barakat, and C.J. Rowe. 1986. 'Is It Normal for Terminally Ill Patients to Desire Death?', *American Journal of Psychiatry* 143, 2: 208–11.

Brown, J.T., and G.A. Stoudemire. 1983. 'Normal and Pathological Grief', *Journal of the American Medical Association (JAMA)* 250, 3: 378–82.

Bugen, L.A. 1977. 'Human Grief: A Model for Prediction and Intervention', *American Journal of Orthopsychiatry* 47: 196–206.

Burack, J.H., D.C. Barrett, R.D. Stall, M.A. Chesney, M.J. Ekstrand, and T.J. Coates. 1993. 'Depressive Symptoms and CD4 Lymphocyte Decline among HIV-infected Men', *JAMA* 270, 21: 2568–73.

Cassens, B.J. 1985. 'Social Consequences of the Acquired Immunodeficiency Syndrome', *Annals of Internal Medicine* 103: 768–71.

Catalan, J. 1995. 'Psychological Interventions in Infection with the Human Immunodeficiency Virus', *British Journal of Psychiatry* 167: 104–11.

———, I. Klimes, A. Day, A. Garrod, A. Bond, and J. Galloway. 1992. 'The Psychosocial Impact of HIV Infection on Gay Men: A Controlled Investigation and Factors Associated with Psychiatric Morbidity', *British Journal of Psychiatry* 161: 774–8.

Christ, G.H., L.S. Wiener, and R.T. Moynihan. 1986. 'Psychosocial Issues in AIDS', *Psychiatric Annals* 16, 3: 173–9.

Chuang, H.T., G.M. Devins, J. Hunsley, and M.J. Gill. 1989. 'Psychosocial Distress and Well-being among Gay and Bisexual Men with Human Immunodeficiency Virus Infection', *American Journal of Psychiatry* 146: 876–9.

Clayton, P.J., J.A. Halikas, and W.L. Maurice. 1972. 'The Depression of Widowhood', *British Journal of Psychiatry* 120: 71–6.

———, M. Herjanic, G.E. Murphy, and R. Woodruff. 1974. 'Mourning and Depression: Their Similarities and Differences', *Canadian Psychiatric Association Journal* 19, 3: 309–12.

Cochran, S.D., and V.M. Mays. 1994. 'Depressive Distress among Homosexual Active African American Men and Women', *American Journal of Psychiatry* 151, 4: 524–9.

Dershimer, R. 1990. *Counselling the Bereaved.* New York: Pergamon Press.

Deutsch, H. 1937. 'Absence of Grief', *Psychoanalytic Quarterly* 6: 12–22.

Engel, G. 1964. 'Grief and Grieving', *American Journal of Nursing* 64: 93–8.

Freud, S. 1917. 'Mourning and Melancholia', in *Standard Edition of Complete Psychological Works of Sigmund Freud*, vol. 15. London: Hogarth.

Glick, I.O., R.S. Weiss, and C.M. Parkes. 1974. *The First Year of Bereavement.* New York: Wiley.

Health Canada. 1997. *AIDS In Canada: Quarterly Surveillance Update.* Ottawa: Division of HIV Disease Surveillance, Bureau of HIV Disease and Sexually Transmitted Diseases, Laboratory Centre for Disease Control, Health Protection Branch, Health Canada, May.

Heaton, R.K., R.A. Velin, A. McCutchan, S.J. Gulevich, J.H. Atkinson, M.R. Wallace, H. Godfrey, I. Grant, and the HNRC Group. 1994. 'Neuropsychological Impairment in Human Immunodeficiency Virus Infection: Implications for Employment', *Psychosomatic Medicine* 56: 8–17.

Herbert, T.B., and S. Cohen. 1993. 'Depression and Immunity: A Meta-analytic Review', *Psychological Bulletin* 113: 472–86.

Hodge, J.R. 1972. 'They That Mourn', *Journal of Religion and Health* 11: 229–40.

Hodgkinson, P.E. 1982. 'Abnormal Grief—The Problem of Therapy', *British Journal of Medical Psychology* 55: 29–34.

Holland, J.C., and S. Tross. 1985. 'Psychosocial and Neuropsychiatric Sequelae of Acquired Immuno-Deficiency Syndrome and Related Disorders', *Annals of Internal Medicine* 103: 760–4.

Kalichman, S.C., and K.J. Sikkema. 1995. 'Psychosocial Sequelae of HIV Infection and AIDS: Review of Empirical Findings', *Clinical Psychology Review* 14, 7: 611–32.

Kavanagh, D.J. 1990. 'Towards a Cognitive-Behavioral Intervention for Adult Grief Reactions', *British Journal of Psychiatry* 157: 373–83.

Kelly, J.A., D.A. Murphy, R. Bahr, S.C. Kalichman, M.G. Morgan, Y. Stevenson, J.J. Koob, T.L. Brasfield, B.M. Bernstein, and St Lawrence. 1993. 'Outcome of Cognitive-Behavioural and Support Group Brief Therapies for Depressed HIV-infected Persons', *American Journal of Psychiatry* 150, 11: 1679–86.

Kübler-Ross, E. 1969. *On Death and Dying*. Toronto: Macmillan.

Lamping, D.L., J. Joseph, B. Ryan, and N. Gilmore. 1992. 'Détresse psychologique chez les personnes atteintes du VIH à Montréal', *Santé Mentale au Québec* 17, 1: 73–95.

Lamping, D.L., and M. Sewitch. 1990. *Review of the Literature on HIV Infection and Mental Health*. Ottawa: Minister of Supply and Services Canada.

Lindemann, E. 1944, 1994. 'Symptomology and Management of Acute Grief', *American Journal of Psychiatry* 151, 6: 155–60.

Lister, L. 1991. 'Men and Grief: A Review of Research', *Smith College Studies in Social Work* 61, 3 (June): 220–35.

Lyketsos, C.G., S.R. Hoover, M. Guccione, W. Senterfitt, M.A. Dew, J.E. Wesch, M.J. Van Raden, G.J. Treisman, and Morganstein. 1993. 'Depressive Symptoms as Predictors of Medical Outcomes in HIV Infection', *JAMA* 270, 21: 2563–7.

Maj, M. 1990. 'Psychiatric Aspects of HIV-1 Infection and AIDS', *Psychological Medicine* 20: 547–63.

Marzuk, P.M., H. Tierney, K. Tardiff, E.M. Gross, E.B. Morgan, M.-A. Hsu, and J. Mann. 1988. 'Increased Risk of Suicide in Persons with AIDS', *JAMA* 259, 9: 1333–7.

Mawson, D., I. Marks, L. Ramm, and R.S. Stern. 1981. 'Guided Mourning for Morbid Grief: A Controlled Study', *British Journal of Psychiatry* 138: 185–93.

Middleton, W., B. Raphael, N. Martinek, and V. Misso. 1994. 'Pathological Grief Reactions', in M. Stroebe, W. Stroebe, and R.O. Hansson, eds, *Handbook of Bereavement: Theory, Research and Intervention*. New York: Cambridge University Press, 44–61.

Morin, S.F., K.A. Charles, and A.K. Maylon. 1984. 'The Psychological Impact of AIDS on Gay Men', *American Psychologist* 39, 11: 1288–93.

Myers, J.K., M.M. Weissman, G.L. Tischler, C.E. Holzer, P.J. Leaf, H. Orvaschel, J.C. Anthony, J.A. Boyd, J. Burke, M. Kramer, and R. Stolzman. 1984. 'Six-Month Prevalence of Psychiatric Disorders in Three Communities, 1980–1982', *Archives of General Psychiatry* 41: 959–67.

O'Dowd, M.A. 1988. 'Psychosocial Issues in HIV Infection', *AIDS* 2, supp. 1: S201–5.

Olders, H. 1989. 'Mourning and Grief as Healing Processes in Psychotherapy', *Canadian Journal of Psychiatry* 34: 271–8.

Ostrow, D., J.H. Atkinson, and I. Grant. 1988. 'Assessment and Management of the AIDS Patient with Neuropsychiatric Disturbances', *Journal of Clinical Psychiatry* 49, supp. 5: 14–22.

Ostrow, D.G., A. Monjan, J. Joseph, M. Van Raden, R. Fox, L. Kingsley, J. Dudley, and J. Phair. 1989. 'HIV-related Symptoms and Psychological Functioning in a Cohort of Homosexual Men', *American Journal of Psychiatry* 146, 6: 737–42.

Parkes, C.M. 1965. 'Bereavement and Mental Illness: A Classification of Bereavement Reactions', *British Journal of Medical Psychology* 38: 13–26.

———. 1972. *Bereavement: Studies of Grief in Adult Life*. London: Penguin.

———. 1980. 'Bereavement Counselling: Does It Work?', *British Medical Journal* 53: 3–6.

———, and R.S. Weiss. 1983. *Recovery from Bereavement*. New York: Basic Books.

Perkins, D.O., R.A. Stern, R.N. Golden, S. Murphy, D. Naftolowitz, and D.L. Evans. 1994. 'Mood Disorders in HIV Infection: Prevalence and Risk Factors in a Non-epicentre of the AIDS Epidemic', *American Journal of Psychiatry* 151: 233–6.

Perry, S., and S. Tross. 1984. 'Psychiatric Problems of AIDS Patients at the New York Hospital: Preliminary Report', *Public Health Reports* 99: 143–7.

Pope, M. 1995. 'The Salad Bowl Is Big Enough for Us All: An Argument for the Inclusion of Lesbians and Gay Men in Any Definition of Multiculturalism', *Journal of Counselling and Development* 73: 301–4.

Potocky, M. 1993. 'Effective Services for Bereaved Spouses: A Content Analysis of the Empirical Literature', *Health and Social Work* 18, 4: 288–301.

Rabkin, J.G., J. Johnson, S.H. Lin, J.D. Lipstiz, R.H. Remien, J.B.W. Williams, and J.M. Gorman. 1997. 'Psychopathology in Male and Female HIV-positive and negative Injection Drug Users: Longitudinal Course over 3 Years', *AIDS* 11, 4: 507–16.

Rabkin, J.G., J.B.W. Williams, R. Neugebauer, R.H. Remien, and R. Goetz. 1990. 'Maintenance of Hope in HIV-spectrum Homosexual Men', *American Journal of Psychiatry* 147, 10: 1322–6.

Ramsay, R. 1977. 'Behavioural Approaches to Bereavement', *Behavioural Research and Counselling* 15, 2: 131–5.

———. 1979. 'Bereavement: A Behavioral Treatment of Pathological Grief', in P. Sjoden, S. Bates, and W.S. Dockens, eds, *Trends in Behavior Therapy*. New York: Academic Press.

Rando, T.A. 1984. *Grief, Dying and Death*. Champagne, Ill.: Research Press Company.

Regier, D.A., J.K. Myers, M. Kramer, L.N. Robins, D.G. Blazer, R.I. Hough, W.W. Eaton, and B.Z. Locke. 1984. 'The NIMH Epidemiological Catchment Program', *Archives of General Psychiatry* 41: 934–41.

Robins, L.N., J.E. Helzer, M.M. Weismann, H. Orvaschel, E. Gruenberg, J.D. Burke, and D.A. Regier. 1984. 'Lifetime Prevalance of Specific Disorders in Three Sites', *Archives of General Psychiatry* 41: 949–58.

Rynearson, E.K. 1987. 'Psychotherapy of Pathologic Grief: Revisions and Limitations', *Psychiatric Clinics of North America* 10: 487–500.

Sadovsky, R. 1991. 'Psychosocial Issues in Symptomatic HIV Infection', *American Family Physician* 44, 6: 2065–72.

Schneiderman, G., P. Winders, S. Tallett, and W. Feldman. 1994. 'Do Child and/or Parent Bereavement Programs Work?', *Canadian Journal of Psychiatry* 39: 215–17.

Schuchter, S.R., and S. Zisook. 1993. 'The Course of Normal Grief', in M. Stroebe, W. Stroebe, and R.D. Hansson, eds, *Handbook of Bereavement: Theory, Research and Intervention*. New York: Cambridge University Press, 23–43.

Siegel, K., D. Karus, and V.H. Ravis. 1997. 'Correlates of Change in Depressive Symptomology among Gay Men with AIDS', *Health Psychology* 16, 3: 230–8.

Sireling, L., D. Cohen, and I. Marks. 1988. 'Guided Mourning for Morbid Grief: A Controlled Replication', *Behavior Therapy* 19: 121–32.

Staudacher, C. 1991. *Men and Grief: A Guide for Men Surviving the Death of a Loved One; A Resource for Caregivers and Mental Health Professionals*. Oakland, Calif.: New Harbinger Publications.

Stroebe, M. 1992–3. 'Coping with Bereavement: A Review of the Grief Work Hypothesis', *Omega: Journal of Death and Dying* 26, 1: 19–42.

———, and W. Stroebe. 1991. 'Does "Grief Work" Work?', *Journal of Consulting and Clinical Psychology* 59, 3: 479–82.

———, ———, and R.O. Hansson. 1988. 'Bereavement Research: An Historical Introduction', *Journal of Social Issues* 44, 3: 1–18.

Stroebe, W., and M.S. Stroebe. 1987. *Bereavement and Health: The Psychological and Physical Consequences of Partner Loss*. New York: Cambridge University Press.

Thompson, S.C., C. Nanni, and A. Levine. 1996. 'The Stressors and Stress of Being HIV-positive', *AIDS Care* 8, 1: 5–14.

Tross, S., and D.A. Hirsch. 1988. 'Psychological Distress and Neuropsychological Complications of HIV Infection and AIDS', *American Psychologist* 43: 929–34.

Weitz, R. 1989. 'Uncertainty in the Lives of Persons with AIDS', *Journal of Health and Social Behavior* 30: 270–81.

Williams, J.B., J.G. Rabkin, R.H. Remien, J.M. Gorman, and A.A. Ehrhardt. 1991. 'Multidisciplinary Baseline Assessment of Homosexual Men with and without Human Immunodeficiency Virus Infection', *Archives of General Psychiatry* 48: 124–30.

Wolcott, D.W., C.A. Maida, R. Diamond, and A.R. Neissenson. 1986. 'Treatment Compliance in End-stage Renal Disease Patients on Dialysis', *American Journal of Nephrology* 6: 329–38.

Worden, J.W. 1991. *Grief Counselling and Grief Therapy: A Handbook for the Mental Health Practitioner*. New York: Springer.

Wortman, C.B., and R.C. Silver. 1989. 'The Myths of Coping with Loss', *Journal of Consulting and Clinical Psychology* 57, 3: 349–57.

Zaiger, N. 1986. 'Women and Bereavement', *Women and Counselling* 4: 33–43.

Part Three

Practice, Policy, and Politics

The Canadian federal government announced a National AIDS Strategy in 1988 that focused on 'education and prevention', 'research', 'care, treatment and support', 'support of non-governmental organizations', and 'coordination and collaboration' (Health and Welfare Canada, 1993: 5–10). The strategy was renewed in 1993 and shifted its focus to 'enhancing partnerships, improving health promotion for people living with HIV, creating supportive social environments, promoting and sustaining healthy behaviours, and recognition of HIV disease as a chronic and progressive condition' (Bouchard, 1993: 1). From a policy point of view, the federal government's ambivalence showed some progressive and bold initiatives, but these were paralleled by inaction and bureaucratic bungling in practice.

One example of a progressive policy is seen in the adoption by Corrections Services Canada of recommendations made by a committee looking at HIV in prisons. In addition to education and awareness, the policy called for the distribution of condoms and bleach to persons incarcerated in federal facilities. As in all cases, however, there can be a great distance between policy and practice. Even though the policy was progressive, the nature and organization of prisons have meant that the practical application has fallen well short of the goal. For example, some prisons have condom dispensers in public areas on 'the range', while in other facilities an inmate must request a condom from a nurse. With the 'everybody knows everything' atmosphere of closed institutions, these practices fall well short of effective, confidential prevention methods.

One of the most well-known practice disasters in the Canadian experience related to the decision on the part of the Canadian Red Cross and governmental bureaucrats to continue to distribute potentially contaminated blood when safer, heat-treated products were available. This led to the Krever Inquiry (1993–7), which, after much legal and bureaucratic obfuscation, finally presented its harshly critical report in late 1997. This resulted in formal apologies from the Canadian Red Cross and the Ministry of Health, as well as recommendations for the compensation of some of the 'tainted blood' victims.

Policy and practice continue to be shaped as the HIV epidemic evolves. In 1997, the Canadian Public Health Association (CPHA) passed resolutions that could lead to developing a standard protocol for dealing with HIV-infected persons who are unable or unwilling to change their sexual behaviour and/or injection drug-using behaviour and who, consequently, continue to put their sexual and/or injection drug partners at risk of HIV infection. One of these resolutions, for example, was to promote the availability of female-controlled methods of HIV prevention, such as female condoms, spermacides, etc. (CPHA, 1997: 7).

The CPHA has also recommended the adoption and implementation of a National Task Force on HIV, AIDS, and Injection Drug Use, to be co-ordinated by the Canadian Centre on Substance Abuse and the CPHA AIDS program (CPHA, 1997: 8; Health Canada, 1997). This plan recommends the use of harm-reduction principles elaborated in Chapter 4 of this book. All of these recommendations, and others, have the effect of profoundly changing the nature of social work practice and challenge social workers to find imaginative solutions and, in some cases, to redefine practice.

In this section, social workers discuss some of the most perplexing practice issues that have been raised by the HIV epidemic. In Chapter 13, Michèle Bourgon looks at the stresses inherent for the social worker dealing with HIV and offers a set of strategies that some workers have found to be beneficial in coping with these stresses and in transforming their clinical practice. The adaptive strategies are drawn directly from experienced practitioners and speak clearly to the need to prepare and support social workers who work with HIV-affected clients.

Sharon Taylor, in Chapter 14, demonstrates how an ethical issue like confidentiality is intensified for social workers in light of HIV. The author reviews the legal and ethical issues and reflects on the limits of the current *Code of Ethics* in helping social workers grapple with clients' rights versus social responsibility.

In Chapter 15, Jack MacDonald, in the format of a case study, presents a sensitive portrayal of a social worker tracing the HIV epidemic in the blood-transfused community. The author's reflections on the implications for policy and practice are especially useful.

Finally, in Chapter 16, Carol Neron examines an issue—assisted suicide and euthanasia—that has divided the general population and social workers alike. The author thoughtfully considers the practice issues and challenges social workers and social work organizations to take an active role in moving the dialogue forward, given the realities facing persons living with HIV.

REFERENCES

Bouchard, B. 1993. 'Message from the Minister', in Health and Welfare Canada (1993).

Canadian Public Health Association (CPHA). 1997. *CPHA Health Digest* 21, 1 (Spring): 7–8.

Health and Welfare Canada. 1993. *National AIDS Strategy: Phase 2 Building on Progress.* Ottawa: Health and Welfare Canada.

Health Canada. 1997. *HIV, AIDS, and Injection Drug Use: A National Action Plan.* Ottawa: Health Canada.

Chapter 13

Integrating the Personal, the Professional, and the Political in HIV/AIDS

MICHÈLE BOURGON

AIDS has added to the troubles on a scene already beset with anger, pain, sadness and high technology. (Bosk and Frader, 1991)

According to Bosk and Frader, AIDS appeared in a health and social service system already besieged by widespread chronic illness, an aging population, and an ideological shift in responsibility, within health care, from the system to the individual. These trends have since become even more apparent, and changes resulting from major cutbacks in public expenditures and the ever-increasing marginalization of entire populations—young people and those over 50 pushed out of the workforce, for instance—have only further complicated the situation.

Social work, as a profession, has been directly affected by these upheavals and changes. In Quebec, for example, social workers are questioning the meaning of their practice more and more within these emerging and difficult contexts. Unfortunately, their workloads rarely allow them the time to address fully the challenges with which they are continually faced.

The experience of social workers in the field of HIV may be helpful to them in this respect. These workers are confronted with sickness, death, social marginalization, deviant behaviour, and taboo subjects on a daily basis. Because of this, they have had to reconsider and, in many cases, radically modify their professional practices. A large majority of the social workers I met in the course of the research for this chapter admit to having been drastically changed by their contact with HIV, which one worker identified as a 'cruel and harsh master'.

Through its impact and coverage in the media, HIV has mirrored the values of our society. It has revealed the limits of the founding myths of that society: primacy given to reason (Saul, 1995) and absolute faith in the progress and benefits of science and technology (Caillé, 1986; Renaud, 1990, 1996). On a more professional level, HIV has shattered our certainties (Olivier, 1994) and underlined our inconsistencies and limitations, as well as emphasized our strengths and our resources (Abramson, 1990).

The literature addressing the impact of HIV on North American social workers does much more than provide information on specific practices in this field: it leads us to position ourselves with respect to the important social issues we are faced with today. This chapter presents this information and enriches it with the experiences of nine social workers who have been working in the field of HIV in

Montreal over the past several years. These workers come from different institutional backgrounds: CLSCs (state-run local community health and social services centres), hospitals, community groups, and private practice. They also work with different clienteles: homosexual, Haitian, drug user, and significant others of people living with HIV. They generously participated in a two-hour discussion group during the winter of 1996, where they talked of their professional practices and shared the joys and the sorrows, the frustrations and the hopes they have been experiencing in their work. I wish to thank them for their collaboration.

This chapter is organized around two themes: the main stressors related to working in the field of HIV and the principal coping strategies that social workers adopt to deal with these stressors. Each theme is developed in the same manner: first, an overview is given of the literature on a specific point, then the statements the social workers made on the same topic are summarized. The chapter concludes by identifying the main issues HIV has forced social work practice to confront in the years to come.

WORKING IN THE FIELD OF HIV: THE STRESSORS

The training sessions and information campaigns aimed at increasing HIV awareness among health-care workers have not produced expected results. An American survey carried out in 1992 revealed that many workers still harboured negatives attitudes towards people living with HIV and continued to worry about having to treat them (Gallup et al., 1992). A more recent Montreal study confirmed this tendency, revealing that one-quarter of participating nurses felt it was their right to refuse to treat this clientele if they so wished (Taggart et al. in Dionne-Proulx, 1994).

But what, in fact, does this reticence tell us? One worker who participated in a study on the experience of friends and family of people living with HIV begins to shed light on a certain explanation when he states:

> Despite all you say, despite all you do, despite all you try to get others to believe, you are alone with AIDS at night when you go to bed. . . . Even if you are surrounded by a million people and that you know that medical science has made great strides in recent years, at night when you go to bed, you are alone in the dark, face to face with your fear. (Bourgon, Desmarais, and Ryan, 1995)

This very basic fear is one of the main stressors facing health-care workers today, yet it is not the only one. The literature identifies seven major stressors inherent to biomedical and social practices in the field of HIV. They are, in order of importance:

1. The fear of infection.
2. The daily contact with death and dying.
3. The specific characteristics of people living with HIV.
4. The ethical dilemmas.

5. The conflicts surrounding professional identity.
6. The difficult working conditions.
7. The pressures from friends and family.

These seven stressors were also mentioned by the social workers who participated in our focus group, though on a different scale of importance. These differences are described below and are outlined in Table 1.

1. THE FEAR OF INFECTION

The stressor most often mentioned in the literature, which it must be said deals mostly with the experiences of nurses and doctors who have direct physical contact with people with HIV, is, without doubt, the fear of infection. Many nurses are terrified by HIV patients because they are convinced or at least strongly suspect that the virus is more easily contracted than is openly stated. Reuther and Northcott (1994) believe that the medical uncertainties surrounding much of the official discourse on HIV in the beginning years contributed greatly to this source of anxiety.

One study, conducted among psychologists in 1990, revealed that many of those questioned were certain that such a deadly virus must be transmitted by air, regardless of medical and epidemiological evidence to the contrary. This opinion was confirmed by another study carried out during the same period with social workers, half of whom believed that scientists would surely discover unknown ways of transmitting the virus in the years to come (Wiener and Siegel, 1990).

This deeply rooted fear is obviously linked to the specific nature of HIV, and health-care workers are in a firsthand position to observe its terrible effects on people's lives. According to Saint-Jarre (1994), caregivers have great difficulty witnessing the physical and psychological pain of those they care for and target this aspect of their work as the most stressful of all. Bosk and Frader (1991) found that the negative reactions of doctors towards HIV patients are often due to their fear of the suffering that would await them should they contract the disease.

On a psychosocial level, health-care workers also frequently witness the rejection, abandonment, and grave discrimination those living with the virus must face on a daily basis (Wiener and Siegel, 1990). Is it any wonder that in such a context HIV provokes terror in many of those who must come into contact with it?

Although the fear of contagion was labelled one of the possible stressors by the social workers of our discussion group, few considered it important in their present-day work experience. Rather, they claimed to be more afraid of contracting opportunist diseases closely associated with HIV, such as tuberculosis. This feeling of relative security towards HIV, however, seemed extremely fragile. This was clearly illustrated when one worker told of an experience she had had with a contaminated syringe that put her at high risk of contracting the virus. Those present strongly reacted to her story. One worker summarized: 'Accounts such as yours remind me that the danger is always there and that rekindles my fear even if I know in my head that the risks are nearly non-existent in my situation.'

Table 1 The Stressors (in order of importance)

According to the Literature	*According to Social Workers of Our Focus Group*
1. *The fear of infection* • Absence of scientific certainties • Fragile sense of security	1. *Difficult working conditions* • Bureaucratic rules and regulations • Insufficient financial resources • Job precariousness • 'Dumping' from colleagues • Lack of consensus on organization's mission and on meaning of buzz-words such as 'ambulatory care' • Lack of formal support and recognition of difficulties inherent to working in field of AIDS
2. *The daily contact with death and dying* • This continually evokes questions of a spiritual nature in a society that lacks such meaning	2. *Characteristics of those affected* • Persons in a great deal of pain are often confrontational, through either violent or 'deviant' behaviour
3. *Characteristics of those affected* • Especially with respect to sexual orientation and perceived promiscuity	3. *Conflicts surrounding professional identity* • In regard to their roles, duties, and limits as social workers • In regard to the expectations of other health-care professionals • In regard to the specificity of their contribution • In regard to the possible dangers of overspecialization
4. *Ethical dilemmas* • Stress arising from not being able to answer person's spiritual needs • Conflict stemming from what to do with request of confidentiality in situation when a third party is at risk	4. *Ethical dilemmas* • To whom does one owe one's foremost allegiance—to those affected by the virus or to one's colleagues? What must one do when one does not agree with actions taken by another team member? • To be the bearer of 35 to 40 secrets at one time is very trying • What must one do when not in agreement with adopted research protocol?

Table 1 The Stressors (in order of importance) (continued)

According to the Literature	*According to Social Workers of Our Focus Group*
5. *Conflicts surrounding professional identity* • Fear of not being able to measure up to clients' expectations and of not being able to set one's limits	5. *The pressure from family members and/or close friends* • Mostly indirect in nature: 'You have to be a masochist to work in that field' or 'Don't talk to me about your work, it's much too depressing.'
6. *Difficult working conditions* • Lack of resources for offering quality services	6. *The daily contact with death and dying* • 'Difficult to let go, the deaths haunt us.'
7. *The pressure from family members and close friends* • Field of work considered dangerous for both mental and physical health • Pressure to not treat people with HIV	7. *The fear of infection* • Fear of HIV mostly latent, greater fear of AIDS-related opportunistic diseases • Fragile sense of security for those who work with intravenous drug users

Although they do not consider the fear of contagion a major stressor in their own experience, all the workers pointed out that, notwithstanding the numerous campaigns and training sessions they have had access to, their 'unspecialized' colleagues still are terrorized of contracting the virus should they have to care for someone who has HIV. One of them stated: 'Very little has really changed regarding the reactions of generic workers from the health and social services network. Those who know the ropes are more at ease, but for the others, it's a different story.' Another added: 'The fear is still very present. . . . If a service request marked HIV arrives tomorrow morning at social services, you can be sure that it will be placed in my box right away! Even if HIV is only suspected, they'll give it to me right away so that they won't be stuck with the test results.'

This refusal of colleagues to work with people living with the virus, as well as with their friends and family, has both negative and positive consequences on the workers we met. We will come back to these consequences when we discuss the problems surrounding overspecialization and expertise.

2. THE DAILY CONTACT WITH DEATH AND DYING

Health and social services professionals in the field of HIV consider having to deal with death and dying on a regular basis as one of the main stressors of their work (Saint-Jarre, 1994; Dunkel and Hatfield, 1986; Rolland, 1994; Bourgon and

Renaud, 1989, 1993). They mention that the contact they develop over the months and years with the people they care for makes these deaths particularly trying since they often feel they have lost a very significant person in their lives.

Questions of a spiritual nature, especially those concerning the meaning of the death of young people, are a great source of tension for workers. According to Fortunato (1987), these questions create tension for three reasons. First, workers often fear having to lie and to create false hopes in order for people to keep on fighting. Second, workers feel confused and uncertain when faced with the change in beliefs people with HIV frequently go through during the course of their illness. And finally, workers often feel incompetent to deal with eschatological beliefs that are fundamentally different from their own.

According to Saint-Jarre (1994), HIV also compels workers to deal with forms of death that are uncommon and unacceptable within our society, such as assisted suicide and euthanasia. These forms of death are particularly trying because they force workers to take a stand on ethical issues that remain problematic within our society. Questions surrounding these ethical issues represent one of the most difficult aspects of the work. In theory, workers are supposedly equipped to deal with such issues; in practice, however, they are often called on to answer specific requests for which they feel totally unprepared (Olivier, 1994).

The numerous bereavements inherent to working in the field of HIV are also hard to accept. According to Rolland (1994), workers experiencing multiple griefs often face a complex psychological barrier that results from having to cope simultaneously with several deaths at a time, extremely high professional demands, and recurring memories of people who have died. For several workers, this barrier translates itself into the presence of HIV victims in dreams, unresolved mourning processes, and a feeling of weariness in all spheres of their lives (Lert and Marne in Dionne-Proulx, 1994).

Although the daily contact with death and dying did not represent a major stressor for the social workers who participated in our focus group, all did underline how difficult it was for them to look back and take stock of the many people they had cared for who had died over the years. 'I have been in my job four years', said one hospital social worker, 'and not one of the people I dealt with four years ago is still alive today . . . 378 deaths in four years, I counted them . . . that's an end to a lot of young lives, a lot of lost dreams, a lot of lost love.'

Some of these deaths are more disturbing than others. Among the most trying are those of children and of persons with whom one shares common characteristics. 'My first student trainee died a few weeks ago', recounted a worker in private practice, 'and I found his death very hard to deal with. He wasn't exactly a friend but we had a lot in common and I was fond of him.'

As in the literature, our participants found the contact with the physical, psychological, and moral suffering of those affected by HIV most difficult. One of them expressed this feeling in the following manner: 'Even after all these years, I still get scared when I receive an HIV referral. I still apprehend the suffering I will have to face. . . . I don't think I'll ever get used to that suffering or the fear it creates in my gut.'

3. THE CHARACTERISTICS OF PEOPLE LIVING WITH HIV

The third stressor identified in the literature concerns the specific character traits of many of the people first affected by the HIV virus in North America, that is, young, middle-class males who were homosexual. The social identity of these men was nurtured by the contemporary values of modernity, such as primacy of the individual and of his intrinsic rights, concern for the body, and total responsibility for one's health and well-being (Pollack, 1988). Many, for example, refused the label of 'patient' or 'sick person', claiming instead the status of 'person living with HIV' still totally in possession of his power and authority. This political stance seduced some health workers but alienated many others, who considered it demanding and threatening (Segalen et al., 1988).

Many health-care workers have also had to deal with a population that traditionally was little inclined to use their services (Ryan, 1989), and this forced contact has worsened two anxieties deeply rooted in homophobic society: fear of others different from self and fear of homosexuality. This has resulted in psychological ghettoization among gay men themselves and in the aggravation of unresolved conflicts for heterosexuals, evoking for those who consider themselves open and tolerant, for instance, the fear of seeming homophobic (Dunkel and Hatfield, 1986).

Characteristics of people living with HIV figure prominently among the stress factors of the workers we met, although homosexuality *per se* was rarely mentioned. Rather, the neurological effects of the virus on behaviour were most often identified as difficult to deal with. One worker gave the following example of a very stressful situation:

> My client was changing before my very eyes. The relationship of trust that we had built over the months had suddenly disappeared. She had become suspicious and violent towards me. She even accused me of killing her daughter (who had died of HIV several months before) and of trying to kill her. I attempted to tell her that I was there to help her but she was lost in her madness and was very hostile. I found that really hard to deal with, couldn't sleep at night, asking myself what I could have done otherwise. . . . It's been three years since she died and I still find it difficult to talk about her.

Another group member recounted: 'In my case, the person came to the hospital to shoot me. . . . Luckily, a worker from a community group notified the head of my department that the person was on his way, but still I was terrified and very disturbed for days.'

Several of the workers we met also felt extremely insecure about the fact that they had to deal more and more with people who used drugs intravenously, 'a very unpredictable and unstable clientele who are often confronted with many other serious problems at the same time'. This clientele's high-risk behaviour is omnipresent and charged with meaning. Pointed out one community worker: 'It's hard to work with someone who is going through a risk-taking period because we can't even come to grips with what the person is doing or why he or she is doing it. . . . It makes me question my values and the vision I have of my work continuously.'

As in the literature, the workers of our focus group were more affected by the experiences of people with whom they shared common traits and felt particularly concerned when these persons belonged to their community, as was the case with the gay men and Haitian participants. Admitted one: 'I am often revolted and ashamed by how members of my community reject those who are HIV infected. . . . It gets to me every time!'

4. THE ETHICAL DILEMMAS

The HIV epidemic has raised an array of ethical issues for professionals working in health and social services. Perhaps the most difficult ethical problem faced by psychologists is not knowing how to protect third parties from becoming infected by a client while respecting the latter's right to confidentiality. Such ethical dilemmas also cause distress and insecurity among social service workers. According to Abramson (1990) they are especially frightened of feeling drained and powerless because of an inability to set their limits, and they are very preoccupied by the serious consequences their decisions might have.

Participants in our focus group considered ethical dilemmas an important stress factor in their work. They often felt torn between their allegiance to the person with HIV and their allegiance to their fellow-workers. One member of our discussion group described this feeling in the following manner: 'I work with Haitian children and am often designated as the legal guardian when the parents die. Sometimes I have to take a stand against the doctor in my team when I feel that a research protocol jeopardizes the interests of the child. This creates enormous conflict and I'm asked whose side I'm on anyway. . . . At these times, I sleep really badly, forever asking myself: am I doing the right thing?'

Workers also point out that being the carrier of 35 to 40 secrets at once can become very tiring and stressful in the long run. This becomes particularly true in instances when the secrets are potentially dangerous for others and/or have far-reaching consequences.

Three important ethical issues not mentioned in the literature were brought up by the social workers in our discussion group. One concerns the dilemma many experience around the question of whether or not they must belong to an affected group to be able to understand and help one of its members: 'Must I be Black, speak Creole, and know voodoo to work efficiently with people with the Haitian community?' Another involves the dilemmas surrounding research funding and protocols. 'High stakes surround our collaboration to research projects and protocols. . . . Nothing gets done if it is not financed by research. If a problem is "researchable", then good, it can be dealt with, but if not, then it simply does not exist. . . . This outlook has forced me to participate in research projects that I ethically don't believe in and I find that hard to accept.' And finally, a third aspect involves having to take a stand when faced with the inappropriate professional behaviour of a colleague with HIV. One worker told how she had been troubled when a co-worker began showing signs of being neurologically affected by the virus but refused to admit the problem: 'I was torn between my friendship towards my colleague and my obligation to tattle on him to our boss.'

5. THE CONFLICTS SURROUNDING PROFESSIONAL IDENTITY

Current social representations of the role and the duties of a professional health-care worker as someone 'who is uncritical, rational, open, friendly and infinitely generous, who listens, understands, and provides care without expectation or ulterior motives, who reacts calmly to attacks and whose morale remains constantly high' come into conflict with the extremely difficult realities of working with very sick and dying people (de Montigny in Olivier, 1994).

Dionne-Proulx and Pépin (1994), for example, identify three myths nurses come to accept as unquestionable truths during their training that later on become enormous sources of stress. These are: (1) nurses significantly influence the lives of their patients; (2) medical research can and will overcome disease and suffering; and (3) nurses are capable of caring equally for all their patients, regardless of their individual characteristics. Since HIV patients are often perceived as contentious and demanding and trigger negative feelings among health-care workers (Dunkel and Hatfield, 1986), it is not difficult to understand why nurses frequently experience conflict when caring for them.

Rolland (1994), on the other hand, states that the majority of training programs offered to health-care professionals tend to promote a stoic attitude that prevents the expression of feelings and perceived inadequacies among colleagues, all the more so if questions of hierarchy further compound the situation. As a result, workers are left on their own to resolve the conflicts surrounding their role and function and to cope with the unavoidable feelings of powerlessness and failure.

This sense of professional helplessness and conflict concerning one's role was among the most important stress factors identified by the participants in our group discussion. Three dimensions of their social work role seemed particularly problematic in this respect: (1) the dangers of overspecialization and the pitfalls of expertise; (2) the conflicts with professionals of other disciplines; and (3) the grey area between friendship and professional assistance.

The Dangers of Overspecialization and the Pitfalls of Expertise

All workers in the focus group mentioned, to varying degrees, the conflicts stemming from their 'HIV specialist' status. The conflict most often reported occurs after a certain time when many begin to feel that their specialization in the field of HIV has deconnected them with the essence of social work practice. Said one worker: 'I have become highly effective in the field of HIV but I sometimes wonder if in doing so I haven't lost my identity as a social worker.'

This specialist status can also result in feelings of alienation from colleagues: 'My fellow social workers always identify me with the HIV team, rarely with the social work team. For instance, they will forget to invite me to their meetings and I often am left out of discussions.' It can also leave them with the impression that they are not progressing in their general social work practice: 'We have become experts, great! But after a while we become limited in our expertise and begin to turn around in circles.'

Another drawback to specialization mentioned in the discussion group related to the fact that those present often felt they were the target of 'dumping' on the part of their less specialized colleagues. Complained one worker: 'Little by little an HIV label becomes stuck to your forehead and everyone is very happy to refer all questions related to the disease to your ballpark.'

Being so closely linked to a social reality as emotionally and politically charged as HIV obviously brings about very particular repercussions for those working in the field. One worker summarized the exchange on this subject by saying: 'I've carried the HIV burden on my shoulders for six years. . . . I'm tired and I'm drained.'

Conflicts with Professionals of Other Disciplines

It is not surprising that in a field as medicalized as HIV, several of the workers in our focus group spoke of the role conflicts they were having with other health-care professionals. These conflicts led them to question the specificity of social work with regards to nursing, for example: 'There are grey areas between our professions. . . . Nurses often feel that they can do psychosocial interventions as well as we can. This creates a lot of tension within our multidisciplinary teams.' The situation is somewhat different with doctors, who often perceive social workers as mere executioners of their decisions: 'I'm expected to make sure the patient meets the m.d.'s expectations. . . . For instance, when someone doesn't show up for an appointment, I'm told: "Why didn't you fix this properly?" '

The Unclear Boundaries between Friendship and Professional Assistance

These unclear boundaries generated a great amount of stress for many of the workers of our group. This was particularly true for homosexual workers, who had to deal with this issue frequently. One of them had some powerful thoughts on the matter:

> The barriers between the 'them' and the 'us' are very difficult to define. These men are my kin. What is a professional relationship and what is a personal relationship in such a situation? Where do I draw the line between the two in order to protect myself? These men become my colleagues, we fight the same battles, struggle for the same social chance. We can be on the same board together for five years and the sixth year, he can become my 'client'. What does professionalism mean in such an instance? The ability to remain objective and untouched by the other's plight? I don't know any more.

6. DIFFICULT WORKING CONDITIONS

Several of the workers quoted in the literature felt that the greatest stressor was the lack of resources needed to provide the quality of care expected of them (Haines, 1987). Caught in an official discourse on the need to humanize care and working conditions that results in the opposite effect, health-care professionals often pay a high price for the systemic contradictions they are forced to manage on a daily basis. Nurses, in particular, complain of the enormous amount of time they must spend doing case-management activities instead of caring for those who need their services (Bennet, 1987). Conditions surrounding social work do not seem much easier. According to Wiener and Siegel (1990), workers rarely have access to the resources they require to meet the psychosocial needs of those who are HIV-positive.

It is not surprising to note, then, as did Bosk and Frader (1991), that in such difficult conditions many doctors in the US are avoiding practising in regions where HIV is endemic and in facilities where a strong percentage of clients show signs of behaviour considered self-destructive, such as drug use. This pursuit of better working conditions causes additional stress for those remaining behind, who often feel that they have been left alone to fend off the demons of job rationalizations and budget cutbacks all on their own. This is particularly the case of nurses working in hospitals, who often feel angry and betrayed by their colleagues who refuse to care for patients with HIV (Haines, 1987).

For participants in our discussion group, increasingly demanding bureaucratic rules, combined with the consequences of diminished funding (job cutbacks and heavier workloads, for example), constituted the most significant stressor. All deplored the effects of decisions made by management without prior consultation with staff and decried the use of trendy buzz-words such as 'ambulatory care', which often are used without prior agreement as to their exact meaning, leaving the door open to contradictory and conflictual interpretations.

Comments made by the social workers in our group reveal the degree of tensions linked to this very important stressor:

> What tires me a lot is having to continually negotiate with hospital personnel. For instance, I had to negotiate for hours in order that staff leave the body of a Hindu patient in the room at least five hours after death since this was extremely important to family and friends. . . . It's incredible the amount of time it takes to revoke a few rules.

> There are many different visions of our organization's mission. For some, we're community-oriented, for others we're not. In the long run, everyone just does his own thing but we lose a lot of time in dead-end discussions.

> The greatest stressor of all? Not knowing whether my position will be renewed or not on a nearly monthly basis. No funding equals no job. So I spend a lot of my precious time lobbying so that our service will continue to be funded.

> I'm sick and tired of continually having to justify my work. I spend half my time doing damn statistics. If I get caught up in my work and forget to do them, then I'm told that it will be my fault if my position is not renewed.

> When I tell my boss I'm swamped with work, I'm told it's because I don't know how to manage my time. That they abolished a position in the department seems irrelevant.

7. PRESSURES FROM FRIENDS AND FAMILY

The last stressor identified in the literature review concerns the pressures many caregivers receive from their friends and family to abandon their work in the field of HIV. These pressures, often insidious in nature, frequently revolve around the fact that workers feel that their loved ones do not want to hear about their difficult experiences. Family members can become jealous of the attention given to HIV patients and believe that the worker has more time for these strangers than for them. This can become particularly true if an illness occurs within the family. In such situations, workers feel even more torn between professional and personal and family obligations and have difficulty making all the pieces fit (Rolland, 1994).

Several of the people in our discussion group felt that their loved ones did not appreciate their working in the field of HIV, considering it a much too depressing and time-consuming environment. Said one person, for example: 'My husband is very much afraid that I'm going to burn myself out and that he'll have to pick up the pieces. I dare not talk about the difficult times because all I'll hear is "quit the damn job." '

REMAINING IN THE FIELD OF AIDS: THE COPING STRATEGIES

Despite all the difficulties, many health-care workers remain deeply committed to their work in the field of HIV. How do they manage to summon up the courage and conviction needed to continue under such difficult conditions? To provide an answer to this question, we refer to the notion of coping strategy.

Coping strategies are the efforts people deploy to manage situations that tax their resources (Lazarus, 1990). The literature identifies eight coping strategies most often adopted by health-care workers in the field of HIV. These strategies, in order of importance, are: (1) denial—i.e., the negation of one's vulnerability or of the possible danger represented by the virus; (2) developing a privileged relationship with the person living with the virus; (3) distancing from those affected; (4) redefining the affected person so that HIV is no longer that person's main characteristic; (5) referring to a new system of belief that allows one to attribute a positive value to the experience; (6) maximizing precautions beyond universal safety guidelines; (7) seeking social support; and (8) redefining the problem in such a way as allow one to feel a certain sense of control over the situation.

Two of these eight strategies—denial and maximizing precautions—were not mentioned by the workers in our discussion group. We will focus on the other six coping strategies (see Table 2). They are, in order of importance to the focus group:

1. Referring to a system of belief that attributes positive value to the experience.
2. Seeking social support.
3. Distancing.
4. Developing meaningful relationships with those affected by the virus.
5. Redefining the person living with the virus.
6. Redefining the problem.

Table 2 The Coping Strategies (in order of importance)

According to the Literature	*According to Social Workers of Our Focus Group*
1. *Denial* • Denial of one's vulnerability and of possible danger	1. *Adopting beliefs that allow one to give meaning to one's experiences* • 'Working with people with AIDS gives meaning to my own pain and suffering.'
2. *Developing significant relationships with affected people* • Creation of bonds that, on the other hand, make loss of person more difficult	2. *Seeking social support* • From support group of other social workers in the field of AIDS, immediate colleagues, supervisors, friends, family, and/or AIDS community groups
3. *Distancing* • Reducing or altogether avoiding contact with people who have AIDS	3. *Distancing* • By setting one's limits and by 'cutting off' at times • Through knowledge of self and of one's more vulnerable aspects
4. *Redefining the person with AIDS* • AIDS is no longer considered the person's most important characteristic: he/she is first and foremost a human being	4. *Developing significant relationships with affected people* • 'It is those relationships we develop with the people who have AIDS that allow us to continue.'
5. *Adopting beliefs that allow one to give meaning to one's experiences* • Referral to rituals and spiritual beliefs that allow one to find meaning in so much suffering and so many deaths	5. *Redefining the person with AIDS* • Through recognition of person's strength and humanity • Through recognition of what the person with AIDS has taught us
6. *Maximizing precautions* • Wearing gloves and masks when uncalled for	6. *Problem-solving* • Reference to professional knowledge and techniques
7. *Seeking social support* • Sharing with health-care workers living similar experiences	
8. *Redefining the problem*	

1. Referring to a System of Belief That Attributes Positive Value to the Experience

According to Elford (1987), the absence of scientific certainty surrounding the HIV virus explains why many health-care workers feel the need to refer to rituals and sometimes near-magical systems of belief to gain a sense of protection and control over their difficult work environment. The use of professional jargon and techniques often plays this role. Workers can also adopt a new school of thought that allows them to extract a positive value from their experiences, and many have found that Eastern philosophy and esotericism fulfil this purpose well (Light, 1988).

All the participants in our focus group attributed positive value to their overall experience in the field of HIV. Here are their most telling comments:

> This very difficult experience has allowed me to redefine myself. I know myself better now and I think I am a better person.
>
> It gives meaning to my personal suffering since it has allowed me to better understand the suffering of others.
>
> My experience with AIDS has forced me to think about my own death. I used to believe death had nothing to do with me, that I could never get sick and die. Now I know that I can and will. . . . The whole experience has made me stronger.
>
> I like the fact that I'm in the forefront of a practice that has yet to be completely institutionalized. It gives me a chance to create and invent, to be spontaneous and maybe, just maybe, it allows me to do a better job.
>
> In the beginning I thought I was Superman. . . . I was doing something no one else wanted to do and it was very self-actualizing, at least for a while. Now what I enjoy most is the opportunity to share the expertise and knowledge I have acquired over the past eight years with others.

2. Seeking Social support

The search for social support was the second most often mentioned strategy in our discussion group. It is also one of the main antidotes to stress identified in the literature (House, 1980; Maslach, 1982; Driedger and Cox, 1991; CASW, 1997).

This support can present itself under different forms; for example, some workers prefer a more silent form of support, expressed through simple respect of one's limitations, while others feel the need for a more active form of support, such as scheduled meetings in which difficult experiences are processed and shared (Wiener and Siegel, 1990; Driedger and Cox, 1991; Segalen et al., 1988). Support from family members and close friends also helps alleviate tensions stemming from the workplace (Maslach, 1982).

The workers of our group stressed that in their opinion, the most significant expressions of support came primarily from the work environment itself. For example:

—*from co-workers:*
On my team, we really, really support each other. . . . We share opinions and difficult cases among ourselves. . . . Without this ongoing sharing, I don't think I could carry on.

My colleague and I have an implicit understanding: when one of us is finding things difficult and is having a hard time managing, we ask the other to take over for a while. It enables us to get back on our feet.

—*from managers:*
My boss insists we take a week off every three months. He recognizes that the work we do is really draining and we need time for ourselves.

I've been lucky to be working for an organization that has made my work a priority and has always supported me in my endeavours. I don't think I could have achieved as much hadn't it been for this recognition.

—*from co-participants in support groups:*
I wasn't getting any support in my work milieu, so I joined a support group outside my organization. This has allowed me to discuss my problems with other social workers who really understand what I'm going through because they've been there themselves.

—*from volunteers and workers in grassroots organizations:*
My contact with the AIDS community network has helped me a lot. I know these people are there and that I can count on their help and support.

3. DISTANCING

The third strategy most often mentioned during our discussion was distancing. In the literature this refers to the behaviours and attitudes adopted by health-care professionals to distance themselves from their patients, whether through the inappropriate wearing of gloves and mask (Amchin and Polan, 1986) or through the refusal of contact with people living with the virus (Driedger and Cox, 1991).

Distancing took on a completely different meaning for the workers in our group. They felt it more aptly described behaviours and attitudes that allowed them to distance themselves, not so much from the people living with HIV but rather from the difficult components of their work. The following statements reveal the meaning the participants attributed to this strategy:

I have developed a way of protecting myself. . . . Alarm bells start to go off in my head when I'm getting too immersed in my work and then I know it's time to back off physically and to ask my colleague to take over for a while.

When several people die within a short period of time, I call my sister and tell her to send me her two young children for the weekend. This allows me to grasp life once again and I can come back to work on Monday morning, physically tired but psychologically replenished.

4. Developing Meaningful Relationships with Those Affected by the Virus

Numerous workers quoted in the literature mention that the relationship they develop with the people they care for is, without a doubt, the most enriching part of their practice (Lamarche, 1994; Olivier, 1994). Participants in our group felt the same way:

> The relationships I have developed over the years with the men and women with AIDS have sustained me in my practice. We have shared many beautiful moments together and I remember many of them with fondness and caring.
>
> The bonds I have created with the children I work with give me the strength to stand up to the doctors and defend their rights.

5. Redefining the Person Living with the Virus

Workers we met did not attribute as much importance to this strategy as the professionals quoted in the literature. According to the latter, redefining the person with HIV seems to play a major function in the modification of their attitude and behaviour towards that person, especially in the beginning of their experience in the field. Reuther and Northcott (1994), for example, recount how some nurses adopted a more discretionary use of precautions once they began to consider the person with HIV otherwise than simply an incarnation of his or her disease. Gallup et al. (1992) also found that this strategy helped hospital staff in Toronto empathize with HIV patients and develop with them relationships based on respect rather than on fear and avoidance.

Once again, this strategy took on a whole different meaning for the workers we met, who, we might recall, had several years' experience in the field. In their case, redefining the person with HIV allowed them to see the positive side of working with people who are marginalized in our society and considered problematic in dominant professional discourse. As such, this played very much the same role as the first coping strategy—referring to a system of belief that attributes positive value to the experience.

> I'm in this field because of the people. They teach me so much about life and make me see things in a different perspective. I'm 36 years old, married, with a home and debts up to my ears and the people I work with help me understand that there's a reality out there that is much more meaningful than mine often is.
>
> The drug user clientele I work with is composed of very colourful individuals. They're extremely imaginative and creative and they all have incredible stories to tell. . . . Sometimes I think I'm reading a novel. I'm always learning about life and living and despite all the pain and suffering, there's a lot of love and joy, too. Many of my 'clients' are like a breath of fresh air in my existence.
>
> When you get to know a person, AIDS loses much of its importance. Sometimes I surprise myself thinking: wow, don't forget this incredibly strong person also has AIDS.

6. Redefining the Problem

This strategy consists of defining the problem in such a way that it generates alternative solutions, which allows one to make informed decisions that bring about a certain sense of control over stressful situations (Lazarus, 1990). According to Driedger and Cox (1991), this is among the strategies most often used by nurses working with HIV patients because it brings them a feeling of security in their work environment and leads them to influence this environment in concrete and positive ways.

Participants in our discussion group underlined the positive function played by professional knowledge and expertise in the use of this particular strategy:

> The knowledge I have acquired of what to do, how to be and what to say in certain situations helps me work with our clientele, which is considered difficult. When someone in front of me is going through a major crisis, I can analyse what's going on, be a good listener, and calm the person down. I am capable of doing this because I feel professionally secure.
>
> My expertise in the field of prevention has allowed me to survive for 12 years. I now know more about how to prevent people from getting sick in the first place and this gives me a sense of control over what is happening.
>
> Three years ago, I would stay awake for nights before making a decision, asking myself if I was doing the right thing. Now, I have a certain expertise and I'm much more confident about the decisions I make.

Conclusion: Where to From Here?

What conclusions can be drawn with regard to the challenges facing the social work profession in the next few years? What lessons can we learn for future practice from the information gathered?

First of all, we must acknowledge that difficult working conditions constitute the most important stressor faced by health-care workers today. Statements from the social workers interviewed emphasize the extent to which current arrangements undermine the morale of those from whom society still expects quality services. And this is exactly where the shoe pinches. On the one hand, workers are subjected to the disastrous effects of the progressive dismantlement of our health and social services system that has been ongoing for nearly 30 years; at the same time, they have to meet the ever-increasing expectations of those around them. The specific case of social workers in the field of HIV illustrates this point well. Confronted with the repercussions of current cutbacks and with a client population more and more assertive and demanding of the services it has come to expect, these workers find their role continually called into question. Although the resources to which they have access are continually being diminished and the people they are meant to help are more and more marginalized and therefore despondent, they nevertheless continue to view themselves as providers of limitless affective and material means.

The harsh reality is that workers carry on their shoulders the inconsistencies and contradictions of a system over which they feel they have little control. At the same time, they receive the implicit message that these difficulties are in fact of their own making and are mainly due to their professional incompetence and inadequacies. Notwithstanding these difficult conditions, many workers still manage to survive and to help those who need them.

This brings us to the second lesson that can be drawn from the experience of practitioners in the field of HIV: the major role that the search for meaning plays in the overall system of professional survival. This search for meaning is in itself very significant in that it reveals to us the total absence of meaning to which our current obsession with technology has inevitably driven us. Trapped as we are in the dominant mould of technocratic professional practice, our work has become a means to an end that we no longer are able to identify. In other words, although we now have access to more techniques, more protocols, and more grids than ever before, we are, paradoxically, less and less capable of saying why we carry out our professional acts. In so doing we reflect a dominant tendency in our society, which Renaud (1996) describes as follows:

> Our society has lost its compass; it is disoriented with regards to its finality and appears to be caught up in a system of means whose sole purpose is to increase overall efficiency. As a result of this, fundamental questions of meaning, of personal and collective identity and of ethics, have disappeared.

When applied to social work, these fundamental questions become, for example: *Why*, instead of how, do we practice the profession in 1998? What type of social rapport do we wish to establish with those who find themselves, often quite unwillingly, in our offices? What type of social actor do we wish to contribute to create? And finally, what values do we wish our interventions to translate on a day-to-day basis? Workers who participated in our discussion group stressed that questions such as these confronted them continually in their practice.

Their experiences also allow us to identify a third dilemma facing social workers today: that of the acceptance or refusal of the double-edged sword of expertise—double-edged because, on the one side, recourse to this expertise, as we have seen, constitutes one of the main strategies that allows workers to cope with the difficulties with which they were faced; on the other side, this expertise also represents a trap that rigidifies their practice, alienates them from their fellow workers, and obscures the generic components of all social work practice. This is a cruel predicament for those who must choose between the security afforded by expertise with the sense of professional alienation that follows or the feeling of belonging yet at the same time being continually confronted with the limitations of professional practice.

Such choices cannot and should not be avoided. As stated in the beginning of this chapter, HIV is a harsh and demanding master that has shown us that technical responses, no matter how efficient they are, cannot shield us from dealing with the ethical dilemmas that life puts before us. Writes Renaud (1996): '*In a world which is becoming more and more dehumanized,* such choices give us the opportunity to once again give meaning to our existence. They are not to be missed.'

REFERENCES

Abramson, M. 1990. 'Keeping Secrets: Social Workers and AIDS', *Social Work* 35: 169–73.

Amchin, L., and H.J. Polan. 1986. 'A Longitudinal Account of Staff Adaptation to AIDS Patients on a Psychiatric Unit', *Hospital and Community Psychiatry* 37: 1235–8.

Bennet, J.A. 1987. 'Nurses Talk about the Challenge of AIDS', *American Journal of Nursing* 87: 1150–5.

Bosk, C., and J. Frader. 1991. 'AIDS and Its Impact on Medical Social Work: The Culture and Politics of the Shop Floor', in D. Nelkin, D. Willis, and S. Parris, eds, *A Disease of Society: Cultural and Institutional Responses to AIDS*. Cambridge: Cambridge University Press, 150–71.

Bourgon, M., D. Desmarais, and W. Ryan. 1995. *Vivre proche(s) du sida: recherche de sens et stratégies adaptatives.* Rapport de recherche soumis au CQRS.

———, and G. Renaud. 1989. 'Sida et travail social un croisement propice à la réflexion', *Le travailleur social/The Social Worker* 57: 43–7.

———, and ———. 1993. 'Paul, Marcel, Gérard et les autres. L'expérience des conjoints gais de personnes atteintes de sida', manuscript.

Caillé, A. 1986. *Splendeurs et misères en sciences sociales.* Paris: Droz.

Canadian Association of Social Workers (CASW). 1997. *Comprehensive Guide for the Care of Persons with HIV diseases*. Ottawa: CASW.

Dionne-Proulx, J. 1994. 'Le sida: droits du client, risques professionnels, mesures préventives', *Canadian Nurse* 90: 43–7.

———, and R. Pépin. 1994. 'Le stress vu de l'extérieur', *Canadian Nurse* 90: 403–43.

Driedger, S., and D. Cox. 1991. 'Burnout in Nurses Who Care for PWAs: The Impact of Social Support', *AIDS Patient Care* 8: 197–203.

Dunkel, J., and S. Hatfield. 1986. 'Countertransference Issues in Working with Persons with AIDS', *Social Work* 31: 114–18.

Elford, J. 1987. 'Moral and Social Aspects of AIDS: A Medical Students' Project', *Social Sciences Medicine* 24: 543–9.

Fortunato, J. 1987. *AIDS: The Spiritual Dilemma.* New York: Perennial Library Press.

Gallup, R., G. Taerk, W. Lancee, R. Coates, and M. Fanning. 1992. 'A Randomized Trial of Group Intervention for Hospital Staff Caring for Persons with AIDS', *AIDS Care* 4: 177–85.

Haines, J. 1987. 'AIDS: New Considerations in Caring', *Canadian Nurse*, 83: 11–12.

House, J. 1980. *Occupational Stress and the Mental and Physical Health of Factory Workers.* Ann Arbor: University of Michigan Press.

Lamarche, C. 1994. 'Soigner, même quand on ne peut guérir', *Les diplômés* 383: 23–4.

Lazarus, R. 1990. 'Stress, Coping and Illness', in H.S. Friedman, ed., *Personality and Disease.* New York: Wiley, 97–120.

Light, D. 1988. 'Toward a New Sociology of Medical Education', *Journal of Health and Social Behavior* 29: 307–22.

Maslach, C. 1982. *Burnout: The Cost of Caring.* Englewood Cliffs, NJ: Prentice-Hall.

Olivier, C. 1994. *L'amour assasin.* Montréal: Stanké.

Pollack, M. 1988. *Les homosexuels et le sida. Sociologie d'une épidémie.* Paris: Éditions A.M. Métaillié.

Renaud, G. 1990. 'Travail social, crise de la modernité et post-modernité', *Revue Canadienne de Service Social* 7: 27–48.

———. 1997. 'L'intervention: les savoirs en crise'. Ed. GGC, Université de Sherbrooke.

Reuther, L., and H. Northcott. 1994. 'Achieving a Sense of Control in a Context of Uncertainty: Nurses and AIDS', *Qualitative Research* 4: 51–71.

Rolland, J.S. 1994. 'Working with Illness: Clinicians' Personal and Interface Issues', *Family Systems Medicine* 12: 149–69.

Ryan, B. 1989. 'Sida: la réponse du milieu', *Le travailleur social/The Social Worker* 57: 53–7.

Saint-Jarre, C. 1994. *Du sida. L'anticipation imaginaire de la mort et sa mise en discours.* Paris: Denoel.

Saul, J. 1995. *The Unconscious Civilization.* Concord, Ont.: House of Anansi.

Segalen, J., C. Charmasson, G. Delzant, and E. Hirsch. 1988. 'Éthique et pratique', *L'information psychiatrique* 64: 687–92.

Wiener, L.S., and K. Siegel. 1990. 'Social Workers' Comfort in Providing Services to AIDS Patients', *Social Work* 35: 18–25.

Chapter 14

Confidentiality/Ethical Issues in Social Work and HIV

SHARON TAYLOR

Responsible professional conduct includes the obligation to balance clients' right to confidentiality with the protection of third parties. (Reamer, 1991: 58)

INTRODUCTION

Throughout history, faced with successive threats to its cohesion, our society has always hesitated between two solutions: the elimination of risk factors and the protection of the most vulnerable members of society. The problem raised by all epidemics, whatever their nature, seems to be the antagonism between the right (or duty) of society to defend itself against the danger of destruction and the rights of infected minority groups to claim protection (Manuel et al., 1991: 31). Measures that protect one group in society may encroach on the rights of others, creating an ethical dilemma. At what cost do we protect society and still maintain confidentiality?

HIV poses major ethical questions for society (Abramson, 1990: 169). The 1995 research report of the Canadian Association of Social Workers, *Social Work Practice and Practice Wisdom in the Field of HIV/AIDS* (Clarke, 1995), indicated that ethical dilemmas arising in practice were one of the foremost concerns noted among respondents, as well as one of the top three emerging trends. The critical ethical issues facing social workers whose professional lives are touched by the HIV crisis concern three major issues: testing for HIV; the confidentiality of information related to HIV; and the delivery of services to persons with HIV, their families, and their partners (Reamer, 1988: 460).

Clients' right to confidentiality is among the most enduring and sacred of social work values (Reamer, 1988: 461). Breach of confidentiality is probably the most serious ethical dilemma facing social workers. This chapter will address the issue of confidentiality as sacred trust versus public safety in the context of professional practice and persons with HIV. Relevant legal precedents, reference to professional codes of ethics, and the implications for practice, including guidelines for social workers, will be presented.

HIV has demonstrated its ability to spread across all geographic, social, cultural, economic, and political borders. It has implications worldwide and is an issue in practice that few professionals have not had to face (Mann, 1992: 246). HIV has an enormous impact on today's society and thus is an issue for social work to respond to (Ontario Association of Professional Social Workers, 1989). Since the first AIDS case was identified in the United States in 1981, social work has been a core profession in the provision of service for people with HIV, from counselling about testing to bereavement work with families (Abramson, 1990: 169).

The moral problems social workers face in their day-to-day practice with people with HIV create distress and uncertainty for practitioners. As an ethical issue, breaching confidentiality forces choices between equally competing values without specific guidelines to provide direction. Because the legal limits to therapeutic confidentiality are not defined and uniform, ethical standards of the helping professions have taken on increased importance (Gray and Harding, 1988: 220). If ethical rules are incomplete and in conflict with each other, they may fail counsellors (Kitchener, 1986: 306), so it is important for social workers to be acquainted with what is currently known about ethical and civil liberties issues that may affect their work related to HIV (Reamer, 1993: 412).

THE TARASOFF DECISION

As a challenge to professional responsibility regarding the issue of limits of confidentiality and public safety or protection, the *Tarasoff* case in the United States has become a legal reference regarding the duty to protect society versus the client's right to confidentiality. Although this is US jurisprudence, the implications of the decision have far-reaching consequences and implications for social workers in all Western societies, including Canada. For this reason, the arguments and decisions related to the *Tarasoff* case will be discussed here.

Consensus has begun to build that the court decision in the *Tarasoff* case may be very relevant to HIV cases (Reamer, 1991: 57). In this case (*Tarasoff v. Regents of University of California*, 1976), a patient (Prosenjit Poddar) revealed to his psychotherapist his intent to kill his ex-girlfriend, Tatiana Tarasoff. The psychotherapist considered a hospital commitment and sought the assistance of campus police. After discussions with Poddar, it was decided that he presented no imminent threat. Poddar then discontinued psychotherapy. Approximately two months later he murdered Tarasoff upon her return from a trip abroad. Tarasoff's parents sued the therapist and other state officials for failure to detain a dangerous patient (Poddar) and failure to warn Tarasoff and/or others likely to have contact with her. The case was initially dismissed in the original court in 1973, was appealed, and was heard again in the Supreme Court of California in 1974. The appeal court ruled that psychotherapists have a duty to warn the intended victim or others likely to have contact with the intended victim when the professional determines, or should determine, with professional skill and knowledge, that such action is necessary to prevent danger. In a final appeal brought by the defendants and heard by the Supreme Court of California, the 'duty to warn' was upheld and broadened to the 'duty to protect'. The issue of individual rights versus the rights of society was highlighted in favour of the protection of society (Lamb et al., 1989: 38).

This 1976 decision established a responsibility for practitioners to protect potential victims of dangerous clients and the need to warn possible victims, stating:

> when a therapist determines, or pursuant to the standards of his profession should determine, that his patient presents a serious danger of violence to another, he incurs an obligation to use reasonable care to protect the intended victim against such danger. The discharge of this duty may require the therapist to take one or more of various steps, depending upon the nature of the case. Thus it may call for him to warn the intended victim or others likely to apprise the victim of the danger, to notify the police, or to take whatever other steps are reasonably necessary under the circumstances. (Weil and Sanchez, 1983: 114)

In California, licensed clinical social workers are included in the statutory definition of psychotherapist and thus are bound by the *Tarasoff* decision (Weil and Sanchez, 1983: 115).

Although the *Tarasoff* ruling occurred five years prior to the first known case of HIV in the US, the principle of the precedent of duty to warn, over confidentiality, raises ethical issues to be addressed in practice with HIV clients. As a professional, one is faced with protecting the confidentiality and right to privacy of the individual when there is the possibility of danger to potential victims or, more generally, a threat to the protection of society. Social workers are thus forced to choose between professional duties that would ordinarily be fulfilled (Gelman and Reamer, 1992: 344). Some social workers argue that in such cases they are ethically bound to protect the client's right to confidentiality. Others, though, argue that the welfare of third parties must take precedence over the client's right to confidentiality. The responsibility to the individual and to society presents an ethical dilemma further complicated by the assessment of serious danger. This acknowledges the responsibility for professionals to determine imminent danger and the obligation to protect the intended potential victims using reasonable care.

REACTION TO TARASOFF

There is considerable research and writing related to the decision in the *Tarasoff* case. Many practitioners have been receptive to the *Tarasoff* position as an acceptable legal solution to an ethical dilemma (Kopels and Kagle, 1993: 101). Knapp, Vande-Creek, and Herzog (1986) are of the opinion that *Tarasoff*, if properly applied by the courts, does nothing to interfere with professional judgements (cited in Lamb et al., 1989: 38). Weil and Sanchez (1983: 120) conclude that the *Tarasoff* decision is an instance of good law supporting responsible professional practice. They further state clearly that when a client threatens the life of another person, the practitioner must make critical decisions regarding what actions are necessary to effect reasonable care to protect intended victims, including (1) whether to warn potential victims; (2) what effect the warning would have on the therapeutic relationship and whether to discuss the warning with the client; (3) how to warn the potential victim(s); (4) whether to contact law enforcement agencies; and (5) whether to initiate hospitalization (Weil and Sanchez, 1983: 115).

Gray and Harding (1988: 221) believe that it is at the expense of uninformed sexual partners' safety to keep information that the client has HIV confidential.

They argue that a sexually active seropositive individual places an uninformed sexual partner at peril, and the situation therefore falls under the legal spirit of the *Tarasoff* case.

Kain (1988) focused on the needs of the client rather than the danger to others as the determining factor whether to breach confidentiality (cited in Lamb et al., 1989: 38). Francis and Chin state that the maintenance of confidentiality is central to and of paramount importance for the control of HIV. They argue that information regarding infection with a deadly virus, sexual activity, sexual contacts, the illegal use of IV drugs, and diagnostic information regarding HIV-related disease is sensitive and that, if released by the patient or someone involved in health care, it could adversely affect a patient's personal and professional life (Reamer, 1991: 57). The issues of harassment, discrimination, and decline in the public's trust possibly affecting willingness to seek out professional help are factors to consider. It is further argued, however, that although these are regrettable consequences, the professional must maintain the goal to deliver competent services and be professionally responsible (Gelman and Reamer, 1992: 347).

Addressing the epidemiological risk to sexual partners, Eth concluded that the moral urgency to respond to specific persons in grave danger outweighs consideration of the perhaps larger number of persons who may be deterred from entering treatment or HIV testing programs because of possible violation of their privacy (Reamer, 1991: 57). The position held by Lamb et al. (1989) considers that if a client merely poses a threat to a third party it is sufficient to rely on *Tarasoff* as a precedent. Reamer (1991: 58) acknowledges the obligation to balance the protection of third parties with the client's right to confidentiality. Gelman and Reamer note that there is a delicate line between meeting professional and societal obligations when social workers must confront difficult if not unresolvable ethical dilemmas. They further argue that there is a moral responsibility to alert those at risk, but it is not a professional or legal responsibility (Gelman and Reamer, 1992: 349).

The Ontario Association of Professional Social Workers released a statement on HIV in 1989 in recognition of the special expertise and skills of the social work profession to respond effectively to HIV. Further confirming the Ontario Human Rights Code that no one can be discriminated against on the basis of or suspicion of HIV infection, the OAPSW statement acknowledged that disclosure can be justified only when an HIV-infected person becomes a danger to himself/herself or to others due to a physical, mental, or emotional condition. It further recognized that the social workers' mandate is to protect the confidentiality of all persons with HIV and that they must facilitate the process of disclosure of information only to those at risk. It does not acknowledge that the public has a right to be informed. The responsibility is placed on the social worker to make a judgement with respect to assessing danger, as based on the *Tarasoff* decision.

The NASW acknowledges that social workers must face breaching confidentiality in order to protect third parties (Gelman and Reamer, 1992: 344). A generalized statement intended to protect society may be unacceptable from an ethical point of view, constituting violation of privacy and anonymity. Such encroachment on the fundamental rights of individuals may cause individuals with HIV to experience discrimination related to employment, housing, admission to schools, immigration restrictions, or screening by insurance companies.

Kopels and Kagle (1993: 103) acknowledge that *Tarasoff* provides an ethically acceptable solution to a real practice dilemma; however, it also presents a danger. The *Tarasoff* ruling indicates that reasonable care should be exercised, but does not mandate automatic or immediate warning of third parties. The decision can easily be misinterpreted as licence to breach confidence impulsively and warn others, with possible serious consequences. This could potentially impede or alter treatment, thereby weakening the trust of the therapeutic relationship. Individuals may avoid seeking counselling or may be resistant to full disclosure of the nature of their relationships and contacts. Some professionals or organizations may refuse treatment to clients suspected of HIV or AIDS to avoid breaching confidentiality or liability. Professionals may even avoid gaining further information about behaviours or intent through exploration of an individual's social history in an effort to avoid negligence. There is always the danger of an individual's inability to assess or to overpredict danger or potential for harm. This may lead to inappropriate use of detainment and confinement or overreporting of clients.

Gelman and Reamer (1992: 353) also raise the issue of risk for the social worker who discloses confidential information, as well as the public's willingness to trust the profession. An individual may be sued for not taking appropriate action to inform to protect third parties, but he or she may also be sued for disclosing confidential information, invading privacy, and breach of contract. These possibilities are not new for the profession—social work has faced these issues in relation to child protection cases and to disclosure in regard to protecting clients from self-harm. However, in these instances, decisions made are supported by the CASW *Code of Ethics*.

This raises the concern that if exceptions to confidentiality currently exist, such as recognizing child abuse as precedence over maintaining confidentiality, then professional codes should address the ethical issues social workers face with HIV clients and the danger to others. The professional codes within counselling, social work, and psychology all emphasize the importance of the confidential therapeutic relationship. The American Association for Marriage and Family Therapy Code of Ethics (1991) requires marriage and family counsellors to break confidentiality to prevent clear and imminent danger (Costa and Altekruse, 1994: 347). The American Association for Counselling and Development (1988) provides the following direction: when the client's condition indicates that there is clear and imminent danger to the client or others, the members must take reasonable personal action to inform responsible authorities. Consultation with other professionals must be used where possible. The assumption of responsibility for the client's behaviour must be taken only after careful deliberation. The client must be involved in the resumption of responsibility as quickly as possible (Gross and Robinson, 1987: 340). The American Psychological Association adopted a resolution in 1991 declaring that a legal duty to protect third parties from HIV infection should not be imposed and specific legislation should permit disclosure on three conditions: there is an identifiable third party who is deemed to be at risk; there is reasonable belief that the third party does not suspect that he/she is at risk; and the client has been urged but has refused or is unable to notify the third party (Costa and Altekruse, 1994: 347).

Codes can be ambiguous and sometimes even offer contradictory advice (Costa and Altekruse, 1994: 347). The *Code of Ethics* of the Canadian Association of Social Workers (1994: ch. 5) states that a social worker shall protect the confidentiality of all information acquired from the client or others regarding the client. There are exceptions, however, as section 26 states that a social worker shall disclose information acquired from a client to a person or a police officer where the information involves a threat of harm to that person. Section 25 further permits disclosure to the client's family where there is a threat of harm to self or others (CASW, 1994). This acknowledgement that sometimes confidentiality must be violated to protect third parties is ambiguous and open to interpretation. It further stresses responsibility to both the client and the community, calling on the social worker to assess and determine threat of harm or imminent danger.

Confidentiality between physicians and patients is ensured by ethical and legal codes; however, physicians in the US and the UK are authorized by their medical associations to inform sexual partners of seropositive individuals. Such steps to protect the public against dangerous patients may not be possible without disclosure of confidential information against patients' wishes (Gray and Harding, 1988: 220). The issue of patients who present a danger to others but insist on confidentiality is also facing the medical community. The Canadian Medical Association provides for physicians in Canada to report to public health authorities when they believe a patient is infected with HIV or has AIDS. Physicians must report positive results to the Ministry of Health area unit for follow-up, including partner notification if this has not occurred. The Canadian Medical Association Code of Ethics for psychiatrists further establishes that it is ethical to reveal confidential information when, in the opinion of the psychiatrist, the patient's behaviour is likely to endanger him/herself and others and no other alternative course will procure their safety. It is within the realm of the medical and public health officials to provide pre- and post-test counselling, presenting an opportunity for preventive education and discussion regarding protection of others and to make referrals for other services and resources.

As indicated, it may be necessary to breach confidentiality despite the harm it will do, providing a preventive balance, in determining risk of an even greater harm of transmission. Mandatory notification of partners and health authorities raises the same issue of protection of society versus the protection of the rights of the individual. Under the Health Protection and Promotion Act of Ontario, the Ministry of Health may issue a written order against a person when there is immediate risk to the health of others. A total of 45 orders were written in Ontario by the end of 1993 prohibiting transmission of HIV, requiring counselling, or revealing names. These section 22 orders can be enforced by the courts (Ontario Advisory Committee on HIV/AIDS, 1995: 9–11). In regard to other provincial jurisdictions, the Health Act in BC, for example, allows for incarceration (quarantine) of individuals who breach public health orders. In two cases involving prostitutes who continued working after testing HIV-positive, the Ministry of Health convinced the Attorney-General that counselling rather than incarceration would better serve both individuals (Ontario Advisory Committee on HIV/AIDS, 1995: 48).

One civil lawsuit in Ontario has been brought against a health-care professional for failure to provide sufficient information to a patient. In *Pittman et al. v. Bain*, a physician was found guilty of negligence and duty to warn. The physician in this case was aware that Mr Pittman received HIV as a result of a blood transfusion. He made no effort to inform the patient's wife, however, assuming the couple was not engaging in sexual intercourse. The physician was found negligent of his duty to warn when Mr Pittman was clearly a threat to his wife, who subsequently became infected.

The HIV crisis has exacerbated the tensions among public health concerns and civil liberties, challenging the professional responsibility of social workers (Gray and Harding, 1988: 221). Kaplan, Sager, and Schiavi (1985, 1986) took a strong stand in proposing guidelines that have ethical implications for counselling and educating AIDS individuals. They contend that a highly specific and harsh procedure is necessary to prevent further infection and that counsellors must confront individuals with the fact that they are carrying a deadly disease in their body fluids and that it is their responsibility to see to it that they do not infect others (cited in Gray and Harding, 1988: 221).

A number of studies have reviewed practitioner's responses to the issue of confidentiality versus the duty to protect. A 1976 survey of California psychotherapists following the *Tarasoff* decision studied the impact of the court ruling. The results indicated that therapists, including social workers, were more likely to seek the counsel of other professionals when issues related to violence, threats, or danger arose with their clients. Further, all respondents felt it was a professional responsibility to protect others regardless of circumstances (Weil and Sanchez, 1983: 116).

A 1981 study with a similar sample group revealed that 78 per cent felt it was their professional responsibility to protect others from potential violence by a client when a serious possibility exists that the client will follow through with the threat. Practitioners, however, revealed reservations about violating confidentiality even when a third party is endangered. Only 6.35 per cent believed confidentiality should be upheld despite any circumstances, while 76.9 per cent believed the protection of society was more important than maintaining strict confidentiality with a dangerous client. With regard to action taken, 65 per cent recognized responsibility to the client, to potential victims, and to the agency, 73.4 per cent would deal with the issue in continued therapy, 70 per cent would notify their supervisors, 71.1 per cent would warn the potential victim, while 67.9 per cent believed they would exercise reasonable care to protect the potential victim. Only 22 per cent thought that warning a potential victim of violence should be left up to each individual practitioner and not mandated. The vast majority (97.5 per cent) agreed that confidentiality is a crucial aspect of the therapeutic process, yet only 6 per cent stated that they always make it a point to discuss confidentiality.

Half of the respondents indicated that they normally discuss the limitations of confidentiality at the outset of treatment, while one-third sometimes discuss it. Over one-third (38.7 per cent) felt discussions regarding disclosure of information would jeopardize the therapeutic process, while 47.5 per cent disagreed and 13.7 per cent were indifferent. With regard to judgement of the client's potential to harm others, social workers would most often consult other professionals, including psychiatrists, other social workers, supervisors, lawyers, ensuring to make notations in the client's file or record (Weil and Sanchez, 1983: 116–20).

The *Tarasoff* position was clear that the protective privilege ends where the public peril begins (Weil and Sanchez, 1983: 124). This decision influenced over one-third of respondents to likely act to warn third parties. The respondents in the latter study had directly experienced the impact of the court decision and identified it as a factor in practice. Compliance with a legal mandate, however, did not form the basis for action. Almost two-thirds of the respondents reported a discrepancy in their actions in most recent cases that does not support the belief system that they claimed required them to act to protect third parties. Among the respondents, professional ethics were stated to be the strongest guide for profession action and responsibility when a client threatens to harm a third party.

A further survey in 1987 underscores the confusion counsellors feel in their duty of respecting confidentiality when clients refuse to share their HIV-positive status with their sexual partners (Gray and Harding, 1988: 219).

Where does one turn for guidance and direction regarding interpretation and action to be taken? The studies support the need for more guidance in professional codes of ethics regarding responsibility in this issue (Weil and Sanchez, 1983: 124). Kitchener (1986: 306) points out that although ethics codes are written to provide ethical guidelines for professionals, they are not meant to provide absolute rules. They do, however, raise awareness of the effects of one's decisions and actions on others.

The California Supreme Court decision in the *Tarasoff* case concluded that 'the public policy favoring protection of the confidential character of patient-psychotherapist communications must yield to the extent to which disclosure is essential to avert danger to others' (Gelman and Reamer, 1992: 345). A number of courts have ruled similarly, concluding that in extreme cases professionals have a duty to breach confidentiality when necessary to protect third parties and a duty to exercise reasonable care to prevent harm. Professionals are expected to disclose confidential information in instances where a client makes a specific threat of violence that is imminent and foreseeable against an identifiable victim. Further, a number of court decisions indicate that a 'foreseeable victim' may involve a class of persons (Reamer, 1991: 57). Questions further arise in determining the client. Is it the individual with the disease, identified potential victims, or society at large?

Following a review of several cases related to or based on the *Tarasoff* case, Fulero (1988: 186) concludes that the *Tarasoff* decision will continue to generate litigation, legislation, and controversy for many years to come. Virtually every state uses *Tarasoff* as a precedent in constructing case law. Three conditions existed in the *Tarasoff* case that led the California Supreme Court to find the therapist had a duty to warn. First, one person had a special relationship either to the person whose conduct needed to be controlled or to the foreseeable victim of that conduct. The therapist-client relationship was just such a special relationship. The second condition required that the determination be made that the client's conduct needs to be controlled. The court found that there was clearly a threat and consideration of danger in this case. The third condition required a foreseeable victim, even when the victim was not specifically named. The court ruled that although the victim was not specifically named by the client, she was a readily identifiable victim of the client and should have been warned (Costa and Altekruse, 1994: 346). These conditions may provide guidance to practitioners in considering the relevance of their position in such cases. Although the criteria for warning a client's potential victim were vague, a precedent was established and additional court rulings have been decided on the basis of *Tarasoff*. The ruling may continue to indicate how other courts decide similar cases, reaffirming the court decision of the duty to exercise reasonable care to prevent harm.

HIV AND CANADIAN CASE LAW

Although the *Tarasoff* case does not set a Canadian precedent, it does raise awareness of similar issues being faced in Canada and, in particular, within social work practice. Within the Canadian Criminal Code, there is no provision for knowingly transmitting a communicable disease. There is, therefore, no HIV-specific criminal legislation that applies to people who knowingly transmit or attempt to transmit HIV, nor is there a requirement for persons with HIV to disclose their status to others who might be in a position of risk (Ontario Advisory Committee on HIV/AIDS, 1995: 23). In a few cases in Canada, however, individuals with HIV have been charged or prosecuted for allegedly infecting others (Ontario Advisory Committee on HIV/AIDS, 1995: 12–14). In Ontario, a 1991 criminal case acquitted Mr Lee on charges of aggravated assault after engaging in consensual sexual intercourse. Evidence was presented that he suspected he was HIV-positive and this was later confirmed. No evidence was presented that the complainant had asked him about the possibility of his being HIV-positive.

The *Ssenyonga* case involved three charges of criminal negligence causing bodily harm. The accused knowingly engaged in sexual intercourse aware that he was infected with HIV. All of the victims, including a 16-year-old female, were subsequently found to be HIV-positive. Three additional charges of aggravated sexual assault were dismissed on the grounds that the complainants voluntarily engaged in unprotected sexual intercourse. Mr Ssenyonga pleaded not guilty to all charges. In this case, physicians and a public health nurse had provided counselling in relation to safer sex practices and HIV transmission as directed under the Ontario public health system. The accused died in July 1993 before the judge delivered his ruling at the conclusion of the trial. The complainants were subsequently awarded $25,000 in an Ontario divisional court in February 1995.

In Alberta, Mr Somner was sentenced on a charge of being a common nuisance. He had not disclosed his HIV-positive status and was alleged to have transmitted HIV to two women through unprotected sexual activity. Similarly, in 1989, on a guilty plea to charges of criminal negligence causing bodily harm, Mr Wenzell was subsequently imprisoned for transmission of HIV through ongoing relationships. The *Mercer* case in 1993 involved infection of two women with HIV as a result of non-disclosure of HIV status to sexual partners without practising safe sex methods. Mr Mercer had previously received counselling in relation to his positive testing yet denied to both women the need to take precautions. He further failed to disclose their names as requested to the medical officer of health. He was charged with criminal negligence causing bodily harm. In these three cases the defendants pleaded guilty. Further relevant provisions of the Criminal Code were not used to prosecute. In the *Mercer* and *Ssenyonga* cases, current measures to educate the men regarding their HIV-positive status and danger of transmission to others were not sufficient to influence them to protect unknowing third parties.

SOCIAL WORK, CONFIDENTIALITY, AND HIV

The *Tarasoff* findings and these cases reflect the obligation of professionals to warn to protect potential victims. They also reflect the limitations of counselling alone to protect and reduce any threat of imminent danger. In other words, additional reasonable steps may need to be taken.

Social workers as professionals are in a position to establish non-judgemental supportive relationships based on trust and openness and to provide consultation, support, and direction to persons diagnosed with HIV or AIDS and their significant others. It is essential that social workers who may be working with HIV clients are knowledgeable about the disease, its effects, and transmission. The opportunity exists to use the relationship and counselling skills to provide pre- and post-testing education about HIV, including safety precautions emphasizing the risks of the disease and transmission to partners and offspring. It is also recognized that sometimes individuals need to be given the information more than once.

Assessment of clear and imminent danger and setting a realistic time frame for the client to come to a decision to make a disclosure are necessary for the protection of others. The underlying reasons for individuals' attitudes and behaviour must be considered when assisting clients to focus on their feelings surrounding risk factors and disclosure, which may include fear of rejection or loss of significant others. The extent of danger of a client declaring to be HIV-positive depends on his/her medical diagnosis, the extent to which the client engages in high-risk behaviours, and the extent of the use of safer sex techniques to reduce possible transmission (Lamb et al., 1989). The obligation is to protect potential victims by using the relationship to work mutually with clients to acknowledge an obligation and responsibility to protect others, to balance the benefits of the risks of disclosure, and to examine ways to protect others, including disclosure. Having justified the protection issue with the client, assistance can be provided to enable clients in planning strategies to approach disclosure. Role-playing a potential emotional disclosure or active support by encouraging disclosure in the presence of the worker may be effective to assist the client (Taylor,

Brownlee, and Mauro-Hopkins, 1996: 15). Maintaining client self-determination and empowering the client in decision-making are retained. Making the right decision to inform may assist the client in future decision-making, acceptance of responsibility, and overall functioning.

It is important to recognize and be sensitive to clients' situations that may present a concern for their own safety. When faced with clients who may place themselves at risk through disclosure, it is imperative to assist the client to develop plans to deal with the issue (Ontario Advisory Committee on HIV/AIDS, 1995: 24). The National Advisory Committee on AIDS (1987) states that partner notification is based on the principle that individuals who may have no reason to suspect that they may have been exposed to HIV should have the opportunity to know that they may have been so exposed (Ontario Advisory Committee on HIV/AIDS, 1995: 8). The issue of protection of the rights of a threatened group at the expense of the rights of the individual to privacy and confidentiality is further confirmed.

Violation of confidentiality with clients who are unwilling or unable to disclose presents a dilemma and a risk for professionals. The purpose of confidentiality is not to conceal the condition but to help clients handle the information with responsibility to themselves as well as to others (Lamb et al., 1989: 41). In the CASW *Code of Ethics*, the primary responsibility is to the client, to respect that person's need for privacy and confidentiality. There are no mandatory reporting statutes to breach confidentiality and to make known the nature of the risk presented either to the authorities or to particular individuals who may be at risk (Gelman and Reamer, 1992: 351).

Social workers must carefully consider whether there are compelling reasons to breach confidentiality without consent, recognizing that the anonymity of individuals with HIV or AIDS is clearly protected, as is the confidentiality of health records. Practitioners are faced with the effort to ensure co-operation among high-risk clients who have the assurance of confidentiality and who know that there should be no repercussions for having sought out service. If the client is unwilling or unable to disclose, and reasonable efforts fail, as a last resort the social worker, at the risk of undermining trust, must assume responsibility to make a disclosure to protect third parties. This should be done by notifying the client of the action to be taken and contacting public health authorities, who are mandated to assume responsibility to establish those considered at risk and to contact individuals specifically identified. This eliminates the need for the social worker to assume the role of detective or investigator. Reporting could also be done through the supervisor or executive director of the agency, based on a thorough assessment of information obtained and consultation with the worker.

It must be further recognized that simply informing third parties will not, of itself, reduce or prevent the risk of transmission. It does, however, allow that individual the opportunity to be aware that he/she may be or may have been at risk. Both testing and possible treatment will be necessary, with subsequent education, counselling, and support recognizing a role for social work involvement.

Social workers need to avoid emotional or panic reactions, but rather should be able to justify their actions based on systematically considering competing obligations and the rights of the parties involved (Gelman and Reamer, 1992: 348). Discussion and obtaining permission through written informed consent assure respect for the client without breaching confidentiality. Discussion regarding the limits of confidentiality at the outset of the relationship as well as disclosure requirements will provide the opportunity to acknowledge professional obligations and the limits of the relationship. The Canadian social work *Code of Ethics*, section 5.22, directs social workers to explain to clients the information disclosure requirements of the law or of the agency before the provision of services.

Responsible actions would include thorough assessments and initial social histories, including a sexual history of the client's activities and extent of contacts, confirmation of the diagnosis, the client's behaviour and impulsive tendencies, and the extent of drug and alcohol use. Ongoing assessment regarding level of risk, behaviour, and attitudes towards the protection of others is essential. Consideration of any applicable laws in the area, reference to professional codes of ethics, and any policies and procedures established by the employing agency or service indicate responsible actions that take account of both obligation and consequences. Consultation and guidance from other professionals, including supervisors and lawyers, provide evidence of professional consensus in the determination of risk of threat of imminent danger and about the action taken. Following such procedures, however, does not ensure that a worker will be comfortable or at ease with a decision or the resultant actions, but she or he must be prepared to live with the decision (Gelman and Reamer, 1992: 349). In some cases, it may mean referral to others who may be more experienced in the field or perhaps more familiar with similar ethical dilemmas. In the process of working through these difficult issues with clients, it is important to keep thorough case notes, including assessments, any actions taken, discussions with clients, and consultation or referrals to others.

What are the implications for social workers in light of opposing views regarding the obligation to protect client confidentiality and society? Unequivocally, social workers have a responsibility to assist in the control of the spread of HIV (OAPSW, 1989: 6). Yet, judgements about the limits of confidentiality in AIDS-related cases are among the most difficult social workers are called on to make (Reamer, 1991: 59). Kitchener presents four principles as a foundation for ethical reasoning in facing such issues in counselling: autonomy or respect for the rights of others to make free choices; non-malfeasance or 'do no harm'; beneficence or engaging in actions that benefit others; and finally, justice or fairness (Reamer, 1993: 416).

Social workers need to base their actions on an ethical analysis of competing values, reasoned clinical judgements based on an awareness of the ethical and professional responsibilities, current laws and statutes with least intrusion of privacy and respecting obligations to confidentiality (Gelman and Reamer, 1992: 353). Although there is agreement in regard to the maintenance of confidentiality and the need to protect third parties, disagreement remains in interpretation of legal, moral, and professional obligations. Social work has a limited responsibility to report, but ethically must report. This is where the difficulty is presented for social workers. How one interprets will determine actions. Social workers need to be aware of the impact of their own attitudes, biases, and prejudices as they may relate to individuals with HIV or those at risk of contracting HIV (Lamb et al., 1989: 41).

Discussions surrounding the issues of breach of confidentiality may be limited to only a small minority of individuals (Ontario Advisory Committee on HIV/AIDS, 1995: 3). However, this does not minimize the extent of the difficulty of the ethical issues and decisions to be made when faced with this client in practice. Decisions made in practice significantly reflect on the profession—balancing moral obligations, values, and beliefs (Reamer, 1991: 59). Clients are protected by confidentiality throughout the medical and social services network, and social workers will not always be informed of clients who are HIV-positive or diagnosed with AIDS. However, in the event that a social worker is given information from a client about the presence of HIV and has reasonable grounds to believe that the client is engaged in activities that may be putting others at risk, the social worker is ethically bound to report this information to the local medical officer of health (OAPSW, 1989: 6). As discussed, it is not without significant efforts to work with the client in a supportive role, providing education, guidance, and direction to facilitate disclosure, that decisions to breach confidentiality are made.

At the agency or service level, social workers can advocate for and influence the development of policies and procedures to be followed when facing dilemmas. Any policy or plan of service must seek to protect third parties without sacrificing the needs and rights of the client (Kagle and Kopels, 1994: 218). Social work is in a position to provide access to resources and to advocate for clients to prevent the consequences that cause clients to feel discriminated against, harassed, or denied service.

At the professional level, although the *Code of Ethics* is recognized as providing guidelines, there is a need for it to reflect more specifically the professional responsibility in the discrepancy between protecting individuals and protecting society. The *Code of Ethics* needs to enunciate clearly the principle regarding protection of potential victims and reasonable care (Weil and Sanchez, 1983: 123). There is an opportunity to influence such changes through debate and open discussions and through professional associations, and, further, to encourage the development of standards for practice that equally protect potential victims and clients.

CONCLUSION

Social work has a long-standing tradition of simultaneous concern with individual well-being and social justice. The HIV crisis provides the profession with a compelling challenge to muster its collective resources to address the ethical and civil liberties issues triggered by this devastating disease (Reamer, 1993: 417). At the legal level, social workers may work towards supporting development of policies, changes in laws, and new legislation that provide a basis for protecting the public and professionals' provision of responsible service.

The tension between society and the individual as reflected in the *Tarasoff* decision is an area of professional ethics to be more carefully studied (Weil and Sanchez, 1983: 123). No solution, of course, will protect the interests of all parties. Social workers face ethical dilemmas confused by the obligations to protect both the confidentiality of the individual and third parties potentially at risk. In the surveys cited, the *Tarasoff* case influenced the decision of the majority of respondents and the decision that many anticipated they would make to protect others. As indicated, professional ethics were stated to be the strongest influence guiding social workers' decisions. This is further supported by Huey (1988), who suggested that interpretation is a function of the counsellor's personal values, beliefs, and attitudes (cited in Gross and Robinson, 1987: 340).

Based on the values of the profession, social work is now challenged to deal with and influence society's response in the face of the reality of HIV and professional practice (Reamer, 1993: 417).

REFERENCES

Abramson, M. 1990. 'Keeping Secrets: Social Workers and AIDS', *Social Work* (Mar.): 169–73.

Canadian Association of Social Workers (CASW). 1994. *Social Work Code of Ethics.* Ottawa: CASW.

Clarke, R. 1995. *Social Work Practice and Practice Wisdom in the Field of HIV/AIDS.* Ottawa: CASW.

Costa, L., and M. Altekruse. 1994. 'Duty-to-warn Guidelines for Mental Health Counsellors', *Journal of Counselling and Development* 72 (Mar.-Apr.): 346–50.

Coughlan, S.G. 1995. 'Patients' Secrets and Threats to Third Parties: Where To Draw the Line', *Health Law in Canada* 15, 4: 91–6.

Fulero, S.M. 1988. '*Tarasoff*: 10 Years Later', *Professional Psychology: Research and Practice* 19, 2: 184–90.

Gelman, S.R., and F.G. Reamer. 1992. 'Is *Tarasoff* Relevant to AIDS-related Cases?', in E. Gambrill and R. Pruger, eds, *Controversial Issues in Social Work.* Toronto: Allyn & Bacon.

Gray, E.A., and A.K. Harding. 1988. 'Confidentiality Limits with Clients Who Have the AIDS Virus', *Journal of Counseling and Development* 66: 219–23.

Gross, D.R., and S.E. Robinson. 1987. 'Ethics, Violence, and Counseling: Hear No Evil, See No Evil, Speak No Evil?', *Journal of Counseling and Development* (Mar.): 340–4.

Hanna, L. 1995–6. 'Continuing Education: The Devastating Consequences of HIV Disease', *Connections* (Faculty of Social Work, Wilfrid Laurier University) (Winter): 1.

Kagle, J.D., and S. Kopels. 1994. 'Confidentiality after *Tarasoff*', *Health and Social Work* 19, 3: 127–222.

Kitchener, K.S. 1986. 'Teaching Applied Ethics in Counselor Education: An Integration of Psychological Processes and Philosophical Analysis', *Journal of Counseling and Development* 64: 306–10.

Kopels, S., and J.D. Kagle. 1993. 'Do Social Workers Have a Duty To Warn?', *Social Service Review* (Mar.): 101–19.

Lamb, D.H., C. Clark, P. Drumheller, K. Frizzell, and L. Surrey. 1989. 'Applying *Tarasoff* to AIDS-related Psychotherapy Issues', *Professional Psychology: Research and Practice* 20, 1: 37–43.

Mann, J.M. 1992. 'AIDS—The Second Decade: A Global Perspective', *Journal of Infectious Diseases* 165: 245–50.

Manuel, C., P. Enel, J. Charrel, D. Reviron, M.P. Larher, P. Auquier, and J.L. San Marco. 1991. 'Ethics and AIDS: The Protection of Society versus the Protection of Individual Rights', *AIDS and Public Policy Journal* 6, 1: 31–6.

Mappes, D.C., G.P. Robb, and D.W. Engels. 1985. 'Conflicts between Ethics and Law in Counseling and Psychotherapy', *Journal of Counseling and Development* 64: 246–52.

Ontario Advisory Committee on HIV/AIDS. 1995. *Reducing HIV Transmission by People Who Are Unwilling or Unable To Take Appropriate Precautions*. Toronto: OACHA.

Ontario Association of Professional Social Workers (OAPSW). 1989. 'OAPSW Statement on HIV/AIDS: A Social Work Perspective'. Toronto: OAPSW.

Reamer, F.G. 1988. 'AIDS and Ethics: The Agenda for Social Workers', *Social Work* 33 (Sept.-Oct.): 460–4.

———. 1991. 'AIDS, Social Work, and the "Duty to Protect"', *Social Work* 36, 1: 56–60.

———. 1993. 'AIDS and Social Work: The Ethics and Civil Liberties Agenda', *Social Work* 38, 4: 412–19.

Schrier, C.J. 1980. 'Guidelines for Record-keeping under Privacy and Open-Access Laws', *Social Work* 25 (Nov.): 452–7.

Taylor, S., K. Brownlee, and K. Mauro-Hopkins. 1996. 'Confidentiality versus the Duty To Protect: An Ethical Dilemma with HIV/AIDS Clients', *The Social Worker* 64, 4: 9–17.

Weil, M., and E. Sanchez. 1983. 'The Impact of the *Tarasoff* Decision on Clinical Social Work Practice', *Social Service Review* (Mar.): 112–24.

Chapter 15

Hemophilia, Blood Transfusion, and Social Work Practice

JACK MCDONALD

BACKGROUND

Sometimes ordinary developments in the history of a profession's involvements in chronic illness care systems become of more than ordinary importance to the population involved and to other populations victimized by unforeseen sets of circumstances. This chapter is written in the form of a case study. While the content is a description of persons and populations served, the intent is to present a case example demonstrative of the social work activities of a practitioner over a 15-year period. What began as a part-time social work role with a chronic condition, as a result of the HIV/AIDS epidemic, became a practice frontier in a rapidly evolving epidemic. The activities and experiences recorded herein reflect the personal and professional activities of the author.

Comprehensive hemophilia[1] care systems[2] evolved in Canada through the 1970s. The introduction of blood product concentrates and home-infusion programs, while groundbreaking advances in hemophilia care, left the hemophiliac population vulnerable to blood-born pathogens. Hemophilia specialists continuously warned of the risks involved. Little did they realize that the most deadly agent would be an unknown virus, the primary mode of transmission for which would be sexual, through mingling of bodily fluids, and secondarily, through transfusions and infusions of contaminated blood or blood products. By July of 1985, through heat treatment of products the blood supply system once again became substantially safe from HIV contamination. By then an estimated 800 Canadians with hemophilia and approximately 275 known blood-transfused persons were HIV-infected (McDonald, Devins, and Poon, 1992).

PERSONAL BEGINNINGS IN THE BLOOD SYSTEM AIDS CRISIS

For this social worker, April 1983 marked beginning awareness of human immunodeficiency virus (HIV) contamination of products used in the Canadian blood supply system. At the annual meetings of the Canadian Hemophilia Society (CHS) held in Toronto, the Medical and Scientific Advisory Committee (MSAC) heard reports from several Canadian hematologists. They had just returned from a Centers for Disease Control meeting in Atlanta, Georgia, and they confirmed that HIV was present in the Canadian blood supply system.

The information left the hemophilia community in a state of shock. This social worker was present at the MSAC and society meetings. What follows may best be stated as a personal narrative.

I remember coming on the plane from Toronto to Calgary. I reflected on my situation. The hemophilia clinic role was a small part of my work. In full-time equivalent terms, it was less than 20 per cent of one FTE. I had an associate professor appointment with the Faculty of Social Work and was the assistant dean for the undergraduate (BSW) program. I had just received a three-year grant to implement a health promotion demonstration project at the Alberta Children's Hospital, a tertiary-care child health centre serving the province of Alberta. I was midway through the application process for admission to an Applied Social Studies doctoral program at the University of Bradford in England. My academic and professional life was full. The extent of the catastrophe was unknown. Over 100 persons were listed with the clinic. The worst-case scenario was that everyone, including partners, could be infected. Should I get out so that someone else could commit the required time from the beginning of the crisis, or should I extend my commitments, let go for the time being of my plan for further study, and stick with the demands that would evolve?

I decided to have a talk with my wife. We had six children, ages 7 to 16. Life at home was also full. As soon as I arrived home we talked. I remember saying that to commit to the crisis could involve a 24-hour approach to professional activities over a number of years. My wife said she would support whatever I chose. She asked what my inclinations were. After some thought I said, 'I think much of my life might be seen as preparation for what is now unfolding.' I was 45 years old. I had had a ten-year career as a priest, eight years as director of a pediatric hospital social work department, experience in strategic planning, clinical practice, a beginning career in research, and years of experience as a self-help resource person for a variety of initiatives, most recently a sudden infant death syndrome chapter and Compassionate Friends (a group for parents whose children had died). I had a strong commitment to self-care and health promotion in chronic illness management. All these experiences seemed to harmonize with key elements of the emerging epidemic. I decided to make the commitment. What follows is a reflection, 15 years later, on the outcomes of that commitment.

The Early Years

Following the April 1983 meeting, events moved rapidly and slowly in paradoxical oscillations characteristic of catastrophic events. The hemophilia community, with its existing care system, took immediate steps in education and spread prevention. In those early months and years, a series of issues confronted persons with hemophilia and their clinic teams. For the social worker several issues in counselling and support existed. They were issues for which there were few established answers, but for which answers were essential.

The months from April 1983 to May 1986, while filled with activity, discussion, and attention to implementation of carefully discussed protocols at the clinic level, might also be described as the denial years. We went about our work. We urged caution in spread prevention. But the full impact of the illness trajectory of HIV disease was slow to emerge, and we slowly came to grips with it. During the early years, I served as chair of the social work committee of the Canadian Hemophilia Society and continued as a member of the MSAC. I moved from these roles to CHS AIDS Task Force membership, later served on the CHS National Program Committee, and served two terms as a member at large on the CHS Board of Directors.

Approximately 54 per cent of the known hemophilia population in Canada were HIV-positive.[3] Fortunately, percentages in Calgary were small—about 15 per cent—or 15 persons—were infected. This number would increase to about 30 persons when the blood-transfused group was added. These people constituted my client HIV/AIDS caseload.

In the early years, no test of viral presence was available. After careful discussion, our clinic recommendations were that all persons who had received blood products must consider themselves HIV-positive. Consequently, it was essential that spread prevention precautions be taken. Many persons with hemophilia were married with families or planning to have families. Many were young single men who were sexually interested and active. Many were in or coming into adolescence. Shock, denial, and experience-based conviction may have influenced the intensity of these behavioural prescriptions. In instances where sexual transmission did take place, the intensity of insistence by professionals on safe and safer sex precautions and the compliance of the community were agonizingly re-examined. Many would raise questions about counselling practices followed and decisions taken (Parsons, 1995; Picard, 1995).[4]

Activation of local, regional, and national hemophilia communities progressed slowly and unevenly. Attempts to meet serious illness and the death-related needs of the first waves of infected and affected persons began. Individuals and families coped as best they could and professionals began to acquire practice-based knowledge and experience of HIV and AIDS. The Social Work Committee met as part of the 1986 CHS annual meeting. Social workers pooled their experiences from across the country. Annual consultations became a method of sharing information and provided mutual support to professionals stressed by new, traumatizing experiences. The 1986 meeting saw publication of a first national newsletter for social workers. It was continued as an annually published *Psychosocial Bulletin*. From 1990 to 1992 this writer authored an *AIDS and Hemophilia Bulletin* (French and English editions) as an official publication of the Canadian Hemophilia Society.

The 1986 annual meeting of the CHS featured the organization's first officially scheduled public activity that addressed HIV issues. An expert panel discussed the impact of the epidemic on the community and its professionals.

Client participants from the audience described their experiences, their grief, and their pain. The denial had ended! The annual meeting was also marked by a significant change in representation on the Board of Directors. The CHS was now structurally poised to begin, in earnest, a national approach to the catastrophe that had brought a terminal illness to the lives of so many of its members.

That summer, working collaboratively with the Calgary region of the Society, I applied for and, in January 1987, received funding for the first federally funded project for education and support in the hemophilia community (McDonald and Dowdle, 1989). The CHS Board of Directors created a Strategic Planning Task Force that met in Ottawa in the spring of 1987 (Parsons, 1995). This small task force charted the course of CHS focus on HIV and set priorities for action in the years ahead. Several areas were targeted: (1) a campaign for catastrophe relief from the federal government; (2) creation of a national office infrastructure to address issues in HIV/AIDS; (3) efforts at activating support and education at the local, regional, and chapter levels; and (4) beginning actions to support front-line professionals in dealing with terminal AIDS illnesses in the Canadian hemophilia population.

As stated, I was involved in several activities. Besides the editing and publishing endeavours, I was principal investigator for the Support and Education Project of the Calgary region (McDonald and Dowdle, 1989); served as a member of the Strategic Planning Task Force; continued as a member of the MSAC; and continued clinical practice roles with the Southern Alberta Hemophilia Clinic. A second follow-up Support and Education Program was funded in 1988 by the province of Alberta (McDonald and Heath, 1989). Each of these support and education programs provided group education through public information meetings and Society-sponsored retreats/workshops. In addition to these local efforts, I provided consultative and workshop facilitative services to the Ontario chapter and its Toronto and Sudbury regions. Nationally, 'Dialogue Days for Hemophilia Professionals', two conferences in central and western Canada sponsored by the federal government, served as the first national efforts at strengthening front-line clinic services (McDonald and Dowdle, 1987). These conferences may well have served as prototypes for two national 'Caring Together' conferences that later served the total HIV/AIDS community.

SOCIAL WORK ROLE EXPRESSIONS

To this point social work practice involved a number of roles described by Mary Romano (Brown, Kirlin, and Watt, 1981, as adapted in McDonald, 1984). The roles and functions listed in Table 1 are further exemplified in the remainder of this chapter.

The roles took place in an existing regional/local clinic structure and within the framework of a national consumer organization, the Canadian Hemophilia Society. Role expression activities on behalf of blood-transfused persons began with no previously existing structures.

Table 1 Social Work Roles

Clinical Roles

1. psychosocial data gatherer
2. psychotherapeutic treatments (individuals, families, groups)
3. consultation
4. conferencing
5. co-ordinating
6. enabler/facilitator
7. educator
8. advocate

Administrative Roles

1. program administration
2. administrative accountability (quality assurance)
3. applied social work research
4. policy development and implementation

Community Development and Action Roles

1. consumer empowerment
2. community development and social action
3. community planning and implementation

ADVOCACY AND SERVICE ON BEHALF OF HIV-POSITIVE BLOOD-TRANSFUSED PERSONS

In March 1988, I was asked to initiate services for persons infected following blood transfusion. An article in *The Social Worker* (McDonald, 1996) provides a description of those activities. A summary of that involvement follows.

Persons transfused with HIV-contaminated blood experienced realities dramatically different from most persons in the hemophilia community. Identification of transfusion-infected persons prior to 1989 was anecdotal. The first Calgary cases were reported in 1986. AIDS case enumeration from provincial and federal reporting sources documented only AIDS cases and carried undifferentiated blood system categories. From one end of the country to the other, persons with transfusion-derived HIV had no organized support, information, or education service. Months and years dragged by, marked by medical and governmental inaction that can accurately be described as a conspiracy of silence. Fear of lawsuits caused many Canadian physicians and institutional officials to hide behind barriers of silence and recording systems often declared to be flawed and inadequate. It would be several years (1993) before the federal government created the Krever Inquiry to investigate the reasons for failures in the Canadian blood supply system, and an additional four years (1997) before recommendations could be made for blood supply system reform.

BEGINNINGS—ADVOCACY, SUPPORT, AND EDUCATION

Two Calgary physicians, John Gill and Deirdre Church,[5] facilitated the beginning of support, education, and advocacy for Canadian HIV blood transfusion-infected persons. Dr Gill, director of the Southern Alberta HIV Clinic, was aware of my own efforts on behalf of the hemophilia community. He telephoned asking for action to meet the needs of persons in the transfusion-infected population. He described the population as isolated, confused, and alienated. He and Dr Church agreed to forward a letter to their transfusion-infected patients. The letter acknowledged the crisis and offered the opportunity to attend a meeting where the wish for confidentiality would be respected. If participants so desired, they would have a chance to create a self-help group for HIV-positive blood-transfused persons.

On 7 May 1988, seven persons attended the inaugural meeting at the Alberta Children's Hospital; five were transfusion-infected and two were spouses. The group agreed to continue meeting and requested that the social worker serve as a professional resource to the newly created group. Since 1988, the group has met an average of 8–10 times per year. Attendance ranges from 6 to 12 persons per meeting. In total, 23 individuals have attended meetings; 15 were HIV-infected and of these, 7 are now deceased. Over the years, meeting locations changed from the hospital, to a member couple's home, to the social worker's home. The professional resource role came to involve most of the functions described above, most particularly group facilitator, advocacy representative, individual clinical practitioner, and applied researcher.

In November 1988, a group-edited letter was sent to the federal Minister of Health and Welfare. Participants were aware of discussions between the government and the CHS concerning catastrophe relief for blood product-infected persons. Through the letter, the minister was apprised of the group's existence. Members requested inclusion in any award that the federal government might make. In January 1989 a letter from the minister stated that the request would be carefully considered (McDonald, Devins, and Poon, 1992). The minister's letter was followed up by a call from the Health and Welfare representative (Greg Smith) charged with catastrophe relief negotiations. He asked to meet with the group, and in April 1989 he came to Calgary for a meeting in the home of a member couple. He assured the group of the minister's concern and interest. Members spoke positively of their support group experiences and expressed concern for the needs of transfusion-infected persons in other parts of the country. In addition to discussion concerning catastrophe relief, they requested financial assistance to determine the extent of transfusion-derived HIV infection in Canada (a population identification study) and to assess needs specific to the population. The group was encouraged to apply for funding. A $15,000 grant application was developed and forwarded to the National Health Research and Development Program (NHRDP). The project was funded immediately.

As national population identification research and blood-transfused community development work progressed, the group continued to meet. It provided mutual support and served as an island of acceptance. In the words of a 70-year-old woman who joined the group in 1988: 'You'll never know, after two years of terrifying isolation, how nice it was to come to a meeting, to be with people suffering the same problems, and to talk about being HIV-positive.'

POPULATION IDENTIFICATION AND COMMUNITY DEVELOPMENT EFFORTS: CHALLENGES AND SUCCESSES

Attempts to enumerate the Canadian HIV-infected, blood-transfused population met with nearly insurmountable barriers. The most formidable obstacles involved health-care institutions, medical personnel, and the confidentiality-based fears of infected persons. Infected persons feared the social stigma that might accompany public knowledge of their HIV status. Self-help group members demanded confidentiality. Hospitals, physicians, physician organizations, and blood agencies saw few benefits in co-operating with a population identification process. The spectre of lawsuits was ever present, and there was little interest in identifying the populations or in offering support to those infected.

A multifaceted approach was taken. An information package was designed, which included the opportunity for infected persons to register with a confidential support and information service administered through a Calgary law office. Letters containing the information packages were sent to hematology departments, HIV/AIDS clinics, and community organizations throughout the country. Physicians and AIDS service workers were requested to forward the package to any person known to be HIV-positive secondary to blood transfusion. Personal telephone contacts were made with many service providers, particularly physicians. While verbal support was frequent, instances of enthusiastic co-operation were rare. Initial efforts yielded meagre results. By February 1990, 15 persons had registered with the embryonic support and information service.

Parallel to population identification efforts, work began on the establishment of support and education services. In October 1989 and January 1990, approaches were made to the Canadian Red Cross and the Canadian AIDS Society (CAS). Requests were made for assistance in sponsoring a national support and education service. The Red Cross, replying to a written request, stated by mail that it was giving the matter serious consideration (McDonald, Devins, and Poon, 1992). No further response was forthcoming. A conversation with the executive director of the CAS revealed that they had no interest in sponsorship. In November 1989 the Canadian government had announced a Catastrophe Relief Program[6] for blood-system infected persons. The CAS representative was simply not interested in helping a group of people who were now eligible for major financial relief. The needs of the gay community were viewed as too great for the CAS to assume a leadership role on behalf of this population, in spite of its official name. It is interesting that with the emergence of the Krever Inquiry, the CAS requested and obtained official standing.

The co-operation of the Canadian Hemophilia Society opened the way to a national program. The Calgary group, communicating through this social worker, made use of personal communications and a letter to request CHS sponsorship for a national support, education, and advocacy service. The executive director of the CHS, Robert Shearer, took the matter to the annual meeting of the CHS board in May 1990. The board gave approval to the request with a proviso that the program not be a financial burden. The federal government's AIDS Community Action Program indicated interest in funding the service. In June, the CHS executive director and the group social worker met in Calgary, at which time we developed a proposal and presented it to a meeting of the self-help group. The group unanimously endorsed the proposal and agreed to provide representatives to a Project Advisory Committee. By the end October, the $150,000 proposal was approved, and by December a project co-ordinator, Robert St Pierre, was working on behalf of the national needs of the blood-transfused and -infected community. A National Support and Education Service for persons HIV-infected secondary to blood transfusion was now in existence.

PRACTICE REFLECTIONS

Social work intervention and group self-help practice principles underpinned the achievement of each of these objectives. My own conviction about the appropriateness of actions taken and the extent of the need and the strategic contacts I had with key individuals were essential in the successes achieved. When a door closed, it was important not to waste time or energy on reasons for refusal. Always, the needs of the group and those who continued to suffer in isolation were the impetus to unrelenting effort at achieving agreed-to ends. The Calgary group, through its quiet yet effective efforts, had to this point gained inclusion in a National Catastrophe Relief Program, obtained funding for a National Population Identification Study, and created a National Support and Education Service.

SUPPORT SERVICE MEMBERSHIP RECRUITMENT

The creation of the National HIV-T Service set the stage for important co-operative action on behalf of the population. The efforts of the same Health and Welfare employee, Greg Smith, removed the barriers. The Federal Catastrophe Relief Program had information on all persons applying under the blood transfusion category. Through the National HIV-T Service, Health and Welfare was asked to forward an information package to transfusion-infected persons. The department agreed to do so. The package informed recipients of the HIV-T Service, listed a 1–800 number, offered opportunity to register, and requested completion of a brief needs-assessment questionnaire. Within days of the mailing, registrations began to arrive. By the end of the project's pilot phase (1993), registrations had reached 150.

By March 1991, through the efforts of the program co-ordinator, Robert St Pierre, self-help groups were operative in Montreal, Toronto, and Vancouver. In addition to face-to-face meetings, self-help group sessions within the BC group used a telephone conference mode. In May 1991, transfusion-infected persons held their first formal national meeting at the Vancouver site of the Canadian AIDS Conference. The remainder of HIV-T Service history is a story in its own right. The project evaluation (McDonald, 1993) describes its pilot phase.

POPULATION IDENTIFICATION

How large was the HIV transfusion-infected population in Canada? An additional request was made to Health and Welfare Canada to analyse a data file created from blood-infected applicants for catastrophe relief. The file contained no personal identifiers; 261 persons were identified through this method, of whom 126 were still living. Based on analysis of these data, a population identification study report (McDonald, Devins, and Poon, 1992) was released in November 1992. The following morning the *Calgary Herald* carried a front-page headline, 'Red Cross blasted on AIDS' (Walker, 1992). The reporter had contacted me in August requesting a copy of the report as soon as it was completed. The report's release and Walker's front-page article served as a spark that ignited media attention across the country. Hemophilia and blood transfusion groups in Montreal and Toronto fanned the emerging flame, and within days a special subcommittee of the Canadian Parliament began hearings into Canada's HIV blood scandal. An outcome of the hearings was the creation of the Krever Inquiry into the Safety of the Canadian Blood Supply System. Members of the HIV-T community were visible and active in many aspects of the Inquiry, with the Canadian Hemophilia Society and the Ontario HIV-T Group eventually having official standing.

In June 1993, as a representative of local blood-transfused persons and as part of national lobby efforts, I joined the Hemophilia Society for a meeting with the Alberta deputy minister of health. Provincial governments had unanimously rejected requests for compensation. A few weeks before, responding to lobbying by Janet and Randy Connors, the government of Nova Scotia broke ranks and announced that it would offer compensation. The Alberta meeting took place a few days before a provincial election. Within a week of the Edmonton meeting, the Alberta government followed suit and all other provinces soon fell into line.[7]

GROUP FUNCTIONING

Meetings of the Calgary Self-Help Group are characterized by a relaxed and informal structure. Participants discuss issues of mutual interest, such as HIV/AIDS problems and stresses, medical and community care systems, healthy living, medication regimes, and advocacy topics. A number of supportive friendships have evolved. The deaths of seven persons (two women and five men) were experienced with participation in ritual observances. The dreaded progressive illnesses and deaths serve as concrete expressions of the toll taken by the disease and how survivors grieve, move on, and remember. Continuance in the group by bereaved partners is helpful to the healing needs of participants. In several instances, uninfected spouses have continued group contact for several years following the death of a partner. The loss of male members has left the group with a preponderance of women, several of whom were unknowingly infected before discovery of their partner's HIV-positive status. A tradition since 1988 is a potluck dinner held in the Christmas season. It serves as a family gathering event. A June barbecue concludes group meetings until September. Occasionally, members reflect on their history together. Sometimes this takes place during introductions of a new member. It becomes a means through which traditions are passed. Recent additions to the group of persons whose infection source is from other at-risk groups has served to unite HIV-T persons with the broader HIV community. Annual national retreat weekends have taken place since 1995. Participants come together, reflect on their history, discuss recent developments, celebrate their continuing survival, and remember the deceased.

REFLECTIONS ON A 15-YEAR EXPERIENCE: THE SPECIALIZED GENERALIST

A principle that guided me through the crises encountered in the epidemic was the importance of understanding and responding to the emerging needs of persons infected, persons affected, and those providing services. For several years prior to the emergence of the epidemic—in social work hospital department administration, personal clinical practice, undergraduate and graduate teaching—I emphasized the concept of the specialized generalist. Within the practice domain of a chronic illness, especially where social work resources are limited to a single practitioner, there must be commitment to delivery of generic social work services. In-depth expertise in specialty areas can be developed as a combination of practitioner interest, talent, and the requirements of the condition, but ability to provide a full range of generic services is critical to the role.

REVISING PERSONAL AND PROFESSIONAL PRACTICE BOUNDARIES

An additional realization gradually emerged through the years of the HIV/AIDS experience. It can now be articulated. The specialized generalist role in HIV/AIDS goes beyond the usual boundaries of generalist roles as experienced in traditional health and illness settings. In these respects, social work practice in HIV/AIDS may well be a model for emerging patterns of practice. Workers now ought to be prepared to embrace equality-based partnerships, stakeholder/employee alliances, and shared governance roles that in their beginnings are often not well articulated. Commitment to collaborative activity derived from client group needs is essential. Practitioners must be prepared to re-examine their personal and professional boundaries in relation to their work world. These changes in practice expression are of growing importance to transformed, reformed, and community-based health and illness care systems. In these models, the practitioner can no longer be considered as aloof and segregated from the population. The practitioner is an integral part of the (care) community, as totally personally involved as those who bear the burden of the condition, those affected, and, indeed, the total community.

PROFESSIONAL TURF ISSUES

Professional turf protection and professional territorial imperialism are negative elements in a multidisciplined, multisectored, humanly diverse HIV/AIDS world.

They are detrimental to the crisis-based needs of populations served and to the professions that struggle to adjust in role-revising and -testing times. In the crisis of an epidemic such as that of HIV/AIDS, it was important to work with positive, synergistic, and affirming elements. It was important not to waste time or effort on pockets of resistance. Always, of primary concern were the needs of those infected and affected. Experience soon taught that those, especially professionals, who were weighed down by fear, denial, and a need to protect status—economic status, social status, professional status, and institutional status—were best avoided. Many, however, functioned from motivations and principles that transcended these concerns. It was these persons who were the best collaborators.

RESEARCH, PROFESSIONAL DEVELOPMENT, AND MUTUAL LEARNING

The scope of the AIDS epidemic and events in the tragedy of contamination of the blood supply system unfolded slowly. Events occurred at a time when the value of qualitative research methodologies was emerging and when participatory action research was in its formative stages. It was a time when sensitivity to feminist and various sexual-orientation constructs was becoming societally acceptable. The importance attached to qualitative, lived experiences related to the epidemic have influenced research activity through the years. In addition, staff development activities were, for the most part, combinations of lived experiences, consultative sharing, and learning with the client population. Partnered approaches to chronic and acute illness care are now standard fare in community-based health care.

THE NEEDS OF CLIENTS AND FAMILIES

Social work with clients and families was the bedrock of efforts related to the epidemic. Existing worker-client relationships, established over several years of clinical practice, became the foundation from which provision of services to the hemophilia community developed. The client community was already in existence; working relationships were in place. Social work practice with the population expanded to include a major focus on HIV/AIDS.

Many persons from the blood-transfused community had no permanently established connections to the health system. While some had chronic illness conditions, many, perhaps most, received blood transfusions as part of a transitory illness or an episodic medical intervention. Many had never had previous contact with social workers and often had had only limited contact with health professionals. Such characteristics are common in present-day health and illness management. For the most part, the population requires supportive, expert assistance. Traditional psychotherapeutic interventions, while continuing to be needed, are often secondary to the self-care and personal responsibility paradigm of the affected communities. This is a marked feature of emerging health- and illness-care regimes. Social workers would do well to reflect on these realities and their future implications.

'THE WORRIED WELL'

In the years that preceded the epidemic I had established, through the annual assessment and review process of the comprehensive care clinic, a condition-focused working relationship with each person with hemophilia and with his nuclear family. This familiarity meant that precious time was not required to establish working relationships.

However, it should be cautioned that such relationships can be, and in some instances perhaps were, detrimental to work that was sorely needed immediately upon awareness of the seriousness and extent of the catastrophe. In some parts of Canada, denial on the part of professionals and a desire not to upset clients and families with gloom and doom are claimed by some to have led to needless infection spread, both from the type of blood products used and by failure to sufficiently warn infected or potentially infected persons of transmission risks.

An unforgettable lesson from those early experiences was the importance of professional activity that was both aware of the crisis and capable of carrying out, clearly and decisively, professional responsibilities that emerged. One could not be overly swayed either by feelings of client protectionism or by fears of possible legal consequences. As one of the only non-hands-on professionals involved, the social worker had to recognize that his/her responsibilities were unequivocal. It was a time for intense commitment to the emerging needs of clients and families.

In the beginning no tests for viral presence existed. Once they did exist, during the first three or four years of the epidemic, no curative or ameliorative treatments were available, and the stigma attached to being known as infected left many persons with little interest in establishing their HIV status (and in many instances they were so advised). Such decisions were complex, technical, and required ongoing supportive counselling, particularly where concerns existed as to potential sexual transmission.

What was previously almost exclusively individual counselling for men with hemophilia, focused on living with a chronic condition, became couples counselling related to life and death realities. Some clients, families, and professionals made this transition well. For others, the transition was filled with emotional crisis, pain, and suffering. Substantial safety in the blood system was not achieved until mid-1985. Worry about continuing infections from the blood system and from sexual transmission was constant in the early years, as was concern about the ultimate effectiveness of what was being done.

Clinical role expressions ranged from education through support to psychotherapeutic interventions. The expression of these interventions could (and often did) take place in individual, couple, or group formats. While the above may seem straightforward by hindsight, each step, each decision-making direction, took place in the vortex of a condition whose nature and course were only slowly unfolding. Correlative with and often evolving from every client and family intervention step was a parallel experience in professional development. This worker carries lifelong regrets for not insisting strenuously enough on a couple's use of safer sexual precautions. Once again, hindsight gives wisdom, but not without immense costs in personal friendship and professional expression.

THE INFECTED POPULATION

At the same time as activities related to 'the worried well' dominated clinical practice, and often even before any confirmations of HIV status were made, people were manifesting illnesses and secondary infections. Individuals and families were living the personalized course of HIV disease. People were dying. Families and the hemophilia community were reeling under the effects of anticipatory, current, and subsequent grief. Social work roles and functions in providing services to persons and families experiencing strange debilitating illnesses, dealing with service systems that were uncharacteristically fearful and knowledge-deprived, were continuous and ongoing. For many social workers in hemophilia care, working in palliative care was not a part of their original practice repertoire. Walking with families through the illnesses, death, and observance rituals for infected persons became a common experience and an essential element of hemophilia and HIV practice.

EMERGENCE OF THE HOLISTIC PARADIGM FRONTIERS FOR HEALTH-CARE SOCIAL WORK

In 1988 the First National Conference on AIDS was held in Toronto. The presentations of two speakers profoundly influenced me in the articulation of social work HIV practice modalities in hemophilia and beyond. The first speaker, a sociologist, presented a commentary on the social co-factor causes of AIDS. These included a homophobic, discriminating North American social structure, the criminalization of intravenous drug use, and the commercialization of the blood system. He declared that without these ideological constructs and their resultant social structures, there would not have been an HIV epidemic. Articulation of these social causalities brought a deepening understanding of the essential role of the social work profession, not only in dealing with the consequences of HIV but also in interventions directly associated with causality. These elements of social causality formed the conduits for HIV transmission. This was one macro expression of the holistic paradigm.

The second, a more micro expression of the holistic paradigm, was couched in a presentation made by Jim St James, who at the time was identified as the person who had lived for the longest time with AIDS in Canada. St James described how, in the absence of a medicinally based physiological cure, he was staying alive by paying careful attention to his personal health in the physiological, psychological, social relationship, and spiritual domains. He argued persuasively for health promotion approaches to strengthening each of the remaining domains.

From the words of Jim St James came further conviction of the importance of social work to the HIV/AIDS epidemic and a framework that was to extend social work practice into important areas of self-care, health promotion, and illness prevention in the physiological, psychological, social, spiritual, and environmental domains. Social work in HIV/AIDS was no longer simply focused on problem intervention. Social work roles had now emerged as essential elements of care, treatment, and support.

Conclusions

Reflection on the history related above reveals a variety of professional roles as expressed throughout the nearly 15 years of social work involvement. Clinical counselling and self-help group support roles have characterized psychotherapeutic functions. Expressed roles include community development work, advocacy, research, scholarship, consultation services, program evaluation, and policy advisory activities. Personal and professional rewards may be concluded by inference from the variety of circumstances described. Most remarkable to me is how a beginning initial professional commitment in one area can, through the years, evolve into processes that carry professional expression far beyond the boundaries of initial expectations.

Work with the hemophilia community and the Canadian blood-transfused population carries many important lessons for social work practitioners. When medical (indeed, any) disasters occur, professional commitments demand attention to the needs of persons directly affected. Failure to act can constitute professional negligence. The Krever Inquiry and the Canadian legal system may eventually decide the reality and the extent of the negligence.

At least one outcome from the experience remains to be fulfilled. It is imperative that psychosocial care protocols be evolved as integral, yet independent, parts of the blood supply system's role in coping with disasters. This realization must be extended well beyond the HIV/AIDS and medical tragedy experiences. The importance of psychosocial protocols being in place to guide responses to the effects of medical tragedies is a significant frontier for social work practice in health care. The field awaits broadening of the experiences related in this chapter, broadening that makes addressing psychosocial need in medical catastrophes a regular part of health- and illness-care procedures. Hopefully, history will record that psychosocial protocol development was a key outcome from Canada's most serious blood system catastrophe.

Notes

1. Hemophilia is a sex-linked congenital, hereditary disorder of blood clotting, which to date is incurable. The person with hemophilia does not produce one of the plasma proteins needed to form a clot. The most common variety of hemophilia is called hemophilia A, or classical hemophilia; the protein missing in hemophilia A is called the antihemophilic factor, or AHF, or factor VIII. The next most common variety is called hemophilia B, or Christmas disease; the protein missing is called PTC or factor IX. There are other varieties, but they are rare. The severity of clotting problems differs greatly from severe to mild. Estimates indicate that one in 10,000 of the male population suffers from severe

hemophilia; all races and socio-economic groups are equally affected. In most cases, if adequately treated by infusion of blood products (or recently developed synthetic products), a stable condition can be maintained (Bittner, 1981; *Hemophilia: A Canadian Handbook*, 1976; Jones, 1984).

2. In North America and Europe two developments in hemophilia care emerged during the 1970s. Home-infusion, self-care programs allowed many persons with severe hemophilia to infuse on a prophylactic basis (regular infusions, two to three times per week to maintain near-normal clotting levels). Second, the emergence of 'comprehensive hemophilia care programs' (Agle, 1977; Deitrich, 1977) provided persons with hemophilia with regionally based, multidisciplinary care systems. Core disciplines for comprehensive care include hematology, nursing, social work, physiotherapy, orthopedics, and dentistry.
3. Dr Chris Tsoukas of Montreal had stored blood samples from Canadian hemophilia clinics. Once a test for the presence of the virus was developed, Dr Tsoukas could test these historically stored samples. The above figure was commonly quoted (Tsoukas, 1987). Percentages varied from clinic to clinic. They ranged from the 15 per cent in Calgary to about 80 per cent in some Canadian hemophilia clinics.
4. Anecdotal reports ranged from those who said they received careful and accurate spread-prevention counselling to those who claimed they were told not to change behavioural practices until more information was available. Where sexual transmission took place, personal and professional regrets became lifetime burdens to be resolved by each person in the best way possible.
5. While it might not seem appropriate to name the physicians, readers might wish to know that these were the only two Canadian physicians known to act in a patient-need advocacy manner as a result of this serious medical tragedy. Several years later Dr Susan King, a Toronto physician, led an active search for transfusion victims who had been patients at the Toronto Hospital for Sick Children.
6. The Catastrophe Relief Program provided $30,000 per year for four years to persons accepted as HIV-infected secondary to blood transfusion or the infusion of blood products.
7. HIV-infected victims were awarded $30,000 per year for life, plus an amount for signing, benefits for surviving partners, and funding for education of dependent offspring.

REFERENCES

Agle, D. 1977. 'Home Care—Psychological Benefits and Hazards', *Scandinavian Journal of Haematology* 30: 65–9.

Bittner, E., ed. 1981. *Your Child and Hemophilia: A Manual for Parents*. New York: National Hemophilia Foundation.

Browne, J., B. Kirlin, and S. Watt. 1981. *Rehabilitation Services and the Social Work Role: Challenge for Change*. Baltimore: Williams and Wilkins.

Deitrich, S. 1977. *Comprehensive Care for the Person with Hemophilia*. New York: National Hemophilia Foundation.

Hemophilia: A Canadian Handbook. 1976. Hamilton: Canadian Hemophilia Society.

Jones, P. 1984. *Living with Hemophilia*, 2nd edn. Lancaster: MTP Press.

McDonald, J. 1984. *Social Work and Chronic Health Conditions: An Orientation Manual with Special Reference to Hemophilia*. Calgary: University of Calgary, Faculty of Social Work.

———. 1991. *Visionshift: Social Work with Blind and Visually Impaired Persons*. Toronto: Canadian National Institute for the Blind.

———. 1993. *HIV Positive Blood Transfused Support and Information Service*. Montreal: Canadian Hemophilia Society. Demonstration Project Final Report.

———. 1996. 'From Fearful Isolation to the Krever Inquiry: A Social Work History of Grassroots Self Help and Social Action Initiatives for Blood Tranfused HIV Positive Persons in Canada', *The Social Worker* 64, 4: 122–8.

———, J. Devins, and M. Poon. 1992. *Canadians HIV Positive Secondary to Blood Transfusion*. Calgary: Faculty of Social Work, Health and Welfare Canada, National Health Research and Development Program, Project # 6609–1694–AIDS.

———, and G. Dowdle. 1987. *AIDS, Hemophilia and Psychosocial Issues: Dialogue Days for Canadian Hemophilia Professionals*. Calgary: Canadian Hemophilia Society and Health and Welfare Canada.

———, and ———. 1989. *Hemophilia, HIV and AIDS: Chronic Illness in Crisis*. Calgary: Calgary Region, Canadian Hemophilia Society. Final Report Demonstration Project #6554–2–74.

———, and J. Heath. 1989. *An HIV and AIDS Education and Support Needs Survey: The Alberta Hemophilia Community*. Calgary: Calgary Region, Canadian Hemophilia Society.

Parsons, V. 1995. *Bad Blood: The Tragedy of the Canadian Tainted Blood Scandal*. Toronto: Lester Publishing.

Picard, A. 1995. *The Gift of Death: Confronting Canada's Tainted Blood Tragedy*. Toronto: HarperCollins.

Tsoukas, C. 1987. Unpublished presentation to the Directors of Canadian Hemophilia Programs, annual meeting of the Canadian Hemophilia Society, Toronto.

Walker, R. 1992. 'Red Cross Blasted on AIDS', *Calgary Herald*, 3 Nov., 1.

Chapter 16

Euthanasia, Assisted Suicide, and HIV/AIDS

Ethical, Legal, and Counselling Considerations for Social Workers

CAROL NERON

Over the last decade, significant developments in the treatment and medical management of HIV and AIDS have increased control over disease progression and allowed persons with AIDS to live longer. Yet to date there is no cure for AIDS. Like other terminal illnesses, AIDS is progressive and can build to a slow, painful death that can include recurring symptoms, physical deterioration, and, in many cases, mental deterioration. The nature and progression of symptoms associated with the illness have raised questions related to the quality of life and death for persons with HIV and AIDS. Many have chosen to improve the quality of their death and the dying process through palliative care, pain relief, counselling and support, and, in some cases, euthanasia and assisted suicide (van den Boom, 1995).

Although research on euthanasia, assisted suicide, and HIV/AIDS is still in its infancy, the few studies in this area have confirmed that some persons with HIV/AIDS are considering or choosing euthanasia and assisted suicide as a way to control some of the circumstances surrounding their death. For example, in two recent Canadian studies, persons with HIV/AIDS who are planning out their deaths and those who have assisted in AIDS-related deaths were interviewed (Neron, 1996; Ogden, 1994). In a Scottish study, it was found that 33 per cent of a sample of persons with HIV/AIDS were considering euthanasia or assisted suicide as a choice in the final stages of their illness (Green, 1995). Other studies have addressed the incidence of euthanasia and assisted suicide among persons with AIDS. Ogden (1994) estimated that the rate of assisted deaths among persons with AIDS in the province of British Columbia is between 10 and 20 per cent. Although similar rates were estimated in one study in the Netherlands (de Wachter, 1991), other more recent Dutch studies have found the rate of euthanasia and assisted suicide among persons with HIV/AIDS to be 22 per cent and 25 per cent (Bindels et al., 1996; Laane, 1995).

Historically, social workers and other mental health professionals have perceived a professional obligation to prevent clients from self-harm. When clients consider euthanasia and assisted suicide, social workers are challenged to balance this obligation with the clients' right to self-determination and death with dignity (Werth, 1996; Goldblum and Moulton, 1989). For the most part, little is known about the frequency with which social workers are confronted with euthanasia and assisted suicide. In the lone Canadian study in this area, it was found that nearly 40 per cent of social workers who worked in medical settings had been consulted by clients about these issues (Ogden and Young, 1998). While it is unknown how often social workers who work in the HIV/AIDS area deal with euthanasia and assisted suicide, it is likely that many will inevitably be confronted with these issues. This chapter will focus on the ethical, legal, and counselling issues that social workers must consider when euthanasia and assisted suicide arise in their work with persons with HIV/AIDS.

DEFINITIONS

In this chapter, 'euthanasia' is defined as an act by one person to a second person that results in the alleviation of suffering and ultimately the death of the second person. Active euthanasia is the administration of treatment or an act that induces death, e.g., lethal injection (Ogden, 1994; Smith et al., 1993), whereas passive euthanasia is the withdrawal or withholding of life-sustaining treatment or nourishment (Smith et al., 1993). 'Assisted suicide' occurs when a person intentionally ends his/her own life with the assistance of another person, such as when medication is provided that is used in a suicide.

Euthanasia and assisted suicide are distinguished by the person who is committing the act. For example, if a physician provides medication to a patient aware that the patient will use the medication to end his/her life and the patient uses the medication to commit suicide, the physician has assisted in a suicide. If a physician administers a lethal injection to a patient who has requested to die, then the physician has participated in active euthanasia.

Other terms used in this chapter include 'assisted death' and 'advance health-care directive'. 'Assisted death' is a broad term that can include euthanasia and assisted suicide. An 'advance health-care directive' is a document that specifies the type and duration of treatment an individual desires, and may include a proxy or power of attorney. An advance directive, sometimes referred to as a living will, takes effect when an individual is no longer capable of making these choices, such as in the case of mental incompetency (Singer, 1994).

ETHICAL ISSUES RELATED TO EUTHANASIA AND ASSISTED SUICIDE

Unlike in the United States, where the National Association of Social Workers (NASW) has published a policy statement defining an appropriate level of social work involvement in end-of-life issues, Canadian social workers do not have a policy to which they can refer when faced with these situations. However, other documents and resources provide some direction for Canadian social workers in this area. The Canadian Association of Social Workers (CASW) *Code of Ethics* (1994a) and the *Statement of Principles on Euthanasia and Assisted Suicide* (1994b) outline various ethical principles inherent to social work that must be considered when addressing euthanasia and assisted suicide.

CLIENT SELF-DETERMINATION

Nicholson and Matross have defined self-determination as 'the basic right of all individuals to act in accordance with their own values, goals and personal choices' (1989: 234). Client self-determination is viewed by many as one of the primary ethical principles of social work (see Abramson, 1985; Callahan, 1994; Nicholson and Matross, 1989; Rothman, 1989; Weick and Pope, 1988). Its importance to social work is illustrated in the CASW *Code of Ethics*: 'Social workers believe in the intrinsic worth and dignity of every human being and are committed to the values of acceptance, self-determination and respect of individuality' (1994a: 7). Self-determination has also been highlighted in the *Statement of Principles on Euthanasia and Assisted Suicide* and is the primary principle upon which the NASW's policy statement on end-of-life decisions is based (NASW, 1994).

While the social work literature related to self-determination affirms the right of clients to determine their own choices, limits, such as those imposed by the law, have been identified when harm to others is apparent and when someone is unable to make rational decisions, as in the case of mental incompetency (Abramson, 1985; Abramson, 1989; Berstein, 1960; Callahan, 1994; Foley, 1994; Kapp, 1988; NASW, 1994; Rothman, 1989; Spicker, 1990; Weick and Pope, 1988). Assisted death has been addressed as an exception to self-determination by Callahan (1994), and other authors have implied or identified suicide as an exception (Abramson, 1985; Berstein, 1960; Kapp, 1988; Rothman, 1989; Weick and Pope, 1988). However, when a large sample of social workers were recently questioned about their beliefs in this area, over 70 per cent agreed that the principle of self-determination should extend to assisted death (Ogden and Young, 1998).

Persons living with HIV/AIDS have also addressed the role of self-determination in end-of-life decisions. In recent studies on HIV/AIDS and assisted death, it was clear that self-determination in end-of-life decisions, including when and how to die, was important to many of the persons with HIV/AIDS who were interviewed (Green, 1995; Neron, 1996; Ogden, 1994).

The CASW (1994b) has stated that a balance between self-determination and the interests of the collective is required with regard to end-of-life issues. For example, it is important that the needs of vulnerable persons be acknowledged and protected in any policy or guidelines related to end-of-life issues. Wesley (1996) echoed this idea by recommending that self-determination and another social work value, promoting the general welfare of society, be equally considered in social work policy and practice related to end-of-life issues. For example, she suggests that 'a social worker working towards harmony between self-determination and the welfare of society may help a terminally ill patient decide what constitutes a decent and acceptable quality of life while concomitantly advocating social policies to enhance the quality of life of all suffering and dying people' (1996: 119).

BEST INTEREST

According to the CASW *Code of Ethics*, the principle of maintaining and being guided by the client's best interest is considered the primary professional obligation of social workers. In practice this means 'that the wishes, desires, motivations and plans of the client are taken by the social worker as the primary consideration in any intervention plan developed by the social worker' (CASW, 1994a: 4). Clearly, this principle is significant to end-of-life decisions and has been highlighted as such in the CASW's *Statement of Principles on Euthanasia and Assisted Suicide*.

Many authors have discussed the importance of determining the client's best interest, and some have implied that this responsibility lies with the social worker and not the client (Callahan, 1994). However, by adopting this approach one can risk negating the important contribution clients can make to determining their own best interest. Should not this determination require that both the social worker and the client actively participate in discussion and reflection on this issue? While the social worker contributes his or her professional knowledge and experience, the client can bring an inner knowledge, wisdom, and perspective that reflect his or her own needs and desires. In emphasizing the importance of recognizing and honouring the client's perspective with regard to best interest, Weick and Pope (1988: 14) state, 'In large measure, the uniqueness of individual expression is attributable to the meaning each individual gives to life events. Despite the apparently broad consensus about many social phenomena, it is the individual who, on the last analysis, determines the meaning that an event holds.'

Other issues must be considered when determining the client's best interest, such as situations in which 'the client's plans are documented to be unrealistic, unreasonable or potentially harmful to self' (CASW, 1994a: 4). It is conceivable that under some circumstances, such as in the case of mental incompetency or severe depression, the client's end-of-life choices or plans may be found to be unrealistic and require that the social worker intervene. When dealing with situations in which the client's plans may be potentially self-harmful, it is important for social workers to consider what constitutes harm. End-of-life choices such as euthanasia and assisted suicide could be interpreted as physically harmful. However, many factors must be considered when assessing harm. Is it more emotionally, spiritually, and physically harmful for someone to end his or her life through an assisted death or to prolong death and suffering? This question cannot be answered without considering individual circumstances.

INFORMED CONSENT

Informed consent is another ethical and legal principle that social workers must consider when dealing with euthanasia and assisted suicide. The doctrine of informed consent is concerned with an individual's right to be given full information on which to make decisions (Mason and McCall-Smith, 1987). It is considered central to client self-determination (Bisman, 1994; CASW, 1994b). Although this principle originated in health care and medicine, more recently it has been applied to the counselling relationship (Reamer, 1987). For consent to be valid, the client must be able to exercise his or her power of choice without any coercion or undue influence, adequate information must be given to the client, and he or she must be considered mentally competent to make decisions

(Reamer, 1987). Any information related to consent must be communicated on a level the client can understand and in a manner that is culturally sensitive (Ferris et al., 1995; Reamer, 1987).

Social workers have two primary professional responsibilities related to informed consent. First, they must ensure that clients are fully aware of their treatment options and the nature and consequences of these options (Bisman, 1994; Reamer, 1987). With regard to end-of-life decisions, this would include a thorough review and discussion of all end-of-life options as well as potentially related issues and concerns such as pain, depression, and the need for medical treatment. Social workers should approach these discussions with an openness that does not promote any particular end-of-life choice and is free from discrimination related to the client's race, ethnicity, gender, age, sexual orientation, disability, religion, or economic status (CASW, 1994b; NASW, 1994).

The second professional responsibility of social workers is to inform their clients of ways in which information about them can be used (Bisman, 1994; Kirst-Ashman and Hull, 1993; Reamer, 1987). This relates to the issue of confidentiality. Clients have a right to be informed of the limits to confidentiality at the onset of counselling and throughout the counselling relationship. Self-harm is often identified as one of these limits (see Werth, 1996: 90). However, the CASW *Code of Ethics* states that any actions or interventions should be taken only if there is reasonable belief that the client will actually benefit from them, and this would include breaking confidentiality. Issues such as the potential benefits to the client and the client's best interest must be thoroughly examined when social workers consider breaking confidentiality in any circumstances, including those related to euthanasia and assisted suicide.

CURRENT LEGAL SITUATION RELATED TO EUTHANASIA AND ASSISTED SUICIDE

In examining their role in relation to euthanasia and assisted suicide, social workers must consider the legal parameters created by statute and case law pertaining to these issues. Although suicide and attempted suicide were abolished as offences in 1972, counselling, aiding, and abetting a suicide have remained offences under section 241 of the Criminal Code of Canada. In 1992, section 241 was challenged by Sue Rodriguez, a woman suffering from amyotrophic lateral sclerosis, commonly known as Lou Gehrig's disease. She argued that section 241(b) of the Criminal Code prohibits a terminally ill person from committing suicide and violates several sections of the Canadian Charter of Rights and Freedoms. Although Rodriguez's petition was eventually denied by the Supreme Court of Canada (*Rodriguez v. British Columbia*, 1993), this case brought much attention to the issue of assisted death in Canada.

While case law indicates that providing the means to commit suicide (e.g., lethal drugs) is considered aiding and abetting, there is less clarity with regard to other actions, particularly those pertinent to the counselling relationship. Goldblum and Moulton (1989) have suggested that actions such as actively encouraging a client to commit suicide or providing information on how to undertake the act would probably be viewed by the courts as assisting in a suicide. They go on to suggest that providing referrals to organizations that offer this information, such as the Right to Die Society of Canada, the Hemlock Society, and Compassion in Dying, would probably not be deemed aiding and abetting when considered with other actions taken by the counsellor. Yet the act of providing this information has not resulted in assisted suicide charges against the members of these organizations. The CASW has not specifically addressed the appropriateness of providing this information to clients in its statement related to assisted death. However, its American counterpart, the NASW, has suggested it is appropriate for social workers to participate in discussions related to assisted suicide or to attend an assisted suicide, if legally permissible (NASW, 1994).

In the event that an assisted suicide case is brought to court, it must be determined that the health-care professional acted negligently; that is, that the standards of care of the particular profession were not followed (Goldblum and Moulton, 1989; Werth, 1996; Wood et al., 1992). To determine the standard of care for social workers, it is likely that the courts would refer to documents such as the CASW's recent statement related to assisted death and to the *Code of Ethics*. However, as noted in the case of *Matthews and Board of Directors of Physiotherapy* (1986), standards of care need not be written down but also may be values and principles generally accepted within a profession. It was also acknowledged in this ruling that some conduct may be the subject of dispute within a profession.

In the United States, where assisted suicide laws are similar to those in Canada, previous legal decisions have promoted the position that counsellors have a duty to prevent suicide (Wood et al., 1992). However, while this traditional standard of care has been pertinent to cases in which the client's mental competency is in question, these standards have not always been applicable when competency was not an issue (Werth, 1996). It has been suggested that professional standards of care must be adjusted to accommodate situations in which suicidal decisions are made by individuals who are competent and rational (Werth, 1996).

In the absence of a Canadian policy that specifically addresses euthanasia, several sections of the Criminal Code have been used in euthanasia cases, including those pertaining to homicide, prohibiting consent to death (s. 14), prohibiting the acceleration of death (s. 226), and administering a noxious substance (s. 245). With regard to the withdrawal and withholding of life-sustaining treatment, often referred to as passive euthanasia, case law in Canada has affirmed the right of competent adults to refuse and consent to medical treatment (Ogden, 1994; Smith et al., 1993). While there is no statute law upholding these rights, several provinces have implemented or proposed legislation that supports patient autonomy in medical decisions (Senate of Canada, 1995). Medical practices such as the withdrawal and withholding of treatment have become widely accepted in recent years, so much so that they are increasingly being referred to as 'appropriate medical care' (Schafer, 1994: 123).

It is entirely realistic to expect that questions and concerns related to medical decisions such as the withdrawal, withholding, and refusal of treatment will arise when counselling persons with HIV/AIDS. This is an area in which the counselling role has been more clearly defined in the social work literature and for which there appear to be no legal contra-indications. There is consensus that it is appropriate for social workers to encourage discussions related to medical decisions; to provide information related to the refusal and consent of treatment, advance health-care directives, and proxy decision-making; to suggest that clients discuss these issues with family members and their doctor; and, if necessary, to act as liaison between the client, the family, and other members of the health-care team (CASW, 1994b; Keigher, 1994; NASW, 1994; Nicholson and Matross, 1989; Osman and Perlin, 1994).

Although our current Canadian criminal laws clearly state that euthanasia and assisted suicide are serious offences, in reality prosecutions have not been common and in the instances when they have occurred, sentences usually have been lenient. There have been several publicized AIDS-related and non-AIDS-related assisted death cases in which formal charges have not been laid due to factors such as judicial discretion or lack of evidence. While health-care professionals such as physicians and nurses have faced euthanasia and assisted suicide-related charges, and as recently as May 1998 a Toronto physician was found guilty of assisting the suicide of an HIV patient, these cases have been largely related to their responsibilities of administering medication or treatment, duties that are not part of the social worker's role. Essentially, laws related to euthanasia and assisted suicide have been largely untested in relation to the counselling relationship. While legal limits of the counselling role are yet to be determined, a sound knowledge of the current legal situation will assist social workers in determining their role in relation to euthanasia and assisted suicide when working with persons with HIV/AIDS.

Counselling Issues Related to Euthanasia and Assisted Suicide

In addition to ethical and legal issues, social workers must consider several counselling issues when euthanasia and assisted suicide arise in their work with persons with HIV/AIDS. Responding appropriately to a client's expressed desire for euthanasia or assisted suicide requires that the social worker thoroughly address these issues to determine if the desire is rational or connected to needs that could be met in other ways, and which interventions, if any, are necessary. This section outlines these counselling issues, many of which are connected to the ethical principles previously discussed.

Can the Desire for Assisted Death Be Rational?

One of the most important issues for social workers to consider is whether or not the desire for assisted death is rational. In much of the literature, authors contend that self-determined deaths such as euthanasia, assisted suicide, and suicide are never or rarely rational but rather the result of depression or mental incompetency (Callahan, 1994; Siegel, 1986; see also Werth, 1996: 27–31). However, a growing body of literature and research suggests that desires and decisions related to these issues can be rational in some cases (Dunshee, 1994; Kain, 1996; Motto, 1994; Werth, 1994, 1996; Werth and Liddle, 1994; Werth and Cobia, 1995), including studies involving persons with HIV/AIDS (Neron, 1996; Ogden, 1994; van den Boom, 1995). In studies conducted by Werth and Liddle (1994) and Werth (1994), over 80 per cent of the mental health professionals surveyed stated they believed that decisions related to suicide can be rational. In the Werth (1994) study, 20 per cent of the respondents stated they had worked with at least one client whose decisions related to suicide were rational.

It has been suggested that mental health professionals should be involved in determining rational decisions related to assisted death and suicide (Dunshee, 1994; Measure 16, 1994; Motto, 1994; Werth and Cobia, 1995); however, to do this they must have a set of guidelines with which to determine rationality (Werth, 1996). In recent years, guidelines have emerged to determine if decisions related to suicide are rational (see Dunshee, 1994; Motto, 1994; Siegel, 1986; Werth, 1994; Werth and Cobia, 1995). These guidelines, many of which are discussed below, are also relevant to euthanasia and assisted suicide decisions (Werth, 1996). The criteria for rational decisions are that the person must have a hopeless condition such as a terminal illness; make the decision free from depression, mental incompetency, and external coercion; and have considered all treatment options, alternatives, and the impact of the decision on significant others (Werth, 1994; Werth and Cobia, 1995).

DEPRESSION AND OTHER MENTAL HEALTH CONDITIONS

The presence of depression or other mental health conditions has been identified as one of the necessary counselling issues to consider when determining if the desire for assisted death is rational (Dunshee, 1994; Motto, 1994; Siegel, 1986; Werth, 1996). This stems from the concern that such conditions can affect one's ability to make rational decisions. For example, depression can affect cognitive perceptions, reasoning, and insight (Beck, 1972).

The literature on suicide and mental health demonstrates a strong link between suicide and depression and other mental health conditions, such as schizophrenia (Callahan, 1994; Siegel, 1986; Werth, 1996). However, not all individuals who take their own lives or think about it are suffering from depression or another mental health condition (Werth, 1996). For example, in a Canadian study of persons with cancer, approximately 40 per cent of those who expressed a desire for death through suicide or assisted death were not depressed (Chochinov et al., 1995).

Although much of the literature on rational suicide states that depression precludes rational thinking, Conwell and Caine (1991) have suggested that mental health professionals consider the severity of depression when assessing rational decisions. When they face issues such as terminal illness, it is probable that clients will experience depression to some degree. It is useful to consider how severe depression must be before it compromises the ability to make rational decisions (Conwell and Caine, 1991).

Callahan (1994) has suggested that social workers operate from the assumption that any desire for assisted death is irrational and probably a result of factors such as depression, regardless if they believe these acts can be rational or not. This approach, however, ignores evidence that not all persons who express a desire for assisted death are experiencing depression. While it is wise for social workers to explore consistently the possibility of depression or other mental health conditions when clients express a desire for euthanasia or assisted suicide, it is important not to assume these connections. In some cases, social workers may want to consider referring clients to a psychiatric colleague for a formal mental health assessment to obtain additional input.

MENTAL COMPETENCY

Another issue that is relevant to determining rationality, and one that must be considered by social workers when addressing euthanasia and assisted suicide, is that of the client's mental competency (Foley, 1994; Motto, 1994; NASW, 1994; Nicholson and Matross, 1989; Werth, 1996). Competency refers to the ability to understand fully and appreciate the consequences associated with a decision, including the benefits and harm; an understanding of the reasons for the decision, the values underlying the decision, and the process associated with the decision-making; and an ability to communicate the above (NASW, 1994; Nicholson and Matross, 1989; Werth, 1996). It is also important, in regard to competency, to consider if the client's desires and decisions are congruent with personal values and spiritual beliefs or out of character (Motto, 1994; Werth, 1996).

Determining competency in persons with HIV/AIDS can be complicated by the fact that some degree of cognitive impairment related to dementia or opportunistic infections is common (Rogers and Britton, 1994; Werth, 1995). However, it is important not to assume cognitive impairment without the confirmation of neurocognitive testing (Reamer, 1987; Werth, 1995). In the event that the competency of a client is in question and neurological testing is needed, the social worker may need to elicit the aid of a psychiatrist or psychologist who can administer the appropriate tests and help to determine the client's competency.

Nicholson and Matross have suggested that the question of competency may be more likely to arise if the client's end-of-life choice is different from that of family members, significant others, or the mental health professional, as it may be easier to 'question a client's competency than recognize a legitimate conflict of values' (1989: 235). The desire for assisted death is not an automatic sign of incompetency and should be subject to the same guidelines for determining competency as other end-of-life choices. Werth (1996) has suggested that mental health professionals base their assessment of competency on the client's decision-making process rather than on the actual decision.

HOPELESS CONDITION

The presence of a hopeless condition is another issue that social workers and their clients should consider when discussing assisted death and other end-of-life choices. The American organization Compassion in Dying has defined a hopeless condition as one in which a person has a terminal illness and is expected to die 'within a reasonable period of time, usually six months' (Dunshee, 1994: 5). Others have suggested that a condition is hopeless when physical or psychological pain cannot be alleviated, when there is no chance of recovery, and when quality of life has sufficiently deteriorated (Motto, 1994; Neron, 1996; Werth and Cobia, 1995).

This issue is an important one for social workers and their clients to consider since HIV/AIDS can be characterized by periods of health deterioration followed by improvements. These changes may lead to some uncertainty as to when a condition is hopeless or if improvement is possible. Thorough health and treatment information is needed to assess adequately a client's probability of improvement. In addition, social workers can encourage clients to consider and define relevant issues such as pain, quality of life, and suffering, which can also contribute to a clearer understanding of this area.

EXPLORING FACTORS RELATED TO THE DESIRE FOR ASSISTED DEATH

Various factors can contribute to the desire for an assisted death. Two of these potential factors, depression and incompetency, have been discussed. Other factors could include loss of dignity, fear of dependency, fear of physical pain, isolation, inadequate hospice or palliative care, witnessing others die of AIDS, wanting to spare loved ones prolonged grief, loss of control, and coercion from others (Callahan, 1994; Dunshee, 1994; Ferris et al., 1995; Green, 1995; Laane, 1995; Motto, 1994; Neron, 1996; Ogden, 1994; Werth, 1996). It is important that the social worker and client examine these factors to come to an understanding of the client's reasons for considering assisted death and to rule out issues that could be resolved through other means.

For example, social workers can explore with their clients any fears associated with physical pain. Discussion of pain control methods and assurance that most pain can be controlled through medication or other means may alleviate related fears and concerns. However, it is important to consider that concerns may extend beyond controlled pain. In a group of persons with HIV/AIDS who were considering or planning assisted death, many were aware that much pain can be controlled through medication and other means; however, pain that cannot be controlled, the side-effects of pain control methods, and the effect on quality of life did concern them (Neron, 1996).

Persons with HIV/AIDS may also have concerns about becoming dependent on others or a burden to loved ones as they become more ill. Exploration of these concerns may require the involvement of family members and other potential caregivers. Other concerns may require that the social worker encourage or facilitate the involvement of family members, such as when a client perceives coercion or subtle pressure from family members to opt for particular end-of-life choices. It is important to ensure that the client's choices are made voluntarily and free from family constraints or external social pressures (Ferris et al., 1995).

EXPLORING END-OF-LIFE OPTIONS

Thoroughly exploring and considering all end-of-life options and alternatives to assisted death is another important issue, which has been previously mentioned as a necessary element of informed consent (Dunshee, 1994; Motto, 1994; Werth and Cobia, 1995). Part of the social worker's role is to encourage this exploration and ensure the client has all information related to the advantages, disadvantages, and probable risks of each treatment option (Reamer, 1987). These options can include palliative care, hospice care, home care, proper pain management, further counselling, and decisions related to advance health-care directives (NASW, 1994). Motto (1994) has suggested that in situations where the desire for assisted death is expressed, mental health professionals can encourage clients to delay any actions, thereby allowing them an opportunity to explore and consider other alternatives without relinquishing the option of assisted death.

It is important to consider that clients may alter their decisions related to euthanasia and assisted suicide. For example, some may decide not to follow through with an assisted death, despite having made plans (Motto, 1994). Others may change the timing of their planned death. In a study involving nine persons with HIV/AIDS who were planning an assisted death, many acknowledged that they could redefine the timing and this in fact had occurred with two of the persons with AIDS (Neron, 1996). Since circumstances and decisions can change, periodic reviews of end-of-life decisions are important.

INVOLVEMENT OF SIGNIFICANT OTHERS

Social workers should encourage clients to consider the impact that their end-of-life decisions may have on significant others, including parents and other family members, children, a spouse or lover, and close friends. Involving significant others at some point in the decision-making process can be beneficial for the client and those whom he or she chooses to involve (Kain, 1996; Motto, 1994; NASW, 1994). This will allow significant others an opportunity to resolve any ambiguous feelings related to the client's decision and prepare for the client's death. Such involvement can also help to build mutual support between the client and his or her significant others (Motto, 1994) and increase knowledge of the client's wishes related to advance health-care directives and proxy decision-making.

After a client's death, the social worker's role may extend to providing support and assistance to significant others during the bereavement process (Kain, 1996; NASW, 1994). In cases of assisted death, survivors may experience guilt or anger or feel they could have done more to prolong the client's life, particularly if they continue to have ambiguous feelings about the client's decision (Werth, 1996). Others may feel relief that the client is no longer suffering.

CONSULTATION WITH OTHER PROFESSIONALS

When dealing with euthanasia and assisted suicide, social workers can consider the option of discussing these issues with a trusted colleague or supervisor. Consultation demonstrates further effort to maintain a standard of care and provides an opportunity for the social worker to obtain confirmation and feedback on his or her view of the situation (Motto, 1994; Werth, 1996). In the *Code of Ethics* it is suggested that in an effort to provide competent service, social workers may obtain advice from other professionals regarding their clients (CASW, 1994a).

As mentioned earlier, there may be times when the involvement of another mental health professional is necessary, particularly when depression or competency is in question. Any referrals should be discussed and explored with the client beforehand. Social workers must consider the biases and views of those with whom they consult and the implications for themselves and their clients. Colleagues who are open to a full discussion of all end-of-life options and related issues would probably most benefit the social worker and the client in these situations.

THE SOCIAL WORKER'S VALUES

Lastly, social workers must consider the impact that personal values and beliefs can have on their approach to dealing with end-of-life choices (Abramson, 1985; Holmes, 1980; Kain, 1996; Werth, 1996). To develop an understanding of this impact, social workers should examine their attitudes and moral and spiritual beliefs related to euthanasia and assisted suicide, and ask themselves if they believe these choices can be rational. It is also helpful to develop an understanding of personal definitions of pain, quality of life, and suffering, including the physical, emotional, psychological, and spiritual components of these issues (Boyle and DuMoulin, 1994).

Social workers must also consider if their attitudes and values towards issues such as race, class, gender, and sexual orientation have any impact on their approach to dealing with end-of-life issues. For example, does a client's race, class, or sexual orientation affect perceptions of his or her ability to make rational decisions? Also, are women viewed as any less competent to make end-of-life decisions (Logue, 1993)? It appears that women have been viewed as less competent by the courts. In a review of US court decisions related to the withdrawal and withholding of treatment of profoundly ill, incompetent individuals, Miles and August (1990) found that legal decisions generally upheld the medical preferences of men, while decisions related to women did not consider or rejected their preferences.

While some authors have suggested that mental health professionals should support persons with HIV/AIDS through the end-of-life decision process regardless of their moral position (Ferris et al., 1995; Kain, 1996), the NASW (1994) has stated that social workers should determine for themselves if they will participate in discussions related to end-of-life decisions, depending on their own beliefs. Social workers who are unable to assist clients with these decisions have a professional obligation to refer clients and their families to competent professionals who can address these issues (NASW, 1994). This approach is reinforced in the CASW *Code of Ethics*. Ultimately, clients need a supportive forum in which they can openly explore their desires for assisted death, as well as other end-of-life options.

CONCLUSION

Due to the nature and extent of their contact with persons with HIV/AIDS, it is likely that social workers and other mental health professionals will be required to participate in end-of-life discussions, which could include those related to euthanasia and assisted suicide. As Wood and his colleagues state, 'counsellors often develop close relationships with clients, and their support may be particularly important in easing the transition from life to death' (1993: 2). As a result, they must be well prepared to deal with the challenges these issues present. This requires an openness to discussing all end-of-life choices and a sound knowledge of the legal, ethical, and counselling issues discussed in this chapter.

The role of social workers can extend beyond supporting their clients through the process of making end-of-life decisions. Social workers may be asked to participate in the development of policy, standards, and guidelines related to euthanasia, assisted suicide, and other end-of-life choices. Apart from providing their own input, social workers can advocate for the involvement of persons with HIV/AIDS and others directly affected by these issues in the development of policy and guidelines (Neron, 1996).

Social workers can consider initiating and participating in research related to euthanasia, assisted suicide, and HIV/AIDS that explores areas such as factors contributing to the desire for assisted death and rational decisions. These issues and other professional concerns can also be explored through education in the form of presentations, workshops, case studies, and publications (Werth, 1996).

The CASW, provincial social work organizations, and Canadian schools of social work can play an important role in increasing knowledge and understanding of euthanasia, assisted suicide, and other end-of-life choices among social workers by encouraging and supporting related dialogue, education, and research, and by continuing to refine guidelines and standards related to these issues.

Acknowledgement
The author acknowledges the assistance of Russel Ogden, Carolyn Krebs, and Joseph Griffin, whose comments were beneficial in the development of this chapter.

REFERENCES

Abramson, M. 1985. 'The Autonomy-Paternalism Dilemma in Social Work Practice', *Social Casework: The Journal of Contemporary Social Work* 66: 387–93.

———. 1989. 'Autonomy vs. Paternalistic Beneficence: Practice Strategies', *Social Casework: The Journal of Contemporary Social Work* 70: 101–5.

Beck, A. 1972. *Depression: Causes and Treatment.* Philadelphia: University of Pennsylvania Press.

Berstein, S. 1960. 'Self-determination: King or Citizen in the Realm of Values', *Social Work* 5: 3–8.

Bindels, P., A. Krol, E. van Ameijden, D. Mulder-Folkerts, J.A. van den Hoek, G. van Griensven, and R. Coutinho. 1996. 'Euthanasia and Physician-assisted Suicide in Homosexual Men with AIDS', *Lancet* 347: 499–504.

Bisman, C. 1994. *Social Work Practice: Cases and Principles*. Pacific Grove, Calif.: Brooks Cole.

Boyle, M., and A. DuMoulin. 1994. 'Euthanasia and Assisted Suicide: British Columbia Association of Social Workers Brief to the Special Senate Committee', *Perspectives* 16, 5: 10–11.

Callahan, J. 1994. 'The Ethics of Assisted Suicide', *Health and Social Work* 19, 4: 237–44.

Canadian Association of Social Workers (CASW). 1994a. *Social Work Code of Ethics*. Ottawa: CASW.

———. 1994b. *Statement of Principles on Euthanasia and Assisted Suicide*. Ottawa: CASW.

Chochinov, H., K. Wilson, M. Enns, N. Mowchun, S. Lander, M. Levitt, and J. Clinch. 1995. 'Desire for Death in the Terminally Ill', *American Journal of Psychiatry* 152, 8: 1185–91.

Cockburn, L. 1991. 'An Act of Courage', *Vancouver Province*, 12 May, 29.

Conwell, Y., and E. Caine. 1991. 'Rational Suicide and the Right To Die', *New England Journal of Medicine* 325: 1100–3.

Criminal Code of Canada. 1995. Aurora, Ont.: Canada Law Book.

DeMara, B., and D. Freed. 1996. 'Doctor Facing Charge in HIV Suicide', *Toronto Star*, 21 June, A1, A4.

Dunshee, S. 1994. 'Compassion in Dying', *Focus: A Guide to AIDS Research and Counselling* 9, 5: 5–6.

Ferris, F., J. Flannery, H. McNeal, M. Morrissette, R. Cameron, and G. Bally, eds. 1995. *The Comprehensive Guide for the Care of Persons with HIV Disease. Module 4: Palliative Care*. Toronto: Mount Sinai Hospital and Casey House Hospice.

Foley, J. 1994. 'Euthanasia and Assisted Suicide: A Social Work Perspective', *Newsmagazine* 21, 4: 1–2.

Goldblum, P., and J. Moulton. 1989. 'HIV Disease and Suicide', in J. Dilley, C. Pies, and M. Helquist, eds, *Face to Face: A Guide to AIDS Counselling*. San Francisco: AIDS Health Project.

Green, G. 1995. 'AIDS and Euthanasia', *AIDS Care* 7, supp. 2: S169–73.

Hoffman, M. 1994. 'Use of Advance Directives: A Social Work Perspective on the Myth versus the Reality', *Death Studies* 18: 229–41.

Holmes, K. 1980. 'Euthanasia: A Social Work Perspective', *Health and Social Work* 5, 4: 5–12.

Kain, C. 1996. *Positive HIV Affirmative Counselling*. Alexandria, Va.: American Counselling Association.

Kapp, M. 1988. 'Forcing Services on At-risk Older Adults: When Doing Good Is Not So Good', *Social Work in Health Care* 13, 4: 1–13.

Keigher, S. 1994. 'Patient Rights and Dying: Policy Restraint and the States', *Health and Social Work* 19, 4: 298–303.

Kirst-Ashman, K., and G. Hull. 1993. *Understanding Generalist Practice*. Chicago: Nelson Hall.

Laane, H.-M. 1995. 'Euthanasia, Assisted Suicide and AIDS', *AIDS Care* 7, supp. 2: S163–7.

Levy, M. 1992. 'Should "Assisted Suicide" Be Legalized?—Yes', *NASW News*: 4.

Logue, B. 1993. *Death and Control in the Elderly in America*. Toronto: Maxwell Macmillan.

Mason, J., and R. McCall-Smith. 1987. *Butterworths Medico-Legal Encyclopaedia*. London: Butterworths.

Matthews and Board of Directors of Physiotherapy. 1986. 54 O.R. (2d), 375.

Measure 16: Oregon Death with Dignity Act. 1994.

Miles, S., and A. August. 1990. 'Courts, Gender and the Right to Die', *Law, Medicine and Health Care* 18, 1–2: 85–95.

Motto, J. 1994. 'Rational Suicide: Then and Now, When and How', *Focus: A Guide to AIDS Research and Counselling* 9, 5: 1–4.

National Association of Social Workers (NASW). 1994. 'Client Self-determination in End-of-life Decisions', in *Social Work Speaks*, 3rd edn. Washington: NASW Press.

Neron, C. 1996. 'Euthanasia, Assisted Suicide and HIV/AIDS: Implications for Social Work', *The Social Worker* 64, 4: 129–36.

Nicholson, B., and G. Matross. 1989. 'Facing Reduced Decision-making Capacity in Health Care: Methods for Determining Client Self-determination', *Social Work* 34, 3: 234–8.

Ogden, R. 1994. *Euthanasia, Assisted Suicide and AIDS*. New Westminster, BC: Peroglyphics.

———. 1996. 'Death Hastening and Canada's Inuit', *Last Rights* 15: 87–93.

———, and M. Young. 1998. 'Euthanasia and Assisted Suicide: A Survey of Registered Social Workers in British Columbia', *British Journal of Social Work* 28: 161–75.

Osman, H., and T. Perlin. 1994. 'Patient Self-determination and the Artificial Prolongation of Life', *Health and Social Work* 19, 4: 245–52.

Reamer, F. 1987. 'Informed Consent in Social Work', *Social Work* 32: 425–9.

Rodriguez v. British Columbia (Attorney-General). 1993. 3 S.C.R., 519.

Rogers, J., and P. Britton. 1994. 'AIDS and Rational Suicide: A Counselling Psychology Perspective or a Slide on the Slippery Slope', *Counselling Psychologist* 22, 1: 645–59.

Rothman, J. 1989. 'Client Self-determination: Untangling the Knot', *Social Service Review* 63: 598–612.

Schafer, A. 1994. Presentation to the Special Senate Committee on Euthanasia and Assisted Suicide, 30 Sept. *Committee Proceedings* 18 (Ottawa: Queen's Printer).

Senate of Canada. 1995. *Report of the Special Senate Committee on Euthanasia and Assisted Suicide*. Ottawa: Minister of Supply and Services Canada.

Siegel, K. 1986. 'Psychosocial Aspects of Rational Suicide', *American Journal of Psychotherapy* 40, 3: 405–18.

Singer, P. 1994. *Living Will*. Toronto: University of Toronto Centre for Bioethics.

Smith, M., S. Alter, and S. Harder. 1993. *Euthanasia and Cessation of Treatment*. Ottawa: Minister of Supply and Services Canada.

Spicker, P. 1990. 'Social Work and Self-determination', *British Journal of Social Work* 20: 221–36.

Taylor, G. 1990. 'AIDS Mercy Killings', *Macleans* (16 July): 14.

Thal, A. 1992. 'Should Assisted Suicide Be Legalized?—No', *NASW News*: 4.

van den Boom, F. 1995. 'AIDS, Euthanasia and Grief', *AIDS Care* 7, supp. 2: S175–85.

de Wachter. 1991. 'In Brief: The Dutch and the Dying', *The Hastings Centre Report*: 2.

Weick, A., and L. Pope. 1988. 'Knowing What's Best: A New Look at Self-determination', *Social Casework: The Journal of Contemporary Social Work* 69: 10–16.

Werth, J. 1994. 'The Effects of Precipitating Circumstances, Stigma, and Social Support on Psychologists' Perceptions of Suicidal Ideators', Ph.D. dissertation, Auburn University.

———. 1995. 'Rational Suicide Reconsidered: AIDS as an Impetus for Change', *Death Studies* 19: 65–80.

———. 1996. *Rational Suicide? Implications for Mental Health Professionals.* Washington: Taylor and Francis.

———, and D. Cobia. 1995. 'Empirically-based Criteria for Rational Suicide: A Survey of Psychotherapists', *Suicide and Life-Threatening Behaviour* 25: 231–40.

———, and B. Liddle. 1994. 'Psychotherapists' Attitudes towards Suicide', *Psychotherapy: Theory, Research and Practice* 31: 440–8.

Wesley, C. 1996. 'Social Work and End-of-life Decisions', *Health and Social Work* 21, 2: 115–21.

Wood, G., R. Marks, and J.W. Dilley, eds. 1993. *Judicious Practice: An Update to AIDS Law for Mental Health Professionals.* San Francisco: AIDS Health Project.

Conclusion

Future Perspectives

In 1989, at the World Conference on AIDS held in Montreal, people with HIV and their supporters stormed the podium at the opening ceremonies and demanded a voice during the proceedings. As thousands of people applauded, for the first time a person with HIV declared the conference open. Organizers of the World Conference on AIDS in Geneva, in 1997, adopted a resolution called the Geneva Principle, which from the very beginning of the planning stage for the conference gave people with HIV one-half of all committee spaces for all tracks in the conference. In the complex world of HIV care, this stands as a metaphor for one of the most important subtexts in the history of the HIV epidemic. For the first time in the history of medicine, those affected by a diagnosis have taken a major and increasingly important role in making decisions about their care and treatment.

In the future all activities in the issue-area of HIV, whether prevention, care and treatment, or policy development, will be articulated on the principle that people with HIV are key players at all levels. Care will be increasingly community-based, because communities provide better care (when they are sustained) and because governments will provide fewer resources in the future. The increasingly chronic nature of HIV infection and the fact that people with HIV will live longer lives means that care will need to be flexible and integrated with the vast array of health and social services as well as community-based organizations.

Clearly, the authors in this book have demonstrated that social workers have provided leadership in many aspects of prevention, care and treatment, and policy development related to HIV. Equally as obvious is the fact that collaboration within and across the health and social service professions is essential. This implies more than multidisciplinary efforts that often amount to confusion for the client and redundancy in service. True interdisciplinary work maintains focus on the client, and commonality among professionals, while respecting each discipline's unique competence.

One such example is seen in the efforts of the health professions to provide interdisciplinary learning experiences where students from medicine, social work, nursing, psychology, physical and occupational therapy, dentistry, and pharmacy study in the same classes and solve problems using the same case examples of people living with HIV infection.

As well, numerous projects across Canada are defining new parameters in prevention, focusing not solely on explicit behaviours, but also on the individual, environmental, and societal determinants of autonomy and health promotion. Observing the epidemiology of HIV infection, in which micro-epidemics among at-risk populations pose new challenges, social workers will embrace and advocate for strategies involving harm reduction and a change in focus from criminilization to health-care provision as a response to injection drug use.

As this book goes to press, the federal government has just announced the Third National AIDS Strategy. This strategy proposes increases in prevention efforts (particularly to young gay men, women, injection drug users, and Aboriginal communities), basic research in treatments, and continued funding to community-based organizations as the front-line response in prevention and care of persons with HIV.

A cure may not be imminent, but after 15 years of responding to the epidemic in Canada, we know the principles of prevention, we know the methods of care and treatment, and we know the critical need for appropriate health and social policy. We have shown our potential. The real test will be to demonstrate our resolve by the programs, services, and policies that we put in place.

Index